Lecture Notes in Computer Science 9805

Commenced Publication in 1973
Founding and Former Series Editors:
Gerhard Goos, Juris Hartmanis, and Jan van Leeuwen

Guoyan Zheng · Hongen Liao
Pierre Jannin · Philippe Cattin
Su-Lin Lee (Eds.)

Medical Imaging and Augmented Reality

7th International Conference, MIAR 2016
Bern, Switzerland, August 24–26, 2016
Proceedings

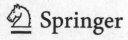 Springer

Editors

Guoyan Zheng
Institute for Surgical Technology
University of Bern
Bern
Switzerland

Hongen Liao
Department of Biomedical Engineering
  School of Medicine
Tsinghua University
Beijing
China

Pierre Jannin
Faculte de Medicine
Universite de Rennes 1
Rennes Cedex
France

Philippe Cattin
University of Basel
Allschwil
Switzerland

Su-Lin Lee
Hamlyn Centre
Imperial College London
London
UK

ISSN 0302-9743   ISSN 1611-3349   (electronic)
Lecture Notes in Computer Science
ISBN 978-3-319-43774-3   ISBN 978-3-319-43775-0   (eBook)
DOI 10.1007/978-3-319-43775-0

Library of Congress Control Number: 2016946309

LNCS Sublibrary: SL6 – Image Processing, Computer Vision, Pattern Recognition, and Graphics

Printed on acid-free paper

This Springer imprint is published by Springer Nature
The registered company is Springer International Publishing AG Switzerland

The original version of the book frontmatter revised:
For detailed information please see Erratum.
The Erratum to this book is available
at 10.1007/978-3-319-43775-0_40

Preface

The 7th International Conference on Medical Imaging and Augmented Reality, MIAR 2016, was held at the University of Bern, Bern, Switzerland during August 24–26, 2016.

The aim of MIAR 2016 was to bring together researchers in computer vision, graphics, robotics, and medical imaging to present the state-of-the-art developments in this ever-growing research area. We also encouraged a broad interpretation of the field: from macroscopic to molecular imaging, passing the information on to scientists and engineers to develop breakthrough therapeutics, diagnostics, and medical devices, which can then be seamlessly delivered back to patients.

Rapid technical advances in medical imaging, including its growing applications to drug, gene therapy, and invasive/interventional procedures, as well as a fusional development of the protein science, imaging modalities, and nano-technological devices, have attracted significant interest in recent years. This is motivated by the clinical and basic science research requirement of obtaining more detailed physiological and pathological information of the body for establishing the localized genesis and progression of diseases. Current research is also motivated by the fact that medical imaging is increasingly moving from a primarily diagnostic modality toward a therapeutic and interventional aid, driven by streamlining the diagnostic and therapeutic processes for human diseases by means of imaging modalities and robotic-assisted surgery.

The impact of MIAR on these fields was reflected by the quality of submitted papers. This year we received 55 full submissions, which were subsequently reviewed by up to three reviewers, selected from the international Organizing Committee. Every review was assessed and ranked by up to three members of the Program Committee to ensure that the reviews were fair, independent, and consistent. The MIAR 2016 Program Committee finally accepted 39 full papers. The meeting consisted of a single track of oral/poster presentations, with each session led by an invited lecture from our distinguished local and international faculty.

Running such a conference requires dedication, and we appreciated the commitment of the MIAR 2016 Program Committee and the MIAR 2016 international Organizing Committee who worked hard in putting together this conference. We were grateful to everyone who participated in the review process; they donated a large amount of time and effort to make this volume possible and insure a high level of quality. We thank the invited speakers: Terry Peters from the University of Western Ontario, Canada, Brad Nelson and Luc van Gool from ETH Zurich, Switzerland, and Dinggang Shen from the University of North Carolina at Chapel Hill (UNC-CH), USA.

It was our great pleasure to welcome this year's MIAR attendees to Bern, the capital of Switzerland, whose old town is a UNESCO World Heritage Site, featured by its six kilometers of arcades — probably the longest weather-sheltered shopping promenades in Europe. Bern is an ideal place for exploring history and culture and for natural beauty. The medieval atmosphere of the city with its many fountains, sandstone facades, narrow streets, and historic towers is unique. The elevated Rose Garden above the Bear Park and the platform of the 101-meter-high cathedral tower offer the best views of the old town around which the River Aare flows. The boutiques, bars, and cabaret stages of the old town, some of which are located in vaulted cellars, and the small street cafes are also a highlight for the attendees.

For those who were unable to attend, we hope that this volume will act as a valuable reference to the MIAR disciplines, and we look forward to meeting you at future MIAR conferences.

August 2016

Guoyan Zheng
Hongen Liao
Pierre Jannin
Philippe Cattin
Su-Lin Lee

Organization

General Co-chairs

Guoyan Zheng   University of Bern, Switzerland
Hongen Liao   Tsinghua University, China

Program Co-chairs

Pierre Jannin   Université de Rennes 1, France
Philippe Cattin   University of Basel, Switzerland
Su-Lin Lee   Imperial College London, UK

International Organization Co-chairs

Xiongbiao Luo   University of Western Ontario, Canada
Junchen Wang   Beihang University, China

Workshop and Tutorial Co-chairs

Stefan Weber   University of Bern, Switzerland
Marcel Lüthi   University of Basel, Switzerland

Local Organization Chair

Lutz-P. Nolte   University of Bern, Switzerland

Program Committee

Adrien Bartoli   Université d'Auvergne, France
Wolfgang Birkfellner   Medical University of Vienna, Austria
Louis Collins   McGill University, Canada
Alejandro Frangi   University of Sheffield, UK
James Gee   University of Pennsylvania, USA
Guido Gerig   New York University, USA
Stamatia Giannarou   Imperial College London, UK
Makoto Hashizume   Kyushu University, Japan
Leo Joskowicz   Hebrew University of Jerusalem, Israel
Ron Kikinis   Harvard Medical School, USA
Shuo Li   The Western University of Ontario, Canada
Cristian Linte   Rochester Institute of Technology, USA
Huafeng Liu   Zhejiang University, China

Jimmy Liu	Institute for Infocomm Research, Singapore
Tianming Liu	University of Georgia, USA
Anthony Maeder	Western Sydney University, Australia
Ken Masamune	Tokyo Women's Medical University, Japan
Leonardo de Mattos	Istituto Italiano di Tecnologia, Italy
Kensaku Mori	Nagoya University, Japan
Nassir Navab	Technical University of Munich, Germany
Yoshito Otake	NAIST, Japan
Dinggang Shen	UNC at Chapel Hill, USA
Li Shen	Indiana University, USA
Pengcheng Shi	Rochester Institute of Technology, USA
Russell H. Taylor	Johns Hopkins University, USA
Theo Van Walsum	Erasmus MC, The Netherlands
Guangzhi Wang	Tsinghua University, China
Stefan Weber	University of Bern, Switzerland
James J. Xia	Weill Cornel Medical College, USA
Yasushi Yamauchi	Toyo University, Japan
Ziv Yaniv	National Institute of Health, USA

International Organizing Committee

Xiao Dong	Southeast University, China
Caroline Essert-Villard	Université de Strasbourg, France
Pascal Fallavollita	Technical University Munich, Germany
Yong Fan	University of Pennsylvania, USA
Michael Figl	Medical University of Vienna, Austria
Germain Forestier	Université de Haute-Alsace, ENSISA, France
Karl Fritscher	UMIT in Hall, Austria
Jaesung Hong	DGIST, Korea
Sanghyun Joung	Kyungpook National University, Korea
Jan Klein	Fraunhofer MEVIS, Germany
Manuela Kunz	Queen's University, Canada
David Kwartowitz	Clemson University, USA
Claudia Lindner	University of Manchester, UK
Valeria De Luca	ETH Zurich, Switzerland
Marcel Lüthi	University of Basel, Switzerland
John Moore	Robarts Research Institute, Canada
Ryoichi Nakamura	Chiba University, Japan
Kilian Pohl	SRI International, USA
Philip Pratt	Imperial College London, UK
Maryam Rettmann	Mayo Clinic, USA
Steffen Schumann	University of Bern, Switzerland
Amber Simpson	Vanderbilt University, USA
Cheol Song	DGIST, Korea
Stefanie Speidel	Karlsruher Institute of Technology, Germany
Danail Stoyanov	University College London, UK

Raphel Sznitman	University of Bern, Switzerland
Tong Tong	Harvard Medical School, USA
Tamas Ungi	Queen's University, Canada
Kirby Vosburgh	Harvard Medical School, USA
Qian Wang	Shanghai Jiaotong University, China
Stefan Wesarg	Fraunhofer IGD, Germany
Guorong Wu	UNC at Chapel Hill, USA
Jue Wu	University of Pennsylvania, USA
Zhong Xue	Weill Cornell Medical College, USA
Pew-Thian Yap	UNC at Chapel Hill, USA
Daoqiang Zhang	Nanjing University of Aeron- and Astron-autics, China
Xiahai Zhuang	Shanghai Jiaotong University, China

Poster Coordination

| Hongen Liao | Tsinghua University, China |
| Philippe Cattin | University of Basel, Switzerland |

Best Paper Award Coordination

| Pierre Jannin | Université de Rennes 1, France |
| Su-Lin Lee | Imperial College London, UK |

Sponsor and Exhibits Coordination

| Karin Nolte | University of Bern, Switzerland |

Local Organizing Committee

Lutz-P. Nolte	University of Bern, Switzerland
Chengwen Chu	University of Bern, Switzerland
Weimin Yu	University of Bern, Switzerland
Dimitrios Damopoulos	University of Bern, Switzerland

Conference Secretariat

| Karin Nolte | University of Bern, Switzerland |

Contents

Computer Assisted Interventions

Augmented Reality and Virtual Reality

Medical Image Analysis

Medical Image Computing

Computer Assisted Interventions

A Novel Computer-Aided Surgical Simulation (CASS) System to Streamline Orthognathic Surgical Planning

Peng Yuan[1], Dennis Chun-Yu Ho[1], Chien-Ming Chang[1], Jianfu Li[1],
Huaming Mai[1], Daeseung Kim[1], Shunyao Shen[1], Xiaoyan Zhang[1],
Xiaobo Zhou[2], Zixiang Xiong[3], Jaime Gateno[1,4],
and James J. Xia[1,4(✉)]

[1] Department of Oral and Maxillofacial Surgery,
Houston Methodist Research Institute, Houston, TX, USA
JXia@houstonmethodist.org
[2] Department of Radiology, Wake Forest School of Medicine,
Winston-Salem, NC, USA
[3] Department of Electrical and Computer Engineering,
Texas A&M University, College Station, TX, USA
[4] Department of Surgery, Weill Medical College, Cornell University,
New York, NY, USA

Abstract. Orthognathic surgery is a surgical procedure to correct jaw deformities. It requires extensive presurgical planning. We developed a novel computer-aided surgical simulation (CASS) system, the AnatomicAligner, for doctors planning the entire orthognathic surgical procedure in computer following our streamlined clinical protocol. The computerized plan can be transferred to the patient at the time of surgery using digitally designed surgical splints. The system includes six modules: image segmentation and three-dimensional (3D) model reconstruction; registration and reorientation of the models to neutral head posture (NHP) space, 3D cephalometric analysis, virtual osteotomy, surgical simulation, and surgical splint designing. The system has been validated using the 5 sets of patient's datasets. The AnatomicAligner system will be soon available freely to the broader clinical and research communities.

1 Introduction

Orthognathic surgery is a surgical procedure to correct dentofacial (jaw) deformities. Each year around the world, a significant number of patients undergo orthognathic surgical procedures. Due to the complex nature of the dentofacial anatomy, it requires extensive presurgical planning. During the past 50 years, the technical aspects of surgery have achieved significant improvements, e.g. rigid fixation, resorbable material and distraction osteogenesis. However, the traditional planning method, e.g., two-dimensional (2D) cephalometry and prediction tracing, hasn't been updated since 1960

P. Yuan and D.C.-Y. Ho—Contributed equally.

© Springer International Publishing Switzerland 2016
G. Zheng et al. (Eds.): MIAR 2016, LNCS 9805, pp. 3–14, 2016.
DOI: 10.1007/978-3-319-43775-0_1

despite there are many well-known problems [1]. Each of them may be minor but all together may result in a surgical outcome that is far away from the ideal [1].

Problems associated with the traditional planning method led us to develop a new computer-aided surgical simulation (CASS) method and its clinical protocol for planning an orthognathic surgery [1, 2]. This protocol has been proven accurate [3, 4]. It is now a new standard of care in this field. However, in order to use the protocol, doctors need to either outsource a commercial service which may significantly increase healthcare cost, or learn to use off-the-shelf computer software which could be extremely difficult for doctors. With the cost-effectiveness and user-friendliness in mind, the purpose of this project was to develop a free and user-friendly CASS system, AnatomicAligner, for planning an orthognathic surgery.

2 System Development

AnatomicAligner system is capable of achieving the following tasks for our streamlined and proven CASS clinical protocol [2]. A composite skull model of a patient can be generated to accurately render skeleton, dentition, and facial soft tissue [5]. In addition, the recorded patient's nature head position (NHP) can be applied to composite skull model [6]. Moreover, for the first time, our innovative 3D cephalometry is incorporated into the planning system [7, 8]. It solves many problems associated with the current 2D and 3D cephalometry [9]. Furthermore, doctors can make any type of virtual osteotomies to simulate any type of orthognathic surgeries. Finally, the surgical splints can be designed within the system.

Our multi-thread computation based AnatomicAligner system includes six modules: (1) Segmentation, (2) Registration/NHP, (3) 3D Cephalometric Analysis, (4) Virtual Osteotomy, (5) Surgical Simulation, and (6) Surgical Splint/Template Design (Fig. 1). The software is programmed with object-oriented programming (OOP) paradigm using Microsoft Visual C++, Visualization Toolkit (VTK), and Insight Segmentation and Registration Toolkit (ITK). The user-interface is wizard-driven. The design principle, data organization and algorithm implementation are described below in details.

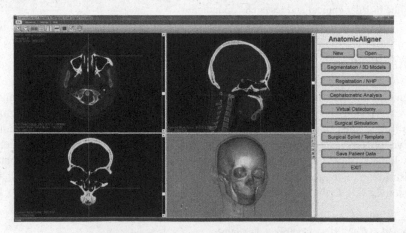

Fig. 1. Main user-interface of AnatomicAligner system.

2.1 Module 1: 2D Image Segmentation and 3D Model Reconstruction

The purpose of this module is to generate a group of 3D models that is capable of displaying an accurate rendition of the skeleton, the teeth and the facial soft tissues for surgical planning. Segmentation tools, including threshold, regional threshold, region growing, manual editing and Boolean operation, are implemented in the system. The resulted masks are used to generate 3D surface models using Marching Cubes algorithm. Note that in order to transfer surgical plan to the patient at the time of treatment (Module 6), 3D surface models, in opposite to volumetric models, are critical to fabricate computer-aided designing/computer-aided manufacturing (CAD/CAM) splints.

In order to plan an orthognathic surgery, at least 4 computed tomography (CT) models are generated: midface, mandible, soft tissue, and fiducial marker [1, 2]. In addition, high-resolution upper and lower digital dental models and their fiducial markers are imported [1, 2]. They are used to generate a composite skull model in the next step. A special feature of the system is that each 3D model has a unique predetermined name following a hierarchical structure. This ensures that the bony segments can be automatically selected, and the hierarchy of the bony segments can be automatically established during surgical planning.

2.2 Module 2: Model Registration and Reorientation of Skull Models to NHP

The first purpose of the Module 2 is to generate a composite skull model. CT is capable of accurately rendering bones and soft tissues. However, its resolution is not accurate enough for teeth rendering. Therefore, the high-resolution digital dental models are merged into the CT midface and mandibular models, replacing the less-than-accurate CT teeth using the corresponding fiducial markers of the two datasets. The resulted model is called a composite skull model, which has an accurate rendition for both bones and teeth. Automatic (iterative closest points), semi-automatic (paired landmarks) and manual registration tools are implemented for registering the 3D surface models. During the registration, a hierarchical structure is automatically formed so the correlated 3D models are automatically grouped and moved/rotated together.

The second purpose of this module is to define a global reference frame (global coordinate system) for the whole head. Due to the nature of human head, correctly positioning the head models into a unique global reference frame is critical for surgical planning. The midsagittal plane should divide the head into right and left halves evenly, while the axial plane should divide the head into upper and lower halves, and the coronal plane should divide the head into front and back halves.

NHP is a routinely used head orientation for clinically evaluation. In this module, NHP is also used to establish a global reference frame for the whole head. It directly reflects the clinical environment in the computer as if a surgeon examines the patient. NHP can be recorded clinically using digital orientation sensor [6], self-leveling laser [4], or standardized photograph method [1]. The clinically recorded NHP (in pitch, roll, and yaw) is applied to the original data space, mapping the entire 2D and 3D datasets into the NHP. Since the transformation matrix is saved in the system, the mapping of

NHP can be adjusted as necessary, or reset to the original data space. Finally, the midsagittal plane is determined based on clinical measurement [2] or mathematical algorithm [10]. Both coronal and axial planes are perpendicular to the midsagittal plane and pass through the midpoint of right and left porion (anatomical landmarks - the most superior point on the external acoustic meatus). From now on, the surgical planning is carried out in the global reference frame.

2.3   Module 3: 3D Cephalometry

Cephalometry, also called cephalometric analysis, is a group of measurements used to quantify the deformity of head and each facial unit (e.g., maxilla and mandible) by maxillofacial surgeons and orthodontists. The measurements are done based on anatomical landmarks. An ideal cephalometry should measure the 5 geometric properties of each facial unit, including symmetry, shape, size, position and orientation [8]. For the first time, our innovative 3D cephalometry is implemented with the 5 geometric properties incorporated into an orthognathic surgical planning system, which has a significant clinical impact (Fig. 4c). Our 3D cephalometry is achieved in 3 steps.

Step 1: To Define Cephalometric Analysis Scheme. Our 3D cephalometric analysis is meant to be modular. The measures are displayed in a grid [8]. Each row displays a different geometric property: object symmetry, shape, size, position and orientation. Each column represents an individual facial unit, such as cranium, maxilla, mandible, chin, etc. The information of each cephalometric analysis, i.e., the name and description of the cephalometric analysis, facial unit category, and measurements and the landmarks used, is stored in a database file.

Symmetry analysis includes both object symmetry and symmetric alignment measurements. In human anatomy, object symmetry refers to the local intrinsic-mirror symmetry that each facial unit should have. The object symmetry of a dental arch, e.g., upper arch, is analyzed by a triangular technique [8] or principal component analysis (PCA) based adaptive minimum Euclidean distances (PAMED, publication pending). The object symmetry of a bone, e.g., mandible, is analyzed by weighted Procrustes analysis [8]. Symmetric alignment refers to the alignment of each facial unit with the respect of the midsagittal plane of the head in the global reference frame. The degree of symmetric alignment of a facial unit is quantified by first measuring the transverse (right-left) deviation to the midsagittal plane, then measuring yaw and roll of the facial unit using 3D orientation measurement (described below).

Shape is an object's geometric property that is not size, position or orientation. Thus, Procrustes analysis is implemented to compare two objects after both have been scaled to the same size, placed in the same location, and rotated to the best possible alignment. For example, the patient's mandible is compared to the averaged mandible of normal population with the same ethnicity, gender and age.

Size is a linear measurement in 3D, e.g., length, width and height. Position is a relative measurement between the local-global or local-local coordinate systems. Both linear and angular measurements are implemented in Cartesian and Cylindrical system, respectively.

Finally, orientation is a relative measurement between the local-global or local-local coordinate systems. A 3D composite angle does not have any clinical meaningfulness. Although there are many ways to measure the orientation in 3D, we implemented the orientation measurement using Tait-Bryan angles following a specific order: first yaw, then roll, and finally pitch. This is because most facial units (i.e., maxilla, mandible and chin) normally have some degrees of pitch, while their ideal roll and yaw are zero. This strategy is helpful to minimize the yaw and roll angles.

Step 2: To Digitize Landmarks and Record Their Initial Coordinates. All the cephalometric measurements are anatomical landmark-based. A library is implemented with built-in 178 frequently used cephalometric landmarks; each has a specific anatomical definition on where it should be located. A template window is also implemented to graphically show where each landmark is located on its corresponding 3D model. This landmark library can be customized that users can add additional landmarks as needed.

In our system, only the landmarks used by the measurements are needed to be digitized. Once digitized, it is attached onto the corresponding 3D model. When a 3D model is cut (medical term: 'osteotomized') into pieces, the attached landmarks will be automatically inherited by the new models. In addition, the landmarks will be automatically moved and rotated along with its corresponding 3D model. This feature is especially important during the surgical planning, where osteotomized bony segments are moved and rotated to a desired position.

Step 3: To Calculate and Report the Results. The resulted measurements are automatically computed once the landmarks are digitized. The results are displayed in a floating window, and automatically updated in real-time when a bony segment and its associated landmarks are moved and rotated to a new location. Finally, a cephalometric analysis report, including both measurements before and after the surgical simulation, can be generated and printed.

2.4   Module 4: Virtual Osteotomy

Virtual osteotomy is a fundamental step in AnatomicAligner system. A typical orthognathic surgery includes a Le Fort I osteotomy (maxillary surgery), a bilateral mandibular sagittal split osteotomy (mandibular body surgery), and a genioplasty (mandibular chin surgery). A virtual knife for osteotomy is first created by defining a group of multi-connected hexahedrons, followed by cutting and separating a single 3D bone model into 2 segments in a hierarchical structure. Finally, the virtual knife is automatically saved. The virtual osteotomy results in the following bony segments: midface, Le Fort I segment and upper teeth, distal segment and lower teeth, chin, and right and left proximal segments. The virtual osteotomy is described below in details.

Step 1: To Form a Virtual Knife. The virtual knife consists of a group of multi-connected hexahedrons. The first step is to manually define the initial shape of the hexahedrons by digitizing a series of landmarks, indicating where an osteotomy should be (Fig. 2a). Two adjacent vertices (landmarks) define the initial position and length of a given hexahedron. Since the initial orientation of the virtual knife is perpendicular to the screen, a second pair of vertices is generated by projecting the first pair 'into' the screen with an initial depth of 70 mm (also for the entire hexahedrons), forming the first (top) face of the hexahedron. The upper face is then vertically extended with an initial thickness of 0.5 mm (also for the entire hexahedron), forming the bottom face and the rest 4 vertical faces of a given hexahedron (Fig. 2b).

The next step is to chain the adjacent individual hexahedrons together, forming a 'curved' virtual knife as defined by the user. If the two adjacent vertical faces of the hexahedrons are parallel (threshold: $1.0e^{-9}$), they are connected directly. If not, the connection between the 2 adjacent top faces of the hexahedrons is always a hinge-axis joint, while the bottom faces are adaptively adjusted, becoming either longer or shorter, depending on the direction of the angle. Finally, 6 control spheres are generated to adjust the length and orientation for each hexahedron (Fig. 2c). A control panel is also implemented to adjust the translation, rotation, and thickness of entire virtual knife.

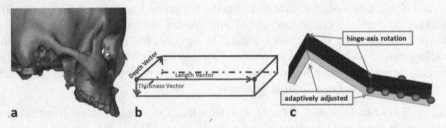

Fig. 2. (a) Red/green dots are the user-defined cutting line. The green dot is the last point. (b) An individual hexahedron. Green dots represent two adjacent digitized points. (c) Four green spheres are used to adjust the size of the hexahedron (one of them is in red, indicating the active operation), and 2 yellow ones are used to adjust the angle between two adjacent hexahedrons. (Color figure online)

Step 2: To Cut and Separate a Single 3D Bone Model into Two Segments.

(1) *To classify triangles that intersect with the multi-connected hexahedrons*
   A surface model is composed of thousands of triangles. The triangles of the target model are classified into 4 types depending on their relationship with the hexahedrons: outside set (completely outside), upper intersection set (intersection at the upper face), lower intersection set (intersection at the lower face), and inside set (completely inside) (Fig. 3a). Since the bone models are usually generated from cone-beam (CB) CT scans, the number of triangles is usually excessive (e.g. 3 million). Therefore, a two-step of coarse-to-fine classification algorithm is implemented to efficiently determine triangle-hexahedron relationship. It is described below in details.

   The first step is to coarsely classify the triangles into the outside set at triangle level using a subdivision-classification algorithm. The bounding box of the target bone model is divided into 64 equally spaced subregions. Each subregion is used as a basic unit during the classification. A mesh collision detection algorithm [11] is used to detect the collision between each subregion and the hexahedrons. The 3 vertices of a triangle are mapped into the corresponding subregions. A bounding box of that triangle is then formed by one or multiple subregions. If all the subregions that form the triangle bounding box are outside of the hexahedrons, this triangle is classified as 'outside' and no further calculation is performed to this triangle.

The next step is to finely classify the remaining of the triangles at vertex level. Each triangle has 3 line segments (l_1, l_2, and l_3) and 3 vertices (v_1, v_2, and v_3). The triangle-hexahedron relationship is determined by vertex-hexahedron relationship. Each vertex of a given triangle is plugged into the plane function set:

$$I(v, f_j) = \begin{cases} + & above\ the\ plane \\ 0 & on\ the\ plane \\ - & below\ the\ plane \end{cases}, for\ j = 1, 2, 3 \ldots 6 \qquad (1)$$

where $I(v, f_j) = Sign(a_j x + b_j y + c_j z + d_j)$ indicates the relationship between v and f_j; $v = (x, y, z)$ represents a vertex of a given triangle; j is one of the 6 planes of a given hexahedron; and, $f_j = a_j x + b_j y + c_j z + d_j$ is one of the 6 plane functions. If all the solutions of $I(v, f_j)$ are negative, this vertex is classified as 'inside' the hexahedron. If any solution is '0', this vertex is classified as 'on' the hexahedron. Otherwise, this vertex is classified as 'outside' the hexahedron. Furthermore, if a triangle is related to multiple hexahedrons, the triangle and its 3 adjacent neighbors are further divided into smaller triangles until each triangle is only related to one hexahedron. Based on the classification of the vertices, the triangles are thus automatically classified into 'outside, 'upper intersection', 'lower intersection' and 'inside' types in relation to the hexahedrons. The outside triangles are not further computed for the virtual osteotomy, while the completely inside triangles are discarded.

(2) *To recreate new triangles replacing the 'broken' triangles*
The multi-connected hexahedrons cut through each of the upper and lower intersection triangles, resulting in a 'broken' triangle with two intersection points, one on each side of the triangle. The 'broken' triangles are fixed by using the following algorithm. If only one vertex of a triangle is outside of the hexahedron, it is used to build a new triangle with the 2 intersection points on the two sides (Fig. 3b). If 2 vertices of a triangle are outside of the hexahedron, they are used to build 2 new triangles with the 2 intersection points on the 2 sides (Fig. 3c). Using this algorithm, the original 'broken' triangles are replaced by the two new sets of triangles.

(3) *To generate a polygon surface along the cutting surface for each bony segment*
The polygon surface along the cutting plane (intersection) for each osteotomized segment is created by first contouring intersection points. Then, polygon surface is reconstructed by a streamlined procedure of reorganizing, simplifying and triangulating each contour, respectively. The polygon surface is used to close the bony segments in the next step.

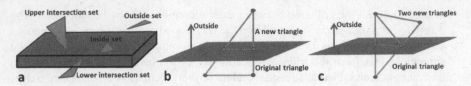

Fig. 3. (a) Relationship between triangles and a hexahedron. (b) Recreating a new triangle (green) from a "broken" original triangle (purple) – showing top surface only. (c) Recreating 2 new triangles (green) from a "broken" original triangle (purple) – showing top surface only. (Color figure online)

(4) *To separate the osteotomized model into two new bone models*
     All the outside, the upper intersection, the lower intersection, and the polygon surfaces are combined together to form a temporary bone model. This temporary model is then separated into two pieces using 3D region growing method. The polygon surface for each segment is finally capped.

2.5 Module 5: Surgical Simulation

Once the deformed jaws are osteotomized into multiple segments as the surgery requires, a doctor needs to plan where the desired positions of these bony segments are. Figure 4 shows the surgical simulation of a typical orthognathic surgery, including Le Fort I osteotomy, right sagittal split osteotomy, left inverted-L osteotomy and genioplasty. The surgical simulation is completed in the following 4 steps.

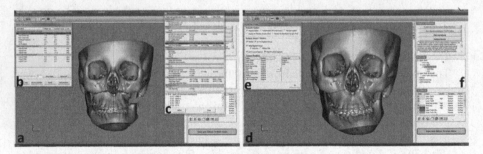

Fig. 4. Surgical Simulation. (a) Planning the surgical movement (showing at final position). (b) Control panel for surgical planning. (c) Real-time 3D cephalometric report. (d) Position review to compare the original and planned positions (showing at original position). (e) Control panel for position review. (f) Automatically formed hierarchical structure for surgical simulation.

The first step is to define a hierarchical structure for the osteotomized bony segments. Each bony segment has a unique name in orthognathic surgery. Therefore, system checks all the required models for a given type of surgery, and automatically forms a customizable hierarchical structure.

The second step is to establish final dental occlusion - to restore the malocclusion to a normal bite. It is a temporary position in which the lower teeth and its 'child' mandibular distal segment are placed to the maximum intercuspation with the corresponding upper teeth, and it is also the desired relation between the maxilla and the mandible. After that, all the bony segments are grouped together as a maxillomandibular combination.

The third step is to move the bony segments to a desired position. Following the clinical protocol [2], the maxillomandibular combination is translated and rotated around the maxillary dental midline point (an anatomical landmark used to determine the upper dental midline) in six-degree of freedom. The surgical planning is achieved in the following sequence: midline correction, yaw correction, roll correction, vertical adjustment, pitch adjustment, and anteroposterior adjustment. During the simulation, the doctor checks the bone collisions and adjusts the movements accordingly as needed. 3D cephalometric measurement report is automatically updated in real-time during the each step of the movement.

The last step is to perform a genioplasty as an option. The chin segment can be osteotomized either before or after the maxillomandibular combination is moved and rotated. The chin segment can also be moved and rotated in 6 degrees of freedom around pogonion (also an anatomic landmark with specific definition).

2.6   Module 6: Designing of Surgical Splints

Surgical splint is a horseshoe-shape teeth-anchored wafer that is placed in-between the upper and lower teeth for transferring the surgical plan to the patient intraoperatively (Fig. 5). In a double-jaw surgery, although both maxilla and mandible are operated in the same procedure, one jaw is always osteotomized first, followed by the opposite jaw. Surgeons usually decide which jaw been operated first based on their clinical assessment, e.g., in a maxillary surgery first procedure, an intermediate splint is used to reposition the Le Fort I segment to the planned position in regard with the intact mandible. The mandible is then osteotomized, and the distal segment is repositioned to the planned position in regard with the already repositioned Le Fort I segment using a final splint. Since the splint is only related to the teeth, only upper and lower dental models are used for designing the splint. Once designed, a .stl file of the splint can be exported for any 3D printer. The process is described below in details.

Step 1: To Select the Type of the Splint to Be Designed. There are 3 types of the surgical splint: immediate splint for maxillary surgery first, intermediate splint for mandibular surgery first, and final splint. During the design, the type of the splint is selected first. The positions of the upper and lower dental arches are then automatically displayed at the corresponding positions. For the intermediate splint of the maxillary surgery first, the upper teeth are at the final planned position while the lowers are at the original position. Vice versa in case of the mandibular surgery first. For final splint, both upper and lower teeth are at the final planned positions.

Step 2: To Autorotate the Lower Dental Arch (An Optional Step) During the intermediate splint design, one jaw is at its final position while the other is at its original position. The upper and lower teeth may collide to each other. In order to avoid the collision, the lower teeth need to autorotate around the center of rotation of the right and left condyles (both are anatomic landmarks) – the same autorotation we do clinically. Autorotation is not required for the final splint.

Step 3: To Design the Horse Shoe-Shaped Raw Model of the Splint. Three landmarks are digitized on the occlusal surface of the upper and lower dental arch respectively, forming a top and a bottom planes for the splint. In order to create enough anchorage between the teeth and the splint, both planes are automatically offset 2 mm away from the occlusal surface. In the next step, the contour for the top face of the splint is manually traced on the top plane using a cardinal spline (Fig. 5a). The contour for the bottom face is created by copying and manually editing the top contour on the bottom plane. Therefore, both top and bottom contours consist of the same numbers of the points. If needed, a top and a bottom contour extension can be created by copying the corresponding contour and positioning it 0.5 mm towards the occlusal surface. The contour extensions serve as transitional layers between the top and bottom faces in case there is a large positional discrepancy between the upper and lower teeth, which often happens during the designing of the intermediate splint (Fig. 5b). Each contour and its extension can be adjusted individually. Furthermore, collisions are automatically detected among the contours to ensure the quality of the raw splint model. Finally, the corresponding points of the each contour are automatically connected and triangulated, forming a surface model of the raw splint (Fig. 5c).

Step 4: To Create the Final Model of the Splint. The final model of the splint is generated by a Boolean operation, subtracting the upper and the lower teeth from the raw splint model (Fig. 5d). The final model of the splint can be exported as a .stl file and printed using any 3D printer that uses United States Food and Drug Administration (FDA) approved biocompatible materials (Fig. 5e). The 3D printed intermediate and final splints are finally used in the operating room during an orthognathic procedure (Fig. 5).

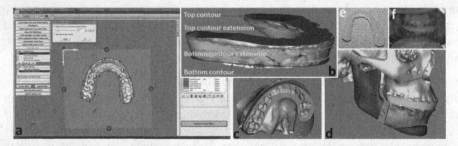

Fig. 5. Designing an intermediate surgical splint. (a) The contour for the top face of the splint is manually traced on the top plane. The plane can be adjusted using 4 spheres and 3-axis. (b) Assembling the raw splint. (c) The splint after Boolean operation. (d) The intermediate splint was placed between the lower jaw at the final position and the uncut upper jaw. (e) 3D printed splint. (f) Intraoperative use of the intermediate splint for repositioning the mandible.

3 Accuracy Evaluation

Five CT datasets in DICOM format of patients with dentofacial deformity were used [IRB(2)1011-0187x]. The accuracy of our AnatomicAligner system was compared to the industrial gold standard - Mimics 17.0 system (Materialise, Leuven, Belgium). The evaluation was done by comparing the accuracy in: (1) segmentation and 3D reconstruction; (2) virtual osteotomy and surgical movement. These were the only 2 key functions that both systems had. Mimics did not have the other functions, including NHP, 3D cephalometry and splint design, thus couldn't be compared.

To evaluate the accuracy of segmentation and 3D reconstruction, CT was imported into both systems. A mask was generated using a predetermined threshold (gray scale: 1250), and manually edited by removing the spine from the image. Region growing was then performed, resulting in a skull mask. Afterwards, a 3D skull model was reconstructed in high resolution (sampling 2:2:1 in x,y,z) using Marching Cubes (AnatomicAligner) and proprietary algorithm (Mimics). The two 3D models were then imported into RapidForm (INUS Technology, Korea). The 3D model generated by Mimics was first registered (translation only) to the AnatomicAligner model, removing the offset between the 2 systems. Finally, errors (absolute mean Euclidean distances) between the 2 models were computed automatically by Rapidform.

To evaluate the accuracy of virtual osteotomy and surgical movement, a whole midface 3D model, generated by AnatomicAligner, was used in both systems. This was to remove the confounding factor of segmentation errors. A Le Fort I osteotomy was performed using "virtual osteotomy" function in AnatomicAligner and "PolyPlane" function in Mimics to cut the whole midface model in 2 segments: a midface and a Le Fort I. Afterwards, the Le Fort I segment was duplicated, translated 5 mm (x), 10 mm (y) and 15 mm (z), and rotated 15° (x), 10° (y) and 5° (z), respectively. Finally, the midface, and both unmoved and moved Le Fort I segments were imported into RapidForm to compute the errors between the 2 corresponding models.

The resulted errors were tabulated and paired. The mean and range (min, max) were calculated for each pair. The results showed an error of 0.41 mm (0.38, 0.43) for the segmentation and 3D reconstruction. The errors were mainly due to the scattering at the margins where the images exceeded field of view during CT acquisition, and the artifacts caused by amalgam and orthodontic bands. They were clinically insignificant. The results also showed an error of 0.01 mm (0.00, 0.03) for both osteotomy and surgical movement, indicating a high degree of accuracy for both operations.

4 Discussion and Conclusion

We successfully developed a CASS system, the AnatomicAligner, for planning orthognathic surgery. The system will be soon available freely to the boarder clinical and research communities. The clinical contribution of our AnatomicAligner system is that it allows doctors to accurately plan orthognathic surgery following our streamlined clinical protocol [2]. In addition, the true 3D cephalometric analysis [8] that includes five geometric properties of orientation, symmetry, position, size and shape is implemented in a surgical planning system for the first time. This is especially important to correctly quantify the deformities and plan the treatment. Finally, the surgical splints can be effectively designed in the system and printed by any in-house 3D printer that uses FDA-approved biocompatible materials. These splints are used at the time of the surgery to accurately transfer the computerized surgical plan to the patient.

The technical contributions include: (1) The user-interface of the system is designed with the perception that the endusers are medical doctors with little knowledge in computer graphics. Necessary prompts and error-checks are also implemented to guide and warn the users. (2) A versatile and efficient virtual osteotomy is implemented, in which doctor can freely design or modify any types of osteotomies. A two-step of coarse-to-fine triangle classification algorithm is developed to significantly improve the efficiency of virtual osteotomy. To our knowledge, there is no similar virtual osteotomy approach implemented in any surgical planning system for orthognathic surgery. (3) During the registration and surgical simulation, all involved bony segments are moved and rotated under an automatically generated hierarchical structure. (4) The design of surgical splint is a guided semi-automatic procedure. To our knowledge, this also has never been implemented before. In a future study, we will investigate a possible learning curve for inexperienced users.

References

1. Xia, J.J., Gateno, J., Teichgraeber, J.F.: New clinical protocol to evaluate craniomaxillofacial deformity and plan surgical correction. J. Oral Maxillofac. Surg. **67**(10), 2093–2106 (2009)
2. Xia, J.J., et al.: Algorithm for planning a double-jaw orthognathic surgery using a computer-aided surgical simulation (CASS) protocol. Part 1: planning sequence. Int. J. Oral Maxillofac. Surg. **44**(12), 1431–1440 (2015)
3. Hsu, S.S., et al.: Accuracy of a computer-aided surgical simulation protocol for orthognathic surgery: a prospective multicenter study. J. Oral Maxillofac. Surg. **71**(1), 128–142 (2013)
4. Bobek, S., et al.: Virtual surgical planning for orthognathic surgery using digital data transfer and an intraoral fiducial marker: the charlotte method. J. Oral Maxillofac. Surg. **73**(6), 1143–1158 (2015)
5. Gateno, J., et al.: A new technique for the creation of a computerized composite skull model. J. Oral Maxillofac. Surg. **61**(2), 222–227 (2003)
6. Xia, J.J., et al.: A new method to orient 3-dimensional computed tomography models to the natural head position: a clinical feasibility study. J. Oral Maxillofac. Surg. **69**(3), 584–591 (2011)
7. Gateno, J., Xia, J.J., Teichgraeber, J.F.: New 3-dimensional cephalometric analysis for orthognathic surgery. J. Oral Maxillofac. Surg. **69**(3), 606–622 (2011)
8. Xia, J.J., et al.: Algorithm for planning a double-jaw orthognathic surgery using a computer-aided surgical simulation (CASS) protocol. Part 2: three-dimensional cephalometry. Int. J. Oral Maxillofac. Surg. **44**(12), 1441–1450 (2015)
9. Gateno, J., Xia, J.J., Teichgraeber, J.F.: Effect of facial asymmetry on 2-dimensional and 3-dimensional cephalometric measurements. J. Oral Maxillofac. Surg. **69**(3), 655–662 (2011)
10. Gateno, J., et al.: The primal sagittal plane of the head: a new concept. Int. J. Oral Maxillofac. Surg. **45**(3), 399–405 (2016)
11. Gottschalk, S., Lin, M.C., Manocha, D.: OBBTree: a hierarchical structure for rapid interference detection. In: Proceedings of ACM Siggraph 1996 (1996)

Computer Assisted Planning, Simulation and Navigation of Periacetabular Osteotomy

Li Liu[1], Timo M. Ecker[2], Klaus-A. Siebenrock[2], and Guoyan Zheng[1(✉)]

[1] Institute for Surgical Technology and Biomechanics,
University of Bern, Bern, Switzerland
{li.liu,guoyan.zheng}@istb.unibe.ch
[2] Department of Orthopedic Surgery, Inselspital,
University of Bern, Bern, Switzerland

Abstract. Periacetabular osteotomy (PAO) is an effective approach for surgical treatment of hip dysplasia in young adults. However, achieving an optimal acetabular reorientation during PAO is the most critical and challenging step. Routinely, the correct positioning of the acetabular fragment largely depends on the surgeons experience and is done under fluoroscopy to provide the surgeon with continuous live x-ray guidance. To address these challenges, we developed a computer assisted system. Our system starts with a fully automatic detection of the acetabular rim, which allows for quantifying the acetabular 3D morphology with parameters such as acetabular orientation, femoral head Extrusion Index (EI), Lateral Center Edge (LCE) angle, total and regional femoral head coverage (FHC) ratio for computer assisted diagnosis, planning and simulation of PAO. Intra-operative navigation is used to implement the pre-operative plan. Two validation studies were conducted on four sawbone models to evaluate the efficacy of the system intra-operatively and post-operatively. By comparing the pre-operatively planned situation with the intra-operatively achieved situation, average errors of $0.6° \pm 0.3°$, $0.3° \pm 0.2°$ and $1.1° \pm 1.1°$ were found respectively along three motion directions (Flexion/Extension, Abduction/Adduction and External Rotation/Internal Rotation). In addition, by comparing the pre-operatively planned situation with the post-operative results, average errors of $0.9° \pm 0.3°$ and $0.9° \pm 0.7°$ were found for inclination and anteversion, respectively.

1 Introduction

Developmental dysplasia of the hip joint is a prearthrotic deformity resulting in osteoarthritis at a very young age. Periacetabular Osteotomy (PAO) is an effective approach for surgical treatment of painful dysplasia of the hip in younger patients [1]. The aim of PAO is to increase acetabular coverage of the femoral head and to reduce contact pressures by realigning the hip joint [2,3]. However, insufficient reorientation leads to continued instability while excessive reorientation correction would result in femoroacetabular impingement (FAI) [4,5]. Therefore, a main important factor for clinical outcome and long-term success of PAO

© Springer International Publishing Switzerland 2016
G. Zheng et al. (Eds.): MIAR 2016, LNCS 9805, pp. 15–26, 2016.
DOI: 10.1007/978-3-319-43775-0_2

is to achieve an optimal acetabular reorientation [6]. The application of computer assisted planning and navigation in PAO opens such an opportunity by showing its potential to improve surgical outcomes in PAO. Before the PAO-specific navigation system was introduced, some commercially available navigation systems were modified and adapted for PAO clinical trials. Abraham et al. [7] presented an experimental cadaver study in order to investigate the utility of pre-operative 3D osteotomy planning and intra-operative acetabular repositioning in the navigated PAO surgery. Hsieh et al. [8] assessed the efficacy of the navigated PAO procedure in 36 clinical cases using a modified version of commercially available navigation program for THA (VectorVision, BrainLab Inc., Westchester, IL). Seminal work has been done by Langlotz et al. [9], who developed the first generation of CT-based customized navigation system for PAO and applied it to 14 clinical cases. However, this system only focuses on navigated osteotomy procedure while reorientation procedure is lack of standard morphological parameters feedback. More recently, Murphy et al. [10] developed a computer assisted Biomechanical Guidance System (BGS) for performing PAO. The system combines geometric and biomechanical feedback with intra-operative tracking to guide the surgeon through the PAO procedure. In this paper, we developed and validated a novel computer assisted diagnosis, planning, simulation and navigation system for PAO. It is hypothesized that the pre-operative plan done with our system can be achieved by the navigated PAO procedure with a reasonable accuracy.

2   Materials and Methods

2.1   System Workflow

The computer assisted diagnosis, planning, simulation and navigation system for PAO consists of three modules as shown in Fig. 1.

- **Model generation module.** 3D surface models of the femur and the pelvis are generated by fully automatic segmentation of the pre-operatively acquired CT data [11].
- **Computer assisted diagnosis, planning and simulation module.** The aim of this module is first to quantify the 3D hip joint morphology for a computer assisted diagnosis of hip dysplasia, and then to plan and simulate the reorientation procedure using the surface models generated from the model generation module. It starts with a fully automatic detection of the acetabular rim, which allows for computing important information quantifying the acetabular morphology such as femoral head coverage (FHC), femoral head extrusion index (EI), lateral centre edge (LCE) angle, version and inclination. This module then provides a graphical user interface allowing the surgeon to conduct a virtual osteotomy and to further reorient the acetabular fragment until an optimal realignment is achieved.
- **Intra-operative navigation module.** Based on an optical tracking technique, this module aims for providing intra-operative visual feedback during acetabular fragment osteotomy and reorientation until the pre-operatively planned orientation is achieved.

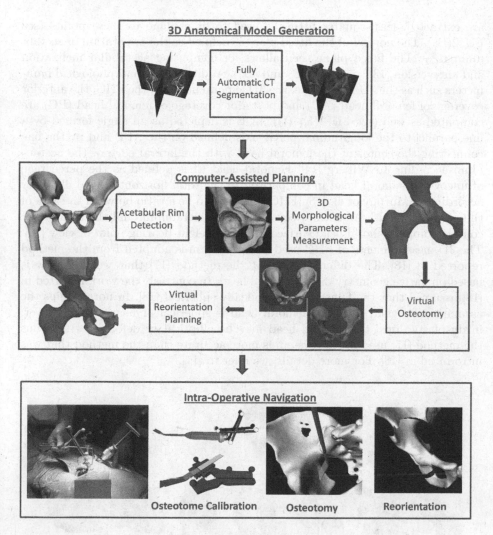

Fig. 1. Schematic view of our computer assisted planning and navigation system for PAO.

2.2   Computer Assisted Diagnosis of Hip Dysplasia

Accurate assessment of acetabular morphology and its relationship to the femoral head is essential for diagnosis of hip dysplasia and PAO planning. After pelvic and femoral surface models are input to our system, the pelvic local coordinate systems is established using anatomical landmarks extracted from the CT data which is defined on the anterior pelvic plane (APP) using the bilateral anterior superior iliac spines (ASISs) and the bilateral pubic tubercles [12]. After local coordinate system is established, a fully automatic detection of the acetabular rim is conducted [11] (see Fig. 2(A)). As soon as acetabular rim points are extracted, least-squares fitting is used to fit a plane to these points (see Fig. 2(B)). The normal of the fitted plane is defined as the orientation of acetabulum n_{CT}. The fitted plane then allows for computing acetabular inclination and anteversion [13] (see Fig. 2(C) and (D)). Additional hip morphological parameters such as the 3D LCE angle, the 3D femoral head EI, the FHC, the anterior coverage of femoral head (AC) and posterior coverage of femoral head (PC) are computed as well (see Fig. 2(E)–(I)). LCE is depicted as an angle formed by a line parallel to the longitudinal pelvic axis defined on the APP and by the line connecting the center of the femoral head with the lateral edge of the acetabulum according to Wiberg [14]. Femoral head EI is defined as the percentage of uncovered femoral head in comparison to the total horizontal head diameter according to Murphy et al. [15]. FHC is defined to be a ratio between the area of the upper femoral head surface covered by the acetabulum and the area of the complete upper femoral head surface from the weight-bearing point of view [16]. The 3D measurements of FHC used in this system is adapted from the method reported in [18]. The difference is that the method [17] that we used now is based on native geometry of the femoral head. In contrast, the work reported in [18] assumed that the femoral head is ideally spherical [18]. In normal hips the assumption is valid since the femoral head is spherical or nearly so. However, in dysplastic hips, the femoral head may be elliptical or deformed [19]. Thus the method [17] used in this system is more accurate than the method that was introduced in [18]. For more details, we refer to [17].

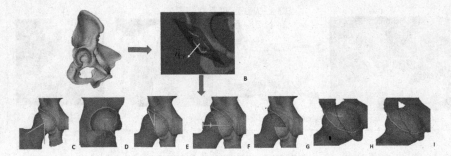

Fig. 2. Computing 3D morphological parameters of the hip joint. (A) Fully automatic acetabular rim detection; (B) Least-squares fitting plane of acetabular rim and the orientation of acetabulum; (C) Acetabular Inclination; (D) Acetabular Anteversion; (E) Lateral Center Edge Angle (LCE); (F) Femoral Head Extrusion Index (EI); (G) Femoral Head Coverage (FHC); (H) Anterior Coverage of Femoral Head (AC); (I) Posterior Coverage of Femoral Head (PC).

2.3   Computer Assisted Planning and Simulation of PAO Treatment

An in silico PAO procedure is conducted with our system as follows. First, since the actual osteotomies do not need to be planned as an exact trajectory, a sphere is used to simulate osteotomy operation. More specifically, the center of femoral

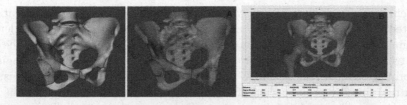

Fig. 3. In silico PAO surgical procedure in our PAO planning system. (A) Virtual osteotomy operation is done with a sphere, whose radius and position can be interactively adjusted; (B) Virtual reorientation operation is done by interactively adjusting anteversion and inclination angle of the acetabulum fragment. The hip morphological parameters (inclination, anteversion, LCE, EI, FHC, AC and PC) are then computed based on the reoriented acetabulum fragment and showed at the bottom of the screen.

head is taken as the center of the sphere whose radius and position can be interactively adjusted along lateral/medial, caudal/cranial, and dorsal/ventral directions, respectively, in order to approximate actual osteotomy operation (see Fig. 3(A)). After that, the in silico PAO procedure is conducted by interactively changing the inclination and the anteversion of the acetabulum fragment (see Fig. 3(B)). During the acetabulum fragment reorientation, 3D LCE angle, EI, FHC, AC and PC are computed in real time based on the reoriented acetabulum fragment and showed at the bottom of the screen (see Fig. 3(B)). Once the morphological parameters of normal hip are achieved (inclination: $45° \pm 4°$, $[37°–54°]$ [22]; anteversion: $17° \pm 8°$, $[1°–31°]$ [22]; LCE $> 25°$ [23]; FHC: $73\% \pm 4\%$, $[66\%–81\%]$ [22]), the planned morphological parameters are stored and subsequently transferred to the navigation module as explained in details in the following section.

2.4 Intra-operative Surgical Navigation

Navigated PAO surgical intervention is described as follow: Before the acetabular fragment is osteotomized, the pelvis is attached with a dynamic reference base (DRB) in order to register the surgical anatomy to the pelvis surface model generated from a pre-operatively acquired CT data (see Fig. 4(A) and (B)). After that, CT-patient registration based on a Restricted Surface Matching (RSM) algorithm [24] is conducted, which is basically divided into two successive steps: a paired point matching followed by a surface matching (see Fig. 4(B)). More specifically, the paired point matching is regarded as an alignment process of pairs of anatomical landmarks. In a pre-operative stage, 4 anatomical landmarks (bilateral ASISs and the bilateral pubic tubercles) are determined on the pelvic model segmented from CT data. In an intra-operative stage, the corresponding landmarks on the patient are digitized using a tracked probe. The digitized points are defined in the coordinate system of the DRB, which is rigidly fixed onto the pelvis. Then the surface matching computes the registration transformation based on 20–30 scattered points around the accessible surgical site that is matched onto a surface of a pelvic model (see Fig. 4(B)). After registration, the osteotomes are calibrated using a multi-tools calibration unit in order to determine the size and orientation of the blade plane (see Fig. 4(C)). The tip of the osteotome is shown in relation to the virtual bone model, axial, sagittal and coronal views of the actual CT dataset. The cutting trajectory is visualized in real time by prolongation of the blade plane of the osteotome. Thus the osteotomies can be performed in a controlled manner and complications such as intraarticular penetration and accidental transection of the posterior column can be avoided [2] (see Fig. 4(D)). After the acetabular fragment is mobilized from the pelvis, another DRB is anchored to the acetabulum area for intraoperative tracking, thereby the acetabular reorientation can be supported by the navigation module. The navigation system can provide interactive measurements of acetabular morphological parameters and image-guidance information, which instantaneously updates the virtual display, current position and orientation parameters of the acetabulum and the planned situation (inclination and anteversion angles) derived from the pre-operative planning module. The surgeon repositions the acetabulum by controlling its inclination and anteversion angle in order to determine whether the current position achieves the pre-operatively planned position or further adjustment is required (see Fig. 4(E)). After successful repositioning, preliminary K-wire fixation and finally definitive screw fixation is conducted [20]. In this sawbone validation study, a 3D articulated arm (FISSO®, 3D Articulated Gaging Arms, Switzerland) is employed to anchor the fragment for navigation accuracy evaluation (see Fig. 4(A)).

2.5 Study Design

In order to validate this newly developed planning and navigation system for PAO, two validation studies were designed and conducted on 4 sawbone models. The purpose of the first study is to evaluate the intra-operative accuracy and reliability of navigation system. The second study is designed to evaluate whether the acetabulum repositioning based on navigated PAO procedure can achieve the pre-operative planned situation by comparing the measured acetabular orientation parameters between pre-operative and post-operative CT data.

In the first study, pre-operative planning was conducted with the PAO planning module. Subsequently the intra-operative navigation module was used to track acetabular and pelvic fragments, supporting and guiding the surgeon to adjust the inclination and anteversion angles of acetabulaum interactively. Acetabular reorientation measured by the inclination and anterversion angles can be planned pre-operatively and subsequently realized intra-operatively without significant difference. In order to assess the error difference between the pre-operatively planned and the intra-operatively achieved acetabular orientation, we compared the decomposed rotation components derived from the acetabular fragment reorientation between the planned and intra-operative situations.

In the following, all related coordinate systems are first defined before the details about how to compute decomposed rotation components will be presented. Pre-operatively all related coordinate systems are defined (Fig. 5) on the virtual

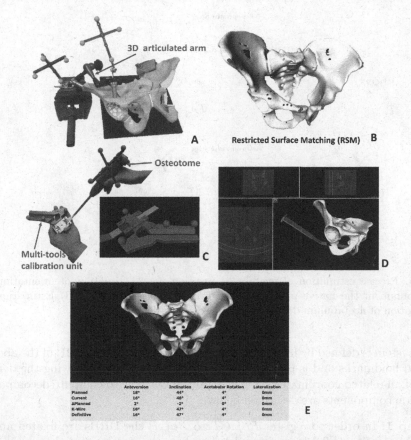

Fig. 4. Intra-operative PAO surgical navigation. (A) Setup of the navigated PAO surgery where two dynamic reference bases (DRBs) with reflective spheres are attached to both the iliac crest and the acetabular fragment; (B) The areas of the pelvis acquired with the tracked probe to perform the RSM registration; (C) Osteotome calibration where the green part represents the blade plane of the osteotome and the yellow part represents the prolongation of the blade plane; (D) Screenshot of CT-based osteotomy guidance where the tip of the osteotome is displayed on axial, sagittal and coronal views of the CT dataset, and a cutting trajectory is displayed on the bony model; (E) Screenshot of navigated reorientation procedure. (Color figure online)

3D model with Ref_CT representing the pre-operative CT data coordinate system of the surface model. $(Ref\_APP)^{Pre}$ represents the local coordinate system established on the APP, which is defined manually by choosing four landmarks (left and right anterior superior iliac spine [ASIS] and left and right pubic tubercle). Using the acetabular rim points extracted in the Ref_CT, acetabular version and inclination can be calculated in relation to $(Ref\_APP)^{Pre}$. Intra-operatively, the Ref_P represents the intra-operative pelvic coordinate system defined on the pelvic DRB, while Ref_A represents the intra-operative acetabulum coordinate system defined on acetabular DRB (Fig. 5(A)). The intra-operative APP coordi-

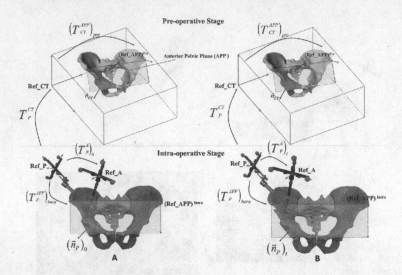

Fig. 5. Precise estimation of acetabular position. (A) Estimation of orientation of acetabulum in the native position before fragment reorientation; (B) Estimation of orientation of acetabulum during fragment reorientation.

nate system is defined by intra-operative paired-point matching [21] of the above-named landmarks and is represented by $(Ref\_APP)^{Intra}$. Following the definition of all related coordinate systems, details about how to compute decomposed rotation components are described below.

- **Step 1:** In order to register Ref_CT to Ref_P the DRBs are fixated and a RSM algorithm [24] is performed before the osteotomies and the acetabular fragment tracking. The transformation $(T_P^{APP})_{Intra}$ between the Ref_P and the $(Ref\_APP)^{Intra}$ can be calculated by Eq. (1).

$$\left(T_P^{APP}\right)_{Intra} = \left(T_{CT}^{APP}\right)_{Pre} \cdot T_P^{CT} \tag{1}$$

where T_P^{CT} is the rigid transformation between the Ref_P and the Ref_CT derived from paired-point matching; $(T_{CT}^{APP})_{Pre}$ is the transformation between the Ref_CT and the $(Ref\_APP)^{Pre}$.

- **Step 2:** Before the fragment is moved, a snapshot of the neutral positional relationship between Ref_A and the Ref_P is recorded (Fig. 5(A)). At this moment, the orientation of the acetabulum $(n_{APP})_{Intra}^{0}$ with respect to the $(Ref\_APP)^{Intra}$ can be estimated by the following equation (Fig. 5):

$$\left(n_{APP}\right)_{Intra}^{0} = \left(T_P^{APP}\right)_{Intra} \cdot (n_P)_0 = \left(T_P^{APP}\right)_{Intra} \cdot \left(T_A^P\right)_0 \cdot \left(T_P^A\right)_0 \cdot T_{CT}^P \cdot n_{CT} \tag{2}$$

where $n_C T$ denotes the orientation of acetabulum measured in the Ref_CT pre-operatively. Equation (2) indicates that one can first compute the orientation of acetabulum $(n_P)_0$ with respect to the Ref_P and then transform it to the $(Ref\_APP)^{Intra}$ through a transformation train.

- **Step 3:** Fragment mobility is measured by the navigation system, which records the instantaneous positional relationship $(T_A^P)_t$ between the Ref_A and the Ref_P. The neutral positional relationship $(T_A^P)_0$ obtained from **Step 2** is used to calculate the orientation of acetabulum $(n_P)_t$ with respect to the Ref_P during motion. The instantaneous orientation of acetabulum $(n_APP)_{Intra}^t$ with respect to the $(Ref\_APP)^{Intra}$ can be calculated by the following equation (Fig. 5(B)):

$$(n_{APP})_{Intra}^t = \left(T_P^{APP}\right)_{Intra} \cdot (n_P)_t = \left(T_P^{APP}\right)_{Intra} \cdot \left(T_A^P\right)_t \cdot \left(T_P^A\right)_0 \cdot T_{CT}^P \cdot n_{CT} \tag{3}$$

Equation (3) indicates that one can first compute the instantaneous orientation of acetabulum $(n_P)_t$ with respect to the Ref_P and then transform it to the $(Ref\_APP)^{Intra}$ through a transformation train.

- **Step 4:** The $(n_APP)_{Intra}^0$ and $(n_{APP})_{Intra}^t$ can then be decomposed into three motion components (Extension/Flexion, External Rotation/Internal Rotation, and Abduction/Adduction) along x-, y- and z axis of the $(Ref\_APP)^{Intra}$.

In the second study, we evaluated post-operatively the repositioning of the acetabular fragment and compared this with the pre-operative planned acetabular orientation parameters. Specifically, the acetabular rim points after reorientation were digitized with a tracked probe and transformed to pre-operative CT space based on the aforementioned registration transformation T_{CT}^P. The transformed acetabular rim points was then imported into the computer assisted PAO diagnosis module to quantify acetabular orientation parameters (inclination and anteversion) and compared them with the pre-operatively planned acetabular orientation parameters.

Table 1. The difference (°) of decomposed motion components between pre-operative planning and intra-operative navigation situations.

Bones	Side	Flex/Ext	Abd/Add	Ext Rot/Int Rot
#1	Left	0.9	0.1	3.6
#1	Right	0.5	0.5	0.7
#2	Left	0.5	0.4	1.1
#2	Right	0.4	0.1	0.2
#3	Left	0.9	0.1	1.2
#3	Right	0.4	0.5	1.2
#4	Left	0.4	0	0.2
#4	Right	1.0	0.3	0.7
Mean $\pm STD$ [Min, max]		0.6 ± 0.3 [0.4, 1.0]	0.3 ± 0.2 [0.0, 0.5]	1.1 ± 1.1 [0.2, 3.6]

3   Results

In the first intra-operative evaluation study, the decomposed rotation components of the acetabular fragment between the pre-operatively planned situation and the intra-operatively achieved situation were compared. According to Table 1, 8 groups of acetabular reorientation data were obtained. It can be seen that the average errors along three motion components (Flexion/Extension, Abduction/Adduction and External Rotation/Internal Rotation) are $0.6° \pm 0.3°$, $0.3° \pm 0.2°$ and $1.1° \pm 1.1°$, respectively.

In the second post-operative evaluation study, the morphological parameters of hip joint between the pre-operatively planned situation and post-operatively repositioned situation were compared. The results are shown in Table 2. From this table, it can be seen that the average errors of acetabular orientation parameters (inclination and anteversion angles) are $0.9° \pm 0.3°$ and $0.9° \pm 0.7°$, respectively. The results are accurate enough from a clinical point of view for PAO surgical intervention and verify the hypothesis that the pre-operatively planned situation can be achieved by navigated PAO procedure with reasonable accuracy.

Table 2. The error of hip joint morphological parameters (IN: Inclination; AV: Anterversion) between pre-operative planning and post-operative evaluation.

Parameter	Stage	#1	#2	#3	#4	#5	#6	#7	#8	Average error
IN (°)	Pre-op	41.4	44.2	44.2	42.6	41.9	40.8	50.4	44.6	0.9 ± 0.3 [0.4, 1.2]
IN (°)	Post-op	42.6	45.3	44.6	43.8	41.1	40.0	49.3	45.3	
AV (°)	Pre-op	13.2	15.1	8.1	8.6	15.3	8.5	10.2	10.3	0.9 ± 0.7 [0.0, 1.7]
AV (°)	Post-op	15.2	16.1	9.6	6.9	15.9	8.5	10.5	10.6	

4   Discussions and Conclusions

In this paper, we presented a comprehensive planning, simulation and navigation system for PAO, and evaluated system efficacy with a sawbone study. Previously, the intra-operative accuracy of the navigation system has been also assessed in a cadaver study in order to investigate the technical feasibility of the pararectus surgical approach [25]. As demonstrated by the results in both sawbone and cadaver studies, the efficacy of navigation system is validated with a reasonable accuracy. Based on the results, we are applying ethics approval for a clinical trial where the efficacy of our system will be further evaluated.

References

1. Murphy, S.B., Millis, M.B., Hall, J.E.: Surgical correction of acetabular dysplasia in the adult: a Boston experience. Clin. Orthop. Relat. Res. **363**, 38–44 (1999)
2. Ganz, R., Klaue, K., Vinh, T.S., Mast, J.W.: A new periacetabular osteotomy for the treatment of hip dysplasias technique and preliminary results. Clin. Orthop. Relat. Res. **232**, 26–36 (1988)

3. Hipp, J.A., Sugano, N., Millis, M.B., Murphy, S.B.: Planning acetabular redirection osteotomies based on joint contact pressures. Clin. Orthop. Relat. Res. **364**, 134–143 (1999)
4. Myers, S., Eijer, H., Ganz, R.: Anterior femoroacetabular impingement after periacetabular osteotomy. Clin. Orthop. Relat. Res. **363**, 93–99 (1999)
5. Ziebarth, K., Balakumar, J., et al.: Bernese periacetabular osteotomy in males: is there an increased risk of femoroacetabular impingement (FAI) after bernese periacetabular osteotomy? Clin. Orthop. Relat. Res. **469**(2), 447–453 (2011)
6. Crockarell Jr., J., Trousdale, R.T., Cabanela, M.E., Berry, D.J.: Early experience and results with the periacetabular osteotomy: the Mayo clinic experience. Clin. Orthop. Relat. Res. **363**, 45–53 (1999)
7. Abraham, C., Rodriguez, J., Buckley, J., Burch, S., Diab, M.: An evaluation of the accuracy of computer assisted surgery in preoperatively three dimensionally planned periacetabular osteotomies. In: ASME 2009 Summer Bioengineering Conference, pp. 255–256 (2009)
8. Hsieh, P.H., Chang, Y.H., Shih, C.H.: Image-guided periacetabular osteotomy: computer-assisted navigation compared with the conventional technique: a randomized study of 36 patients followed for 2 years. Acta Orthop. **77**(4), 591–597 (2006)
9. Langlotz, F., Bächler, R., Berlemann, U., Nolte, L.P., Ganz, R.: Computer assistance for pelvic osteotomies. Clin. Orthop. Relat. Res. **354**, 92–102 (1998)
10. Murphy, R.J., Armiger, R.S., Lepistö, J., Mears, S.C., Taylor, R.H., Armand, M.: Development of a biomechanical guidance system for periacetabular osteotomy. Int. J. Comput. Assist. Radiol. Surg. **10**(4), 497–508 (2014)
11. Chu, C., Bai, J., Wu, X., Zheng, G.: MASCG: multi-atlas segmentation constrained graph method for accurate segmentation of hip CT images. Med. Image Anal. **26**(1), 173–184 (2015)
12. Zheng, G., Marx, A., et al.: A hybrid CT-free navigation system for total hip arthroplasty. Comput. Aided Surg. **7**(3), 129–145 (2002)
13. Murray, D.: The definition and measurement of acetabular orientation. J. Bone Joint Surg. (Br.) **75**(2), 228–232 (1993)
14. Wiberg, G.: The anatomy and roentgenographic appearance of a normal hip joint. Acta Chir. Scand. **83**(Suppl. 58), 7–38 (1939)
15. Murphy, S.B., Ganz, R., Müller, M.: The prognosis in untreated dysplasia of the hip. A study of radiographic factors that predict the outcome. J. Bone Joint Surg. **77**(7), 985–989 (1995)
16. Konishi, N., Mieno, T.: Determination of acetabular coverage of the femoral head with use of a single anteroposterior radiograph. A new computerized technique. J. Bone Joint Surg. **75**(9), 1318–1333 (1993)
17. Cheng, H., Liu, L., Yu, W., Zhang, H., Luo, D., Zheng, G.: Comparison of 2.5D and 3D quantification of femoral head coverage in normal control subjects and patients with hip dysplasia. PLoS ONE **10**(11), e0143498 (2015)
18. Liu, L., Ecker, T., Schumann, S., Siebenrock, K., Nolte, L., Zheng, G.: Computer assisted planning and navigation of periacetabular osteotomy with range of motion optimization. In: Golland, P., Hata, N., Barillot, C., Hornegger, J., Howe, R. (eds.) MICCAI 2014, Part II. LNCS, vol. 8674, pp. 643–650. Springer, Heidelberg (2014)
19. Steppacher, S.D., Tannast, M., Werlen, S., Siebenrock, K.: Femoral morphology differs between deficient and excessive acetabular coverage. Clin. Orthop. Relat. Res. **466**(4), 782–790 (2008)
20. Olson, S.A.: The bernese periacetabular osteotomy: a review of surgical technique. Duke Orthop. J. **1**(1), 21–26 (2010)

21. Lavallee, S.: Registration for computer-integrated surgery: methodology. In: Computer-Integrated Surgery: Technology and Clinical Applications, p. 77 (1996)
22. Dandachli, W., Kannan, V., Richards, R., Shah, Z., Hall-Craggs, M., Witt, J.: Analysis of cover of the femoral head in normal and dysplastic hips new CT-based technique. J. Bone Joint Surg. (Br.) **90**(11), 1428–1434 (2008)
23. Zou, Z., Chávez-Arreola, A., et al.: Optimization of the position of the acetabulum in a ganz periacetabular osteotomy by finite element analysis. J. Orthop. Res. **31**(3), 472–479 (2013)
24. Bächler, R., Bunke, H., Nolte, L.P.: Restricted surface matching numerical optimization and technical evaluation. Comput. Aided Surg. **6**(3), 143–152 (2001)
25. Liu, L., Zheng, G., et al.: Periacetabular osteotomy through the pararectus approach: technical feasibility and control of fragment mobility by a validated surgical navigation system in a cadaver experiment. International Orthopaedics (2016, in press)

FEM Simulation with Realistic Sliding Effect to Improve Facial-Soft-Tissue-Change Prediction Accuracy for Orthognathic Surgery

Daeseung Kim[1], Huaming Mai[1], Chien-Ming Chang[1],
Dennis Chun-Yu Ho[1], Xiaoyan Zhang[1], Shunyao Shen[1], Peng Yuan[1],
Guangming Zhang[2], Jaime Gateno[1,3], Xiaobo Zhou[2],
Michael A.K. Liebschner[4], and James J. Xia[1,3(✉)]

[1] Department of Oral and Maxillofacial Surgery,
Houston Methodist Research Institute, Houston, TX, USA
JXia@houstonmethodist.org
[2] Department of Radiology, Wake Forest School of Medicine,
Winston-Salem, NC, USA
[3] Department of Surgery, Weill Medical College, Cornell University,
New York, NY, USA
[4] Department of Neurosurgery, Baylor College of Medicine,
Houston, TX, USA

Abstract. It is clinically important to accurately predict facial soft tissue changes following bone movements in orthognathic surgical planning. However, the current simulation methods are still problematic, especially in clinically critical regions, e.g., the nose, lips and chin. In this study, finite element method (FEM) simulation model with realistic tissue sliding effects was developed to increase the prediction accuracy in critical regions. First, the facial soft-tissue-change following bone movements was simulated using FEM with sliding effect with nodal force constraint. Subsequently, sliding effect with a nodal displacement constraint was implemented by reassigning the bone-soft tissue mapping and boundary condition for realistic sliding movement simulation. Our method has been quantitatively evaluated using 30 patient datasets. The FEM simulation method with the realistic sliding effects showed significant accuracy improvement in the whole face and the critical areas (i.e., lips, nose and chin) in comparison with the traditional FEM method.

1 Introduction

Facial appearance impacts human's social life. Orthognathic surgery is a surgical procedure of treating patients with dentofacial deformity to improve jaw functions and facial aesthetics. It is a bone procedure in which the jaws are cut into pieces and then repositioned to a desired position (called osteotomy), resulting in a significant facial appearance change. To date, only the osteotomy can be accurately planned prior to surgery [1]. The facial soft-tissue-change following the osteotomies cannot be accurately predicted even though it is a direct result of an osteotomy. The major challenge of accurately predicting facial soft-tissue-change is due to the complex nature of the

© Springer International Publishing Switzerland 2016
G. Zheng et al. (Eds.): MIAR 2016, LNCS 9805, pp. 27–37, 2016.
DOI: 10.1007/978-3-319-43775-0_3

facial soft tissue anatomy. Traditionally, the soft-tissue-change simulation is based on bone-to-soft tissue movement ratios, which has been clinically proven inaccurate [2]. There are a few published reports on three-dimensional (3D) facial soft tissue prediction. The most common methods are finite element method (FEM) [3, 4], mass-spring model [5] and mass tensor model [6–8]. FEM is reported to be the most accurate and biomechanically relevant method [5, 7]. Nonetheless, the prediction results are still less than ideal. This is especially true in the nose, lips and chin regions, which are extremely important for orthognathic surgery. Therefore, there is an urgent clinical need to have a reliable method of accurately predicting soft tissue changes following osteotomies.

Traditional FEM for facial soft tissue simulation assumes that the FEM mesh nodes move together with the contacting bone surfaces without considering sliding movement [3]. The nodes contacting the corresponding bone surfaces are first acquired and then translated the same amount as the bone movement. However, this assumption can lead to significant errors when a large amount of bone movement and occlusion changes are involved. In human anatomy, the cheek and lip mucosa are not directly attached to the bone and teeth; they slide over each other. However, the traditional FEM does not consider this sliding movement, which we believe is the main reason for inaccurate prediction in the lips and chin.

Implementing the realistic sliding movement into FEM is technically challenging. It requires high computational power and long time because the sliding mechanism in human mouth is a dynamic interaction between two surfaces. The second challenge is that even if the sliding movement with force constraint is implemented, the simulation results may still be inaccurate, because there is no strict nodal displacement boundary condition applied to the sliding area. The soft tissues at sliding surfaces follow the buccal surface profile of the bones and teeth. Thus, it is necessary to consider the strict displacement boundary condition for sliding movement. The third challenge is that the mapping between the bone surface and FEM mesh nodes needs to be reestablished after the bony segments are moved to a desired planned position. This is because the bone and soft tissue relationship is not constant before and after the bone movement, e.g., a setback or advancement surgery may either decrease or increase the total soft tissue contacting area to the bones and teeth. This mismatch may lead to the distortion of the resulting mesh. The fourth challenge is that the occlusal changes, e.g., from preoperative (preop) cross-bite to postoperative (postop) Class I normal bite, may distort the mesh in the lip region where the upper and lower teeth meet. Therefore, a more advanced sliding effect method is required to increase the prediction accuracy in these critical regions.

In this study, we have successfully solved these technical problems. We developed a FEM simulation method of realistic sliding effects. The facial soft tissue changes following the bony movements were simulated with an extended sliding boundary condition to overcome the mesh distortion problem in traditional FEM simulations. The nodal force constraint was applied to simulate the sliding effect of the mucosa. Next, strict nodal displacement boundary conditions were implemented in the sliding areas to accurately reflect the postop bone surface geometry. The corresponding nodal displacement for each node was recalculated after reassigning the mapping between the mesh and bone surface in order to achieve a realistic sliding movement. Finally, our simulation method was evaluated quantitatively using 30 sets of preop and postop computed tomography (CT) datasets from the patients with dentofacial deformity.

2 Our FEM Simulation Algorithm with Realistic Sliding Effects

Our facial soft-tissue-change simulation incorporated with realistic sliding effects, which was applied by sequentially satisfying a nodal force and displacement boundary conditions. In this algorithm, a patient-specific FEM model was generated using a previously developed FEM template model [9]. Subsequently, post-operative bone movement according to the surgical planning was applied to the FEM model together with a sliding effect with nodal force constraint to simulate the facial change. Next, sliding effect with strict nodal displacement condition was implemented to efficiently mimic the realistic sliding of the soft tissue. More sophisticated boundary condition and mapping method were developed to implement a realistic sliding movement for prediction accuracy improvement in critical areas.

2.1 Tissue Property for FEM Model

In our study, homogeneous material FEM model was used for computational efficiency. This was based on the results of previous studies investigating optimal tissue properties for facial soft tissue simulation. They found that the effect of tissue property on facial tissue deformation was minimal even if the tissue property changed tremendously [10, 11]. The average prediction error varied less than 0.02 mm when Poisson's ratio varied within 0 and 0.5 [11]. Moreover, the selection of value for Young's modulus is irrelevant to the FEM model deformation for homogeneous material model under displacement boundary condition. Therefore, we utilized 3000 (Pa) for Young's modulus and 0.47 for Poisson's ratio for tissue properties.

2.2 Boundary Condition Assignment for Sliding Effect

Nodes of the FEM mesh were classified into the boundary nodes and free nodes (Fig. 1). The nodal displacement of the free nodes (GreenBlue in Fig. 1b and c) was determined by the displacements of the boundary nodes using FEM. The boundary nodes were further classified into fixed, moving and sliding nodes. The fixed nodes did not move during the surgery and FEM simulation (red in Fig. 1), thus, having zero nodal displacement. The lower posterior regions of the soft tissue mesh were assigned as free nodes for the sliding effect simulation with nodal force constraint. This boundary condition, together with the sliding effect of the partial ramus, ensured the soft tissue flexibility and smoothness in the posterior and inferior mandibular regions when an excessive mandibular advancement or setback occurred.

The nodes on the mesh inner surface contacting movable bony segments were designated as the moving nodes. The moving nodes were assumed to move along with the bony segments during the simulation (blue in Fig. 1a). The corresponding moving nodes on the mesh were determined by finding the closest nodes from the vertices of the .STL bony segments using a closest point search algorithm. The movement vector of each bone segment according to the surgical planning was then applied to the moving nodes as a nodal displacement boundary condition. Additionally, the nodes corresponding to the area where two bony segments (proximal and distal) collided each other after bone repositioning (actually removed in real surgery) were excluded from the moving nodes and reassigned as the free nodes. Together with the sliding effect of the partial ramus, this reassignment further solved the mesh distortion problem at the mandibular inferior border when an excessive mandibular setback movement involved. Furthermore, the soft tissue geometry change from a scar formation was considered in the simulation. The regions degloved intraoperatively were selected as a moving boundary (green in Fig. 1a) and the corresponding nodes were shifted in anterior direction by 2 mm by the nodal displacement boundary condition.

The sliding nodes (pink in Fig. 1a) were selected on the mesh inner surface of the mouth (mucosa), including the cheek and lips, to simulate the sliding movement of the soft tissue. The sliding boundary condition in mucosa area was adopted from [7, 8, 12]. In our study, the definition of the sliding nodes was further extended to partial inferior ramus, preventing mesh deformation problem in posterior of the mandible.

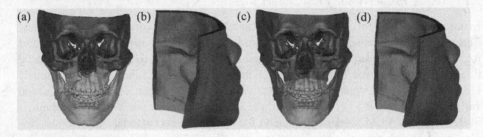

Fig. 1. Boundary condition. (a) Mesh inner surface (illustrated on bones) for the sliding effect with nodal force constraint. (b) Mesh volume and fixed boundary condition for the sliding effect with nodal force constraint. (c) Mesh inner surface (illustrated on bones) for the realistic sliding effect with nodal displacement constraint. (d) Mesh volume and fixed boundary condition for the realistic sliding effect with nodal displacement constraint. **Fixed nodes**: *red*; **Moving nodes**: *Blue*; **Sliding nodes**: *pink*; **Free nodes**: *GreenBlue*; **Scar tissue**: *green*. (Color figure online)

2.3   Implementation of Sliding Effect with Nodal Force Constraint Using Iterative FEM Solving Algorithm

First, the sliding movement of mucosa was implemented by applying nodal force constraint on the sliding nodes. An iterative FEM solving algorithm was developed to solve the FEM with nodal force boundary condition. The general form of global FEM equation is:

$$K\delta = f \tag{1}$$

where K is a global stiffness matrix, δ is a global nodal displacement vector, and f is a global nodal force vector. The above equation can be rewritten as:

$$\begin{pmatrix} K_{11} K_{12} \\ K_{12}^T K_{22} \end{pmatrix} \begin{pmatrix} \delta_1 \\ \delta_2 \end{pmatrix} = \begin{pmatrix} f_1 \\ f_2 \end{pmatrix} \tag{2}$$

where δ_1 is the displacement of the moving and fixed nodes, δ_2 is the displacement of the free and sliding nodes to be determined by FEM, f_1 is the nodal force of the moving and fixed nodes, and f_2 is the nodal force of both free and sliding nodes. Stiffness matrix (K) was reorganized accordingly. The nodal force of the free nodes was assumed to be zero, and only tangential nodal force along the contacting bone surface was considered to determine the movement of the sliding node [7, 8, 12].

The final value of δ_2 was calculated by iteratively updating δ_2 using Eq. (3) until the converging condition was satisfied [described after Eq. (6)].

$$\delta_2^{(i+1)} = \delta_2^{(i)} + \delta_{2_{update}}^{(i)}, (i = 1, 2, \ldots, n) \tag{3}$$

The details of $\delta_{2_{update}}$ calculation was as follows. Equation (4) was derived from Eq. (2) to acquire current value of f_2. f_2 was composed of nodal force of the sliding nodes ($f_{2\,sliding}$) and the free nodes ($f_{2\,free}$). At the first iteration ($i = 1$), the initial δ_2 was randomly assigned and substituted for δ_2 to solve Eq. (4) and f_2 was calculated by substituting current δ_2 into Eq. (4).

$$f_2 = K_{12}^T \delta_1 + K_{22} \delta_2 \tag{4}$$

Then, f_2 was further processed by transforming only the nodal force corresponded to the sliding nodes ($f_{2\,sliding}$) among f_2 using Eq. (5).

$$f_{2\,sliding}^t = f_{2\,sliding} - (f_{2\,sliding} \cdot N) N \tag{5}$$

where $f_{2\,sliding}^t$ is tangential component of nodal force of the sliding nodes, and N is a normal vector of the bone surface corresponding to the sliding nodes. Now, f_2^t composed of the nodal force of the free nodes ($f_{2\,free}$) and a tangential component of the nodal force of the sliding nodes ($f_{2\,sliding}^t$).

Finally, the nodal displacement to update the current δ_2, $(\delta_{2_{update}})$, was calculated from $f_{2_{update}}$. $f_{2_{update}}$ was the required nodal force to make $f_{2\,free}$ zero and calculated by the difference between f_2^t and f_2 ($f_2 - f_2^t$). $\delta_{2_{update}}$ was acquired using Eq. (6):

$$\delta_{2_{update}} = -K_{22}^{-1} (f_{2_{update}} + K_{12}^T \delta_1) \tag{6}$$

Then, δ_2 was updated using Eq. (3). The iteration continued until the maximal absolute value of $f_{2_{update}}$ converged below 0.01 N ($i = n$). The final values of δ (δ_1 and δ_2) represented the displacement of all mesh nodes after the bone repositioning and the sliding effect application with nodal force constraint. The resulted δ was designated as $\delta_{intermediate}$.

2.4   Implementation of Advanced Sliding Effect with Nodal Displacement Constraint

A strict nodal displacement boundary condition was further applied to the result of the iterative FEM solution. Nodal force constraint had limited control on the nodal displacement. Thus, the result of the iterative FEM solution might have geometrical discrepancy between the mesh inner surface and the bone surface (Fig. 2). In real clinical situation, the mucosa should exactly match to the geometry of the teeth and buccal surface of the bone. Therefore, it was necessary to apply strict nodal displacement condition to enhance the iterative (intermediate) result of the nodal force constraint. It was also necessary to redefine the boundary condition mapping between the bone surface and mesh nodes in the sliding area. This was because the relationship between the bone surface vertices and the mesh nodes was changed after the bony segment was repositioned. Moreover, clinically the postop lower teeth were always located inside of the upper teeth (as a normal bite) despite of the preop occlusal relationship. Therefore, more advanced sliding effect with redefinition of boundary condition and strict nodal boundary condition was required to improve the accuracy of the result of sliding effect with nodal force constraint (intermediate simulation).

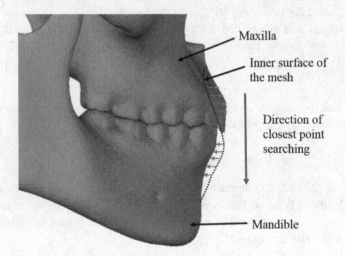

Fig. 2. Assign nodal displacement. The dot line depicts an artifact gap between mucosa and teeth after the sliding effect with nodal force constraint is applied.

The sliding effect with nodal displacement constraint was implemented as follows. First, classification of boundary nodes was redefined. The free nodes at the infero-posterior surface of the soft tissue mesh were assigned as fixed nodes unlike the previous assignment. Then, the nodes on the mesh inner surface corresponding to the maxilla and mandible were assigned as the moving nodes (blue in Fig. 1c). The rest of the nodes are assigned as the free nodes (GreenBlue in Fig. 1c and d). Unlike the previous boundary assignment, there were no sliding nodes.

The nodal displacement for the moving nodes was assigned from superior to inferior direction by finding the closest bone surface vertex from the each of the moving node (Fig. 2), instead of finding correspondence from the bone to the mesh. Once the mapping between the vertex and nodes was computed, the vector between each node and its corresponding closest vertex on the bone surface was assigned as the nodal displacement of the moving nodes. This sequential assignment of nodal displacement prevented the two different nodes from having the same nodal displacement. The reestablishment of boundary condition mapping between the nodes and vertex solved the aforementioned postop mismatch problem between the bone surface and corresponding inner mesh surface due to the bone repositioning and occlusal relationship change.

In Eq. (1), the global stiffness matrix (K), the nodal displacement (δ) and the nodal force (f) were reorganized according to the new boundary conditions. The result was acquired by directly solving redefined Eq. (2) without iterative method. Here, the nodal force of the free nodes, f_2, was assumed to be zero. The nodal displacement of the free nodes, δ_2, was calculated by reorganizing Eq. (2) with this assumption:

$$\delta_2 = -K_{22}^{-1} K_{12}^T \delta_1 \tag{7}$$

Then, the resulted δ (δ_1 and δ_2) was designated as δ_{final}. The final simulation result with realistic sliding effects was acquired by integrating the resulted nodal displacements of the intermediate ($\delta_{intermediate}$) and the final (δ_{final}) FEM simulations.

3 Prediction Accuracy Evaluation

Thirty patients with dentofacial deformities were randomly selected from our datasets [IRB0413-0045]. Both preop and postop CT scan datasets were used for facial tissue prediction and its accuracy evaluation. The soft tissue prediction was completed using 2 methods: (1) traditional FEM without considering the sliding effect; and (2) our FEM method with the realistic sliding effects.

The patient-specific FEM mesh was generated from a template mesh, instead of manually segmenting the tissue volume from CT dataset. The template mesh was previously created from a Visible Female dataset [9]. Both inner and outer surfaces of the template mesh were registered to the patient's skull and facial soft tissue surface respectively using anatomical landmark-based thin-plate splines (TPS) technique. Finally, the total mesh volume of the template was transformed to the patient data by interpolating the surface registration result using TPS again [9].

The actual movement vector of each bony segment was computed from the preop and postop CT datasets. First, the postop patient's bone and soft tissue 3D CT models were registered to the corresponding preop data respectively by matching the surgically unchanged part (the cranium). Then, the osteotomies were performed on the preop models according to the postop CT data. The actual movement vector of each bony segment was calculated by moving each osteotomized segment from its preop original position to the postop position [13]. These vectors were used by both FEM methods as a moving boundary condition.

Finally, the simulated results were evaluated quantitatively. In order to acquire the error of each methods, displacement errors (absolute mean Euclidean distances) were calculated between the nodes on the simulated facial mesh and their corresponding points on the postop model. The evaluation was completed for the whole face and 8 sub-regions (Fig. 3). Repeated measures analysis of variance and its post-hoc tests were used to detect the statistically significant difference.

The results of the quantitative evaluation showed that our FEM method with realistic sliding effects significantly improved the accuracy of the whole face and the critical areas (i.e., lips, nose and chin) comparing to the traditional FEM method, although the chin area only showed a trend of improvement. The malar region also showed a significant improvement due to the modeling of scar tissue. The improvement rates over the traditional FEM simulation were presented in Table 1 sliding.

Table 1. Error of the traditional method (mean ± SD) and improvement of the realistic sliding effects simulation over the traditional FEM method (mm).

Region	Absolute error		Accuracy improvement
	Traditional FEM	Realistic sliding FEM	Rates
Entire face	1.58 ± 0.33	1.51 ± 0.33	4.5*
1. Nose	1.16 ± 0.31	1.06 ± 0.28	8.4*
2. Upper lip	1.36 ± 0.41	1.23 ± 0.41	9.2*
3. Lower lip	1.66 ± 0.60	1.49 ± 0.44	10.2*
4. Chin	1.86 ± 0.81	1.80 ± 0.76	3.6
5. Right malar	1.21 ± 0.30	1.14 ± 0.26	6.2*
6. Left malar	1.41 ± 0.53	1.28 ± 0.49	8.8*
7. Right cheek	1.70 ± 0.53	1.68 ± 0.50	1.3*
8. Left cheek	2.07 ± 0.61	2.05 ± 0.62	1.4*

*Significant difference compared to the traditional method ($P < 0.05$)

In addition to the quantitative accuracy evaluation, the predicted results were also observed visually. The traditional FEM simulation without the sliding effect resulted in a mesh distortion problem in the mandibular inferior border region in the patient underwent severe amount of mandibular movement (Fig. 4(a)). The collision between the two bony segments (proximal and distal) led to the distortion of the mesh in corresponding area, which was clinically unrealistic. On the other hand, the result of our realistic sliding effects clearly solved the mesh distortion problem by showing smooth inferior boarder (Fig. 4(b)).

Figure 5 illustrates the predicted results of a typical patient. Using the traditional FEM method, the upper and lower lip moved together with the underlying bone segments as a whole without considering the sliding movement (1.4 mm of displacement error for the upper lip; 1.6 mm for the lower). This resulted in large displacement errors (Fig. 5(a)), apparently clinically unrealistic. The sliding effect with nodal force constraint moderately improved the accuracy in the upper lip, while the lower lip still showed a larger error. The upper and lower lips were in a wrong relation. In addition, the mesh inner surface and anterior surface of the bony segment were also mismatched that should be perfectly matched clinically (Fig. 5(b)), apparently also unrealistic. Finally, the result of our realistic sliding effects achieved the best prediction results, accurately predicting clinically important facial features with a correct lip relation (the upper lip: 0.9 mm of the error; the lower: 1.3 mm) (Fig. 5(c)), apparently clinically realistic.

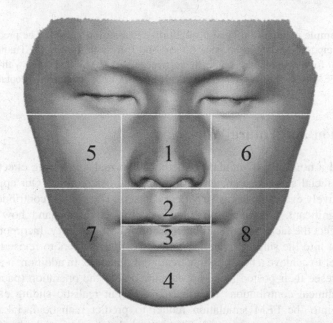

Fig. 3. Sub-regions (automatically divided using anatomical landmarks)

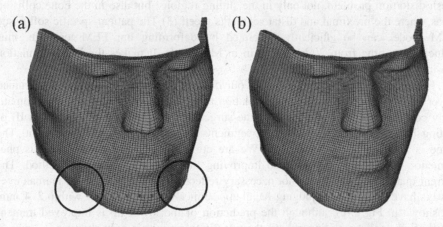

(a)   (b)

Fig. 4. An example of mesh distortion after bone repositioning (inside of circle). **(a)** Mesh collision in inferior border of the mandible in the traditional FEM simulation without sliding effect. **(b)** Smooth inferior border line of the mandible of our method with the realistic sliding effects.

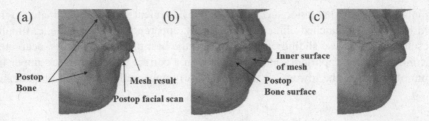

Fig. 5. An example of quantitative and qualitative evaluation results. The predicted mesh (pink) is superimposed to the postop bone (green) and soft tissue (grey). **(a)** Traditional FEM (1.6 mm of error for the whole face, clinically not acceptable). **(b)** Sliding effect with nodal force constraint. **(c)** FEM with realistic sliding effects (1.4 mm of error, clinically acceptable). (Color figure online)

4   Discussion and Future Work

We developed a novel FEM simulation method with realistic sliding effects to accurately predict facial soft tissue changes following the osteotomies. Our approach has been quantitatively evaluated using 30 patient datasets. The clinical contribution of this method is significant. Our approach allows doctors to understand how the bony movements affect the facial soft tissues changes prior to the surgery. Incorporating such prediction tool into the surgical planning will also allow doctors to revise the plan as needed in order to achieve a best-possible treatment outcome. In addition, it also allows patients to foresee their postop facial appearance before the operation (patient education). The technical contributions include: (1) Efficient realistic sliding effects were implemented into the FEM simulation model to predict realistic facial soft tissue changes following the osteotomies. (2) The extended definition of the boundary condition and the ability of changing node types during the simulation clearly solve the mesh distortion problem, not only in the sliding regions, but also in the bone collision areas where the proximal and distal segments meet. (3) The patient-specific soft tissue FEM model can be efficiently generated by deforming our FEM template, thus reducing the time from 20 h to 10 min in MATLAB. It makes the FEM simulation feasible for clinical use.

There are still some limitations in our current approach. Preoperatively strained lower lip is not considered in the simulation. The strained lower lip can be automatically corrected to a reposed status in the surgery by only advancing (for Class II) or setting back (for Class III) the bony segments without any vertical movement. The same is not true in the simulation. We are currently working on solving this phenomenon. In addition, we are also improving the accuracy evaluation method. The current quantitative results do not necessary reflect the visualized results. Human eyes always have tolerances in judging facial appearance changes, usually within 2–4 mm. As shown in Fig. 5(c), although the prediction of the lower lip is improved tremendously with realistic sliding effects, the quantitative analysis only shows a 0.2 mm of improvement, which is a clinically nonsignificant improvement. Moreover, the prediction error of the lower lip using the traditional FEM is only 1.6 mm in quantitative analysis - an error also does not have any clinical significance. Nonetheless, Fig. 5(a) and (c) indicate the otherwise. Ultimately, our two-stage FEM simulation is the first step towards achieving a realistic facial soft-tissue-change prediction following osteotomies. In the near future, it will be fully tested in a larger clinical study.

References

1. Hsu, S.S., et al.: Accuracy of a computer-aided surgical simulation protocol for orthognathic surgery: a prospective multicenter study. J. Oral Maxillofac. Surg. **71**(1), 128–142 (2013)
2. Bell, W.H., Ferraro, J.W.: Modern practice in orthognathic and reconstructive surgery. Plast. Reconstr. Surg. **92**(2), 362 (1993)
3. Koch, R.M., et al.: Simulating facial surgery using finite element models. In: Proceedings of the 23rd Annual Conference on Computer Graphics and Interactive Techniques, pp. 421–428. ACM (1996)
4. Chabanas, M., Luboz, V., Payan, Y.: Patient specific finite element model of the face soft tissues for computer-assisted maxillofacial surgery. Med. Image Anal. **7**(2), 131–151 (2003)
5. Keeve, E., et al.: Deformable modeling of facial tissue for craniofacial surgery simulation. Comput. Aided Surg. **3**(5), 228–238 (1998)
6. Cotin, S., Delingette, H., Ayache, N.: A hybrid elastic model for real-time cutting, deformations, and force feedback for surgery training and simulation. Vis. Comput. **16**(8), 437–452 (2000)
7. Kim, H., Jürgens, P., Nolte, L.-P., Reyes, M.: Anatomically-driven soft-tissue simulation strategy for cranio-maxillofacial surgery using facial muscle template model. In: Jiang, T., Navab, N., Pluim, J.P., Viergever, M.A. (eds.) MICCAI 2010, Part I. LNCS, vol. 6361, pp. 61–68. Springer, Heidelberg (2010)
8. Kim, H., et al.: A new soft-tissue simulation strategy for cranio-maxillofacial surgery using facial muscle template model. Prog. Biophys. Mol. Biol. **103**(2–3), 284–291 (2010)
9. Zhang, X., et al.: An eFace-template method for efficiently generating patient-specific anatomically-detailed facial soft tissue FE models for craniomaxillofacial surgery simulation. Ann. Biomed. Eng. **44**(5), 1656–1671 (2016)
10. Mollemans, W., Schutyser, F., Nadjmi, N., Maes, F., Suetens, P.: Parameter optimisation of a linear tetrahedral mass tensor model for a maxillofacial soft tissue simulator. In: Harders, M., Székely, G. (eds.) ISBMS 2006. LNCS, vol. 4072, pp. 159–168. Springer, Heidelberg (2006)
11. Zachow, S., Hierl, T., Erdmann, B.: A quantitative evaluation of 3D soft tissue prediction in maxillofacial surgery planning. In: Proceedings of CARAC, pp. 75–79 (2004)
12. Roose, L., De Maerteleire, W., Mollemans, W., Maes, F., Suetens, P.: Simulation of soft-tissue deformations for breast augmentation planning. In: Harders, M., Székely, G. (eds.) ISBMS 2006. LNCS, vol. 4072, pp. 197–205. Springer, Heidelberg (2006)
13. Xia, J.J., et al.: Accuracy of the computer-aided surgical simulation (CASS) system in the treatment of patients with complex craniomaxillofacial deformity: a pilot study. J. Oral Maxillofac. Surg. **65**(2), 248–254 (2007)

CathNets: Detection and Single-View Depth Prediction of Catheter Electrodes

Christoph Baur[1]([✉]), Shadi Albarqouni[1]([✉]), Stefanie Demirci[1], Nassir Navab[1,2], and Pascal Fallavollita[1]

[1] Computer Aided Medical Procedures (CAMP),
Technical University of Munich, Munich, Germany
{c.baur,shadi.albarqouni}@tum.de
[2] Whiting School of Engineering, Johns Hopkins University, Baltimore, USA

Abstract. The recent success of convolutional neural networks in many computer vision tasks implies that their application could also be beneficial for vision tasks in cardiac electrophysiology procedures which are commonly carried out under guidance of C-arm fluoroscopy. Many efforts for catheter detection and reconstruction have been made, but especially robust detection of catheters in X-ray images in realtime is still not entirely solved. We propose two novel methods for (i) fully automatic electrophysiology catheter electrode detection in interventional X-ray images and (ii) single-view depth estimation of such electrodes based on convolutional neural networks. For (i), experiments on 24 different fluoroscopy sequences (1650 X-ray images) yielded a detection rate $> 99\%$. Our experiments on (ii) depth prediction using 20 images with depth information available revealed that we are able to estimate the depth of catheter tips in the lateral view with a remarkable mean error of 6.08 ± 4.66 mm.

Keywords: Convolutional neural network · Catheter detection · Depth prediction · Electrophysiology · Interventional imaging

1 Introduction

In electrophysiology procedures such as treatment of ventricular tachycardia and atrial fibrillation, surgeons usually place ablation catheters inside the patients heart under guidance of C-arm fluoroscopy. Surgeons first steer the catheters through the vessels to the target location inside the heart under X-Ray imaging support. In addition to fluoroscopy, more precise and robust 3D localization can be achieved with the help of commercial electro-anatomic mapping systems such as CARTO and CARTOMerge (Biosense Webster), NavX (St. Jude Medical) and RPM (Cardiac Pathways-Boston Scientific). In fact, these systems reduce fluoroscopy times and radiation exposure. In the last years, several groups within the community have focused their efforts in developing algorithms for optical catheter detection, tracking [10,16,18,19,23,24] as well as 3D reconstruction [2,10,11] from these X-ray images. Prior to any tracking or 3D reconstruction,

© Springer International Publishing Switzerland 2016
G. Zheng et al. (Eds.): MIAR 2016, LNCS 9805, pp. 38–49, 2016.
DOI: 10.1007/978-3-319-43775-0_4

detecting the catheters with high precision is of upmost importance. However, this is not a trivial task because of low SNR in the images, the complex shapes of some catheters as well as overlapping catheters [18]. Nonetheless, the community has managed to come up with great detection algorithms yielding detection rates above 95 %. However, state-of-the-art methods either require a large amount of preprocessing and heavy optimizations, such that realtime requirements can hardly be met, or need careful parameter selection.

Our contribution is two-fold. First, inspired by the recent success of convolutional neural networks in many vision tasks, we propose a fully automatic optical catheter detection method with realtime capabilities. Our method is based on a fully convolutional neural network architecture trained on only a small number of X-ray images with the help of a class balancing loss function. In contrast to previous methods, ours does not require any preprocessing, is free of any user interaction and can detect tips and electrodes of multiple, overlapping catheters at once. Our method can act as a substitute to time-consuming, search-space reduction preprocessing or as a standalone 2D multi catheter component detector. Besides catheter electrode detection, we also present our work on catheter electrode depth prediction from single views. The work of Fallavollita [8] showed that depth of catheter tips can be regressed from monoplane X-ray images alone. Recent work on depth prediction from single views [6] based on CNNs showed outstanding results and left us confident that with help of deep learning, the depth of all catheter electrodes can be estimated more precisely.

The remainder of this manuscript is organized as follows: In Sect. 2 we give a brief overview of preceding work on catheter detection, tracking and 3D reconstruction as well as their depth prediction. Afterwards, we present our methodology and the different CNN architectures. This is followed by a section on our experiments for both contributions. Section 5 concludes the manuscript.

2 Related Work

A first attempt towards the automatic detection of catheter tips in X-ray images was made by Franken et al. [9] in 2006. Their method, however, was computationally expensive and lacked robustness. In 2010 Schenderlein et al. [20] proposed a catheter detection method based on 3D snakes (active contours) and the minimization of 2D reprojection errors onto biplane X-ray images. In parallel, Brost et al. [4] developed a 2D-3D registration method for 3D reconstruction of lasso catheters from biplane X-ray data for the purpose of detecting respiratory motion, however also requiring manual seeding of catheter electrodes. Concurrently, Ma [17] developed an algorithm for coronary sinus catheter detection involving blob detection and cost function minimization, however requiring multiple user interactions and careful parameterization depending on the X-ray images. In 2011, Wu et al. [22] proposed a method for coronary sinus catheter tracking which chooses most likely catheter hypotheses with help of a bayesian framework. One year later, Yatziv et al. [24] proposed a different detection method based on background removal. Unfortunately, their method only worked with temporal image sequences and required user interaction. A variety of ablation catheter detection methods based on traditional blob detection were published in 2013. For instance, Ma et al. [16] proposed an automatic detection method based on fast blob detection, shape-constrained searching and model-based detection for different types of catheters. Milletari et al. [19] proposed an ablation catheter detection algorithm also based on fast blob detection, but with a focus on detecting multiple overlapping catheters in single images. A year later, Milletari et al. [18] were able to considerably improve their detection results by replacing their simple cost function optimization with a sparse coding methodology, yielding a very robust detector. Their method is however limited to ablation catheters. The method introduced by Hoffmann et al. [12] in 2015 employs a graph search for catheter detection after manually clicking on the desired catheter in each view, and in succession a subsequent 3D reconstruction of the entire catheter sheath is performed with triangulation.

In the realm of catheter depth prediction, the literature is very sparse. A very first approach for depth estimation of catheter tips was made by Fallavollita [8] in 2010. In his experiments, he exploited the geometrical properties of catheter tips and the projective geometry of X-ray systems in order to turn depth estimation into a linear regression task. However, the work solely focused on the depth estimation in single-views of the catheter tip in a limited amount of datasets. Afterwards, only a few attempts to extract useful information from single-view X-ray images have been made for 3D stent recovery from single views by Demirci et al. [5] in 2013, and single-view X-ray depth recovery using dictionary learning by Albarqouni et al. [1] in 2016.

3   Methodology

3.1   Catheter Detection

Our catheter detection methodology is inspired by the recent work of Long et al. [15], who employ a fully convolutional neural network architecture for the task of semantic segmentation with great success. We also leverage the high computational efficiency of such network design for the purpose of catheter electrode detection. Our architecture was empirically determined, inspired by other successful architectures [13,14,21]. We first carefully chose our training data sampling strategy, and afterwards tweaked the architecture, e.g. adjusted the depth and parameters of our architecture, until we obtained satisfying results. The architecture of our detection network is depicted in Fig. 1. We first apply batch normalization immediately to the input data. This is followed by two convolutional blocks with larger 5×5 kernels, batch normalization and ReLu activation. The resulting feature maps are downsampled with max pooling and two similar blocks of convolution, now at a 3×3 kernel size are employed. Finally, another max pooling and another two convolutional blocks of the same size are applied before the feature maps enter the classification stage consisting of three 1×1 convolutional blocks. The final layer is either a softmax classifier, or a loss function for the training phase.

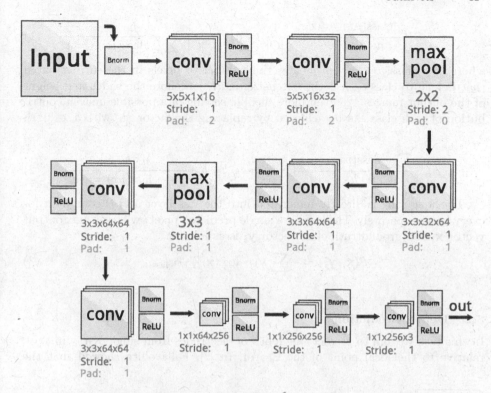

Fig. 1. Our deep fully convolutional architecture for catheter detection consisting of 6 convolutional blocks with batch normalization and ReLU activation, two max-pooling layers and 3 layers with 1×1 convolutional blocks with batch normalization and ReLU activation. For training, we attach a class weighted softmax cross entropy loss to the last ReLU output. For testing, we replace the loss with a softmax classifier.

Particularly important for the success of our method is the choice of the loss function. In order to accurately detect catheters, we have to precisely distinguish between background pixels and electrodes. Thus it is neccessary for the network to learn a large variety of background appearances. For this purpose we train the network from large image patches at the size of 192×192 px. Within these patches however, the catheter electrodes are dramatically underrepresented. Without any class balancing, our model initially tended to classify every pixel as background since a few incorrectly classified pixels hardly influenced the loss function. To cope with this problem, we introduced the Class-Weighted Softmax Cross-Entropy Loss:

Given an image $I \in \mathbb{R}^{h \times w}$ and a set of classes $C = \{c_{bg}, c_{tips}, c_{electrodes}\}$, we aim to ensure a fair influence of all the classes of the pixels in the current batch to the loss function, and more importantly to the weight update. For each class c_i, we therefore introduce the class balancing factor

$$\alpha_{c_i} \cdot \frac{\sum_{px} \text{class}(px) == c_i}{n \cdot h \cdot w} = \frac{1}{|C|} \Leftrightarrow \alpha_{c_i} = \frac{n \cdot h \cdot w}{|C| \cdot \sum_{px} \text{class}(px) == c_i} \qquad (1)$$

where $\sum_{px} \text{class}(px) == c_i$ denotes the number of pixels in the current batch that belong to class c_i, n is the batchsize and h, w denote the width and height of the output images. An even more flexible setting of a possible uneven contribution of each class can be achieved by replacing the factor $\frac{1}{|C|}$ with $b_i \in [0;1]$, $\sum_i b_i = 1$:

$$\alpha_{c_i} \cdot \frac{\sum_{px} \text{class}(px) == c_i}{n \cdot h \cdot w} = b_i \Leftrightarrow \alpha_{c_i} = b_i \cdot \frac{n \cdot h \cdot w}{\sum_{px} \text{class}(px) == c_i} \qquad (2)$$

The weighting is directly integrated into the loss layer and is computed for every batch separately. The loss for a single predicted pixel i with softmax output vector $\mathbf{x}_i$ and groundtruth class vector $\mathbf{y}_i$ is as follows:

$$\mathcal{L}(\mathbf{x}_i, \mathbf{y}_i) = -\sum_j \mathbf{y}_{ij} \cdot \log(\mathbf{x}_{ij}) \cdot \alpha_{\text{class}(i)} \qquad (3)$$

3.2 Depth Prediction

In this task we aim to predict the depth of electrodes from single X-ray images, relative to the focal point of the C-arm. In [7], Fallavollita showed that the

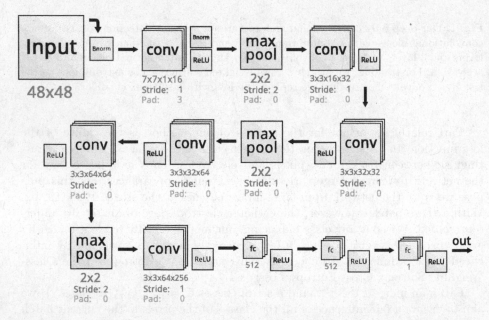

Fig. 2. Our architecture for depth prediction consisting of 6 ReLU-activated convolutional blocks, three max-pooling layers and three ReLU activated fully connected layers. For training, we employ the Tukey loss. During testing, the last ReLU unit immediately outputs the regressed depth in mm.

width & area of a catheter tip electrode is inversely proportional to the distance of the object from the focal plane. Various success stories for single-view depth prediction in interventional imaging [1,5] and computer vision [6] left us confident that we can tackle this problem with a CNN, which would inherently learn to determine the appropriate features for depth regression directly from raw input patches. For this purpose we developed the architecture depicted in Fig. 2. We started off with a network design based on our detection architecture and, again, made adjustments until we were satisfied with the results. Similar to our detection network, the architecture starts with alternations of ReLU-activated convolutional blocks and pooling layers. However, we only rarely made use of batch normalization since we noticed that its excessive utilization in this case hampered proper learning of the weights. At the end of the network, we employ three traditional fully connected layers since we always regress from input patches of the same size. Our choice of loss function was the tukey loss which is well suited for regression tasks, robust to outliers and speeds up convergence [3]. In fact, in early experiments we employed the euclidean loss, but it was clearly outperformed by the tukey loss.

4   Experiments

4.1   Dataset

For our experiments we utilized two distinct datasets. The first dataset consists of 20 pairs of co-registered monoplane X-ray images from the lateral (LAT) and posterior-anterior (PA) view of a mongrel dog heart. The specimen was sedated and three different catheters, i.e. a reference, a pacing and an 8-french ablation catheter were positioned inside its heart. Multiple sequences from the two views were acquired with a Philips Integris Allura C-arm during one intervention. With help of the algorithm proposed in [7], pairs of corresponding images from both views were selected. Groundtruth annotations of catheter electrodes were provided by two experts. Using the intrinsic geometry of the C-arm, 3D groundtruth locations of the catheter electrodes were reconstructed via triangulation. We utilized all of the 20 image pairs for training our detector, but used only 10 image pairs for the training stage of our depth prediction network. Consequently, we chose the other half of the dataset for testing our depth prediction model. Arguably, the size of our training data for both tasks seems very small. But given the facts that (a) ablation catheter appearances in these X-ray images are highly constrained and (b) we perform extensive data augmentation, we consider the size of our training dataset to be sufficiently large for training our models.

The second dataset stems from the same image acquisition setup with the same specimen. Additional 24 fluoroscopy sequences, each containing more than 50 frames, were acquired from the LAT and the PA view during the same intervention. This dataset consisting of 1650 images with groundtruth annotations was solely used for testing our electrode detector.

In order to ensure variability within the data, the X-ray intensity was varied between 70 and 92 keV for both datasets. All images have a resolution of 512×512 pixels at a pixel spacing of 0.44 mm.

4.2 Catheter Detection

Training: We trained two distinct models of the previously presented architecture from images at full scale (512×512 px) and at half the image resolution (256×256 px). The models were trained for 23 and 20 epochs respectively, stopping when the error did not decrease any further, and afterwards evaluated on the 1650 testing images comprising 23,100 electrodes in total. We evaluated the models with regard to detections that are within 5 px distance to the groundtruth annotations (and 2.5 px for the network operating at half scale, respectively). The achieved detection rates for different electrode types and views are reported in Table 1 (Fig. 3).

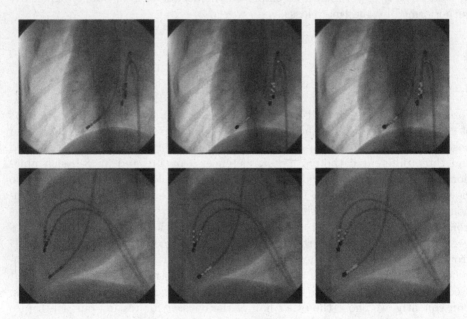

Fig. 3. Electrode detection examples from PA and LAT view from different scales. The left image shows the original X-ray image, the middle image shows the same image with an overlay of the detection results and the right image is an upsampled version of the detection at half the image scale. Blue blobs visualize catheter tips and green blobs show electrode detections. A few false positives are visible in the images where the catheter tubes intersect. (Color figure online)

Speed: Computing the net response for an image at full scale took approximately 1000 ms on a commodity PC (Intel Core i5 2600K) using MATLAB. Inference at scale 0.5 was much faster, operating at 200 ms on the same machine.

Table 1. Comparison of catheter electrode detection rates of a network trained at full scale, a network trained at half the image size and the results from Milletari et al. [18] for all electrodes, tip electrodes and non-tip electrodes ("Elecs") in the PA and LAT view.

Model	All (PA)	Tips (PA)	Elecs (PA)	All (LAT)	Tips (LAT)	Elecs (LAT)
Ours (Full scale)	**99.92 %**	99.92 %	**99.92 %**	99.14 %	**100.0 %**	98.91 %
Ours (Half scale)	99.77 %	**99.95 %**	99.73 %	**99.49 %**	100.0 %	**99.35 %**
Milletari' 2014	97.75 %	-	-	95.77 %	-	-

Table 2. False positive rates of our two different models for all electrodes, tip electrodes and non-tip electrodes in the different views.

Model	All (PA)	Tips (PA)	Elecs (PA)	All (LAT)	Tips (LAT)	Elecs (LAT)
Ours (Full scale)	0.210 %	0.042 %	0.180 %	0.120 %	0.044 %	0.091 %
Ours (Half scale)	0.360 %	0.110 %	0.250 %	0.570 %	0.037 %	0.540 %

Results: Our models trained from both full and half scale images achieve detection rates above 99 % and clearly outperform the method presented in [18]. We compare to this method for two reasons: the authors also try detect the same type of overlapping catheters and it can be considered state-of-the-art. Other methods either focus on different catheter types or do not report the same metrics. In the lateral view the networks were even able to correctly identify 100 % of the catheter tips. Remarkably, the detection rates at lower scale are comparable to the performance of the full scale model, however at the cost of an increased false positive rate (FPR) as reported in Table 2. These false positives (FP) mainly occur in regions where two catheter tubes intersect. We believe that such FP in both models are related to our training data sampling strategy. Catheter tube intersections are not labeled and thus not explicitly sampled from the images, hence potentially underrepresented within the training data.

4.3   Electrode Depth Prediction

Training: We trained a model for depth prediction from 48×48 px sized patches in batches of 200 for 30 epochs. We performed the standard data augmentation of in-plane rotations (in steps of $30°$) and scaling (from 0.7 to 1.3 in steps of 0.01), yielding a total of approximately 470,000 patches.

Results: We evaluated the model on 20 unseen images with a total of 280 electrodes in terms of the mean depth error and standard deviation in millimeter. Our results are listed in Table 2. Figure 4 shows the depth predictions of each of the 280 electrodes compared to groundtruth. By visual inspection, a certain trend can be recognized within the regression results which coarsely approximate the groundtruth data. We also observe a few strong outliers, which we can relate to foreshortened catheters and motion blur in the respective images. Similarly to Fallavollita, we also report best performance for the lateral view

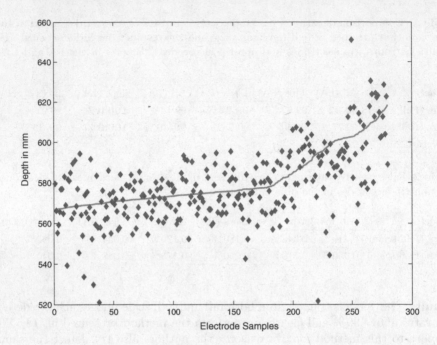

Fig. 4. The depth predictions for each of the 280 testing electrodes, sorted by increasing groundtruth depth. The red line shows the groundtruth depth and blue diamonds the corresponding regression result. (Color figure online)

Table 3. Depth prediction results using our model in millimeters for all electrodes, tip electrodes, non-tip electrodes, all electrodes in PA view and all electrodes in LAT view

View	All	Tips	Non-tips
PA	13.46 ± 11.50	14.11 ± 15.45	13.28 ± 10.25
LAT	**8.24 ± 6.20**	**6.08 ± 4.66**	**8.83 ± 6.45**
Combined	10.85 ± 9.59	10.01 ± 12.02	11.06 ± 8.83

of 6.08 ± 4.66 mm for the tip electrodes and 8.83 ± 6.45 mm for the remaining ones. The worse performance in the PA images is due to a considerable amount of foreshortened catheters for which the network obviously cannot appropriately predict depth.

4.4   Discussion

Commercial electro-anatomic mapping systems like CARTO only track the catheter tips and provide the clinician with a volume in which the tip resides. Usually, the tracking error in these systems lies within 15 to 20 mm due to cardiac and respiratory motion. In this context, our depth predictions match up quite well. Yet, we believe that results can be further improved with more training data. In a clinical application, the predicted depth information, in conjunction with x,y coordinates from the detection, can be used to localize the catheters relative to the C-arm or inside the anatomy after e.g. registration to preoperative data. At the moment our detection model is trained to detect electrodes of ablation catheters, but it can easily be extended for other types of catheters by retraining or training entirely new models. Besides being very robust, our detection method is also free of any parameters and does not require any preprocessing, as opposed to e.g. gaussian blob detectors. The latter are usually heavily dependent on scale-space parameterization and do not intelligently involve any larger context, leading to a high number of FP detections all over the X-ray images. While theoretically possible, there is no guarantee that the models for both detection and depth prediction will work on other C-arm devices out-of-the-box. In future work, this should be examined further. Additionally, our experiments were conducted on X-ray images of a dog, but we also expect our method to work on human X-ray data. However, in human X-ray interventions, the radiation dose is typically lower, leading to lower contrast and more noise in the images. Thus, robustness of our method should also be verified on human X-ray data in future experiments. Apart from that, there is no evidence that our architectures resemble the best choices. Unfortunately, determining the best architecture is still an unresolved problem in deep learning. At the moment, a sophisticated strategy to find better architectures involves grid searches in both model and parameter space. This however requires tremendous computational resources. Another limiting factor for our work is the lack of a publicly available dataset for catheter detection, which would allow us to do meaningful comparisons among different detection methods in general (Table 3).

5   Conclusion

Our experiments showed that convolutional neural networks also live up to their expectations in the tasks of catheter electrode detection and depth regression in X-ray images. Especially the electrode detector turned out to be very accurate and robust to variations in X-ray intensity and noise. Yet, there is room for improvement in both presented tasks. The number of false positives in the detection task should be further decreased and the robustness of the depth prediction needs to be improved. Future work will also involve using the detection output for determining electrode centroids and actually discovering catheter models. Further, both the detection and the depth prediction could be lined up in order to yield a combined automatic detection and depth prediction framework.

References

1. Albarqouni, S., Konrad, U., Wang, L., Navab, N., Demirci, S.: Single-view X-ray depth recovery: toward a novel concept for image-guided interventions. Int. J. Comput. Assist. Radiol. Surg. **11**(6), 873–880 (2016)
2. Baur, C., Milletari, F., Belagiannis, V., Navab, N., Fallavollita, P.: Automatic 3D reconstruction of electrophysiology catheters from two-view monoplane C-arm image sequences. Int. J. Comput. Assist. Radiol. Surg. **11**(7), 1319–1328 (2016)
3. Belagiannis, V., Rupprecht, C., Carneiro, G., Navab, N.: Robust optimization for deep regression (2015). arXiv preprint arXiv:1505.06606
4. Brost, A., Liao, R., Strobel, N., Hornegger, J.: Respiratory motion compensation by model-based catheter tracking during EP procedures. Med. Image Anal. **14**(5), 695–706 (2010)
5. Demirci, S., Bigdelou, A., Wang, L., Wachinger, C., Baust, M., Tibrewal, R., Ghotbi, R., Eckstein, H.-H., Navab, N.: 3D stent recovery from one X-Ray projection. In: Fichtinger, G., Martel, A., Peters, T. (eds.) MICCAI 2011, Part I. LNCS, vol. 6891, pp. 178–185. Springer, Heidelberg (2011)
6. Eigen, D., Puhrsch, C., Fergus, R.: Depth map prediction from a single image using a multi-scale deep network. In: Advances in Neural Information Processing Systems, pp. 2366–2374 (2014)
7. Fallavollita, P.: Acquiring multiview C-arm images to assist cardiac ablation procedures. J. Image Video Process. **2010**, 1–10, Article ID: 3 (2010). doi:10.1155/2010/871409
8. Fallavollita, P.: Is single-view fluoroscopy sufficient in guiding cardiac ablation procedures? J. Biomed. Imaging **2010**, 1–13, Article ID: 631264 (2010). doi:10.1155/2010/631264
9. Franken, E., Rongen, P., van Almsick, M., ter Haar Romeny, B.M.: Detection of electrophysiology catheters in noisy fluoroscopy images. In: Larsen, R., Nielsen, M., Sporring, J. (eds.) MICCAI 2006. LNCS, vol. 4191, pp. 25–32. Springer, Heidelberg (2006)
10. Hoffmann, M., Brost, A., Jakob, C., Bourier, F., Koch, M., Kurzidim, K., Hornegger, J., Strobel, N.: Semi-automatic catheter reconstruction from two views. In: Ayache, N., Delingette, H., Golland, P., Mori, K. (eds.) MICCAI 2012, Part II. LNCS, vol. 7511, pp. 584–591. Springer, Heidelberg (2012)
11. Hoffmann, M., Brost, A., Jakob, C., Koch, M., Bourier, F., Kurzidim, K., Hornegger, J., Strobel, N.: Reconstruction method for curvilinear structures from two views. In: SPIE Medical Imaging, p. 86712F. International Society for Optics and Photonics (2013)
12. Hoffmann, M., Brost, A., Koch, M., Bourier, F., Maier, A., Kurzidim, K., Strobel, N., Hornegger, J.: Electrophysiology catheter detection and reconstruction from two views in fluoroscopic images (2015)
13. Ioffe, S., Szegedy, C.: Batch normalization: accelerating deep network training by reducing internal covariate shift (2015). arXiv preprint arXiv:1502.03167
14. Krizhevsky, A., Sutskever, I., Hinton, G.E.: Imagenet classification with deep convolutional neural networks. In: Advances in Neural Information Processing Systems, pp. 1097–1105 (2012)
15. Long, J., Shelhamer, E., Darrell, T.: Fully convolutional networks for semantic segmentation. In: Proceedings of the IEEE Conference on Computer Vision and Pattern Recognition, pp. 3431–3440 (2015)

16. Ma, Y.L., Gogin, N., Cathier, P., Housden, R.J., Gijsbers, G., Cooklin, M., O'Neill, M., Gill, J., Rinaldi, C.A., Razavi, R., et al.: Real-time X-ray fluoroscopy-based catheter detection and tracking for cardiac electrophysiology interventions. Med. Phys. **40**(7), 071902 (2013)

17. Ma, Y.: Real-time respiratory motion correction for cardiac electrophysiology procedures using image-based coronary sinus catheter tracking. In: Mori, K., Sakuma, I., Sato, Y., Barillot, C., Navab, N. (eds.) MICCAI 2010, Part I. LNCS, vol. 6361, pp. 391–399. Springer, Heidelberg (2010)

18. Milletari, F., Belagiannis, V., Navab, N., Fallavollita, P.: Fully automatic catheter localization in c-arm images using ℓ1-sparse coding. In: Golland, P., Hata, N., Barillot, C., Hornegger, J., Howe, R. (eds.) MICCAI 2014, Part II. LNCS, vol. 8674, pp. 570–577. Springer, Heidelberg (2014)

19. Milletari, F., Navab, N., Fallavollita, P.: Automatic detection of multiple and overlapping EP catheters in fluoroscopic sequences. In: Mori, K., Sakuma, I., Sato, Y., Barillot, C., Navab, N. (eds.) MICCAI 2013, Part III. LNCS, vol. 8151, pp. 371–379. Springer, Heidelberg (2013)

20. Schenderlein, M., Stierlin, S., Manzke, R., Rasche, V., Dietmayer, K.: Catheter tracking in asynchronous biplane fluoroscopy images by 3D B-snakes. In: SPIE Medical Imaging, p. 76251U. International Society for Optics and Photonics (2010)

21. Simonyan, K., Zisserman, A.: Very deep convolutional networks for large-scale image recognition (2014). arXiv preprint arXiv:1409.1556

22. Wen, W., Chen, T., Barbu, A., Wang, P., Strobel, N., Zhou, S.K., Comaniciu, D.: Learning-based hypothesis fusion for robust catheter tracking in 2D X-ray fluoroscopy. In: 2011 IEEE Conference on Computer Vision and Pattern Recognition (CVPR), pp. 1097–1104. IEEE (2011)

23. Wen, W., Chen, T., Strobel, N., Comaniciu, D.: Fast tracking of catheters in 2D fluoroscopic images using an integrated CPU-GPU framework. In: 2012 9th IEEE International Symposium on Biomedical Imaging (ISBI), pp. 1184–1187. IEEE (2012)

24. Yatziv, L., Chartouni, M., Datta, S., Sapiro, G.: Toward multiple catheters detection in fluoroscopic image guided interventions. IEEE Trans. Inf. Technol. Biomed. **16**(4), 770–781 (2012)

Inference of Tissue Haemoglobin Concentration from Stereo RGB

Geoffrey Jones[1](✉), Neil T. Clancy[2,3], Simon Arridge[1], Daniel S. Elson[2,3], and Danail Stoyanov[1]

[1] Centre for Medical Image Computing, University College London, London, UK
geoffrey.jones.12@ucl.ac.uk
[2] The Hamlyn Centre, Institute of Global Health Innovation,
Imperial College London, London, UK
[3] Department of Surgery and Cancer, Imperial College London, London, UK

Abstract. Multispectral imaging (MSI) can provide information about tissue oxygenation, perfusion and potentially function during surgery. In this paper we present a novel, near real-time technique for intrinsic measurements of total haemoglobin (THb) and blood oxygenation (SO_2) in tissue using only RGB images from a stereo laparoscope. The high degree of spectral overlap between channels makes inference of haemoglobin concentration challenging, non-linear and under constrained. We decompose the problem into two constrained linear sub-problems and show that with Tikhonov regularisation the estimation significantly improves, giving robust estimation of the THb. We demonstrate by using the co-registered stereo image data from two cameras it is possible to get robust SO_2 estimation as well. Our method is closed from, providing computational efficiency even with multiple cameras. The method we present requires only spectral response calibration of each camera, without modification of existing laparoscopic imaging hardware. We validate our technique on synthetic data from Monte Carlo simulation and further, *in vivo*, on a multispectral porcine data set.

1 Introduction

Intraoperative imaging is critical for guiding surgical procedures, especially in minimally invasive surgery (MIS) where the surgeons' access to the surgical site is indirect and restricted [9]. Current white light imaging is mostly limited to providing information from tissue surfaces and does not help the surgeon to identify structures within the tissue such as blood vessels. Laparoscopic images contain only macroscopic structural and radiometric information, that does not directly highlight tissue function or characteristics which may be used to identify malignancy. Pathological signals such as oxy and de-oxy haemoglobin (HbO$_2$, Hb) concentration, often correspond to tissue structure [18] or viability [6] and are detectable by their characteristic attenuation of light in the visible wavelength range. Detecting and displaying this information *in vivo* could provide a powerful tool to the surgeon, but current imaging solutions often demand modification the laparoscopic imaging hardware or protocols.

© Springer International Publishing Switzerland 2016
G. Zheng et al. (Eds.): MIAR 2016, LNCS 9805, pp. 50–58, 2016.
DOI: 10.1007/978-3-319-43775-0_5

MSI is an attractive modality for intraoperative surgical imaging because it is non-ionising and compatible with laparoscopic instrumentation. It can be used to measure ischeamia *in situ* [16] and in MIS to measure the oxygenation of tissue or to identify malignant tissue, where the increased vascularisation causes a local increase in THb [8]. Bowel perfusion assessment [5] and uterine viability post-transplantation [6] have been achieved by measuring the oxygenation saturation and total haemoglobin in the transplanted organ. Central to these type of techniques is a liquid crystal tunable filter (LCTF) which is used to serial capture band limited images, giving a high spectral resolution with the trade off of blur and misalignment when imaging dynamic tissue [7]. Rapid filtering with maximally discriminative filter set can still enable estimation of the haemoglobin concentration from fewer measurement, but requires hardware modifications [19]. Fast capture techniques directly utilising RGB images are possible via use of Wiener filtering to estimate the latent multispectral information [17]. Hybrid approaches using several multi bandpass filters can capture full multispectral data at high frame rates [13]. This technique tailors the filters to a specific RGB sensor so would require a break in surgery to switch imaging hardware. Temporal analysis of tissue using RGB video can also be used for estimation of oxygen saturation [14]; however this is not an instantaneous approach, requiring sufficient time to detect periodic pathological processes.

With this paper, we develop a method for estimating THb and SO$_2$ by using the RGB sensors in stereo laparoscopes, which are already the prime imaging modality robotic MIS. The calibrated sensors' response curves define the mapping of the latent multispectral into RGB space we invert this process using a

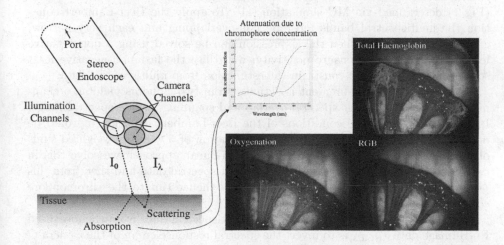

Fig. 1. A stereo RGB endoscope acquires images of the tissue surface under white light illumination. Inside the tissue light is attenuated due to the process of scattering and absorption to a greater, or lesser, degree depending on wavelength and concentration of HbO$_2$ Hb. These concentrations can be calculated and presented to the surgeon in the form of information overlays that map THb or SO$_2$ within tissue.

Tikhonov regularisation scheme to preserve smoothness. This reduces the problem into a two step process with the first of step having a closed form solution, enabling rapid processing of full frame stereo data. We validate our technique using synthetic data generated from Monte Carlo (MC) simulation to evaluate the robustness to sensor measurement noise. We further validate the method on *in vivo* data by using the multispectral derived result [7] as the ground truth, showing our method is a close approximation of full MSI analysis. Our results are promising and suggest that it may be possible to provide additional information during surgery simply by resolving the existing imaging signal.

2   Method

Given a multispectral measurement comprising many non-overlapping band limited individual measurements I_λ, and a corresponding vector of initial illumination $I_{0,\lambda}$, the estimation of the concentration parameters α is a straight forward least squares fitting. Where λ corresponds to the wavelengths of the band centres. This result is simply from rearranging the Beer-Lambert equation as such for an individual wavelength:

$$- log(\frac{I_\lambda}{I_{0,\lambda}}) = \xi\alpha \tag{1}$$

The attenuation coefficients ξ for the chromophores of Hb and HbO_2 are dependant on scattering and absorption characteristics which are often given in the context of transmission. For computational efficiency, and to convert this to a backscattering context, we composite these into a single attenuation factor (Fig. 1) determined via MC simulation [11]. To apply the Beer-Lambert equation the multispectral bands must be non-overlapping and each very narrow, given these conditions then this expression can be solved using a non-negative least squares solver to ensure positivity: we utilise the fast non-negative least squares method of [4] to constrain the estimation from multispectral data.

In our case the measurement is actually from two cameras yielding 6 channels each with significant spectral overlap and spanning a wide spectral range. In order to preserve the conditions of the Beer-Lambert equation it would be necessary to pose the solution as the minimisation of 6 variably weighted sums of exponential terms. Instead of a direct non-linear approach we solve this in two steps, initially we estimate the latent multispectral data and then from this perform the standard least squares fitting to then estimate the chromophore concentrations.

The naïve approach of estimating the multispectral data from the measured RGB image data I_{RGBs} is to invert the spectral response curve of the camera C solving the linear system though a least squares minimization such as:

$$I_\lambda = \arg\min_{I_\lambda} \|CI_\lambda - I_{RGBs}\|^2 \tag{2}$$

where $\|\cdot\|$ is the L^2 norm. This yields a poor estimation of the true multispectral data due to the problem being vastly unconstrained. I_λ can have an order of

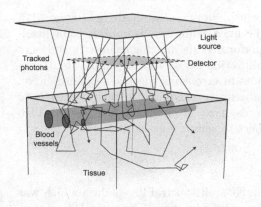
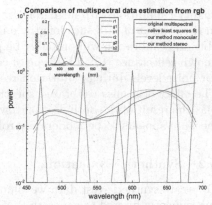

Fig. 2. (L) The synthetic model used for Monte Carlo simulation of test data comprising variable diameter blood vessels embedded within soft tissue. (R) Three estimates of the multispectral data from RGB. Stereo sensor response inset.

magnitude more entries then I_{RGBs}, thus the naïve solution, while correct, is often a metamerism of the true multispectral data for the given C, as shown in Fig. 2. To constrain the estimation we impose a prior (Γ) on I_λ, this is imposed using a Tikhonov regularization:

$$I_\lambda = \arg\min_{I_\lambda} \|CI_\lambda - I_{RGBs}\|^2 + \|\gamma\Gamma I_\lambda\|^2 \qquad (3)$$

The strength of the prior is regulated by the scalar $\gamma = 0.01$. This is typically solved implicitly as:

$$I_\lambda = (C^T C + \Gamma^T \Gamma)^{-1} C^T I_{RGBs} \qquad (4)$$

where Γ is often the identity matrix thus minimising the overall size of I_λ. However we use a Laplacian matrix for Γ to penalise non-smooth I_λ, the Laplacian matrix is formed of ones on the leading diagonal and negative half on the first super and sub diagonals. This choice of Γ is made because we expect the multispectral data to be similar to that predicted by the Beer-Lambert relationship, which is mostly smooth across the visible wavelength range for ξ comprising attenuation due to oxy and de-oxy haemoglobin.

Our method can also be applied to a monocular imaging context by reducing the number of columns in C and the length of I_{RGBs}. This allows concentration estimation to either happen jointly utilising data from 2 or more cameras or independently for each camera.

3   Experiments and Results

3.1   Camera Spectral Response Dependency

Our method is dependant on having available an accurate spectral response calibration for the camera sensor(s), protocols do exist for capturing very high quality calibration with negligible error using a monochromatic light source [1]. In the context of MIS such lengthy and refined calibration is unlikely to be available and calibration will probably be performed via imaging coloured patches of known reflectance [15]. This type of calibration is less accurate and at high sensor noise levels during calibration results in erroneous spectral response curve. The effect of a miss calibrated spectral response acquired in this manner is to bias the result of the optimisation towards deoxy haemoglobin however the THb measure appears to be moderately robust to sensor miss-calibration.

3.2 Synthetic Evaluation

To create synthetic test data we simulated multispectral image data which was subsequently filtered to generate RGB camera responses. The optical characteristics of blood and colonic submucosa (soft tissue) were compiled from [3] and [2] respectively. The synthetic phantom model comprised a homogeneous block of soft tissue with three superficial vessels containing either oxygenated or deoxygenated blood. The three blood vessels had different uniform diameters of 2 mm, 1 mm and 0.5 mm and the top edge of each vessel was at the same depth below the surface of the tissue at a depth of 1 mm.

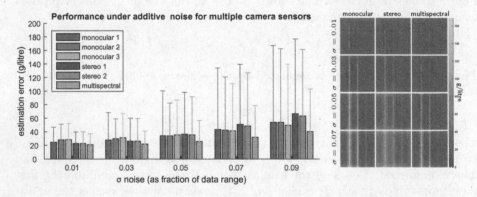

Fig. 3. (L) The absolute concentration estimation error for HbO_2 and Hb combined across both test cases, showing mean absolute error and one standard deviation. For reference typical total haemoglobin concentration for whole blood in an adult male is approx. 145 g/litre. Noise σ is shown generally as for floating point image data, in a typical 8 bit sensor $\sigma = 0.09$ corresponds to $\sigma_{8bit} = 23.04$. (R) The mean concentration estimation error for monocular, stereo and multispectral at four noise levels. (Color figure online)

We used the mesh-based MC (MMC) framework of [12] with the digital phantom model shown in Fig. 2. For the MMC simulation photons were generated at intervals of 10 nm across the range 400 nm to 900 nm. To detect the backscattered light photon momentum was recorded for all photons leaving the bounds of the meshed region. Photons that did not exit through the side of the mesh that was illuminated were discarded as were photons leaving at angles to the surface too oblique to be detected by a detector placed at 10 mm away from the illuminated surface. To simulate multispectral camera images of the scene the photons arriving at the detector were filtered into spectral bands. RGB images were generated by filtering the multispectral data with the response curves corresponding to RGB cameras, a stereo response curve is inset in Fig. 2. Noise was added to the multispectral data by adding zero mean normally distributed vales to each channel, for the RGB noise was generated correlated based on the response curve of the camera.

The performance of our method as seen in Fig. 3 is close to the estimation from full multispectral data as the noise level increases. Also at low noise levels the stereo (6 channel) version of our method outperforms the monocular (3 channel) version. However at high levels of noise the stereo version underperforms due to the increased likelihood of over or under saturated pixel data in the six channels compared to the three of the monocular version. The impact of over or under saturated measurement data is more significant in our method compared to a multispectral approach because each channel in our method corresponds to wide wavelength range, which in the presence of the smoothness prior on the I_λ causes large global under or over chromophore concentration estimation. The presence of a few saturated outliers has less impact on the multispectral method as it is directly fitting against the multispectral data, and the effect of a saturated outlier is localised to an individual wavelength band.

3.3   In Vivo Validation

Multispectral data from a porcine study was used to create a ground truth Hb and HbO_2 concentration maps and corresponding RGB images. Multispectral data sets M comprised 24 non-overlapping 10 nm wide band limited images over the spectral range 460 nm to 690 nm. Multispectral haemoglobin estimation using the method of [7] was performed on these data to establish a best case ground truth and the coefficient of determination (CoD) of this fit was calculated. We masked a subset $\hat{M}$ of the original multispectral data where the CoD was over 0.5 creating a multispectral data set where we have high confidence in the ground truth concentration. From the 58 multispectral data sets we generated corresponding RGB images from typical RGB camera response curves.

We ran both the monocular and stereo version of our method on $\hat{M}$ and comparison was then made against the multispectral derived the ground truth. Concentrations of Hb and HbO_2 were then converted into the total haemoglobin and oxygen saturation measures since these are the markers that would then be used to clinical evaluate a surgical site. As shown in (4) the use of stereo significantly improves on the estimation of total haemoglobin with an overall mean absolute error of less then 3 g/litre when using 6 channels from two cameras compared to over 6 g/litre for a 3 channel monocular approach. The standard deviation of the error for each method remains close yet is slightly lower for the 6 channel variant. Given that total haemoglobin concentration of whole blood is in the region of 145 g/litre this indicates a high degree of accuracy when

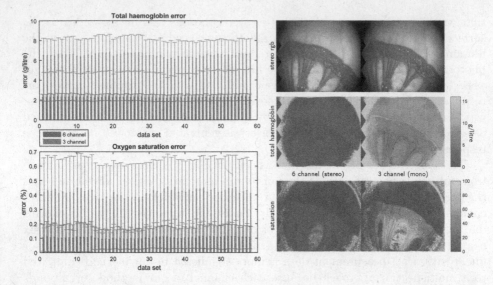

Fig. 4. (L) Estimation error for each of the 58 data sets comparing stereo (blue) and monocular (red) against multispectral derived ground truth. Clearly visible is the improved precision of the stereo method especially for the correct evaluation of the oxygen saturation. (R) A registered stereo view of a surgical site with. Maps of the estimation error for saturation and total haemoglobin computed from stereo and monocular data. (Color figure online)

imaging for the purposes of perfusion mapping. Oxygen saturation estimation shows the most marked improvement when using stereo over monocular with an overall saturation estimation error of 10.27 % down from 41.71 % for the stereo and mono variants respectively. In evaluating the *in vivo* performance, results that corresponded to a THb concentration greater than 200 g/litre were considered outliers this enumerated as less than 0.1 % of the results being rejected as outliers.

In both cases our method produces highly similar results to those from multispectral inference, and the error is typically located in areas not corresponding to vasculature. This is illustrated in Fig. 4 where a section of bowel is exposed on a gauze background. For the stereo case the error in THb estimation is very low across the view however the SO_2 estimation performs less well in areas of low THb. This is to be expected as the oxygen saturation is a ratio of Hb and HbO_2 and when both are at low concentration small errors in estimation of either in either become amplified in the aggregate saturation measure.

4   Discussion

We have presented a novel estimation tool for measuring the concentration of Hb and HbO_2 directly from laparoscopic RGB video. The method provides greater accuracy when applied to stereoscopic data as typically found in robotic assisted MIS. We have shown that the method performs well on synthetic data and is comparable to the result from raw MSI data acquired using modified imaging hardware such as a LCTF camera. Our method's only requirement is to have a calibration of the laparoscopic sensors and light source to capture the response curve of each channel. This makes our technique very applicable to a wide range of MIS procedures and easily to integrate in the operating theatre. The success of our stereo method is going to be strongly linked to the quality of the registration of the two camera views, while this remains an open problem there exist effective techniques specifically targeted at registration for multispectral inference [7,10]. Our method also requires imaging to be at a constant distance from the tissue surface, integrating the stereo acquired depth information may provide was to normalise for these global changes in irradiance.

References

1. EMVA standard 1288: Standard for Characterization of Image Sensors and Cameras. European Machine Vision Association (3.0) (2010). www.emva.org/wp-content/uploads/EMVA1288-3.0.pdf
2. Bashkatov, A.N., Genina, E.A., Kochubey, V.I., Rubtsov, V.S., Kolesnikova, E.A., Tuchin, V.V.: Optical properties of human colon tissues in the 350–2500 nm spectral range. Quant. Electron. **44**(8), 779–784 (2014)
3. Bosschaart, N., Edelman, G.J., Aalders, M.C.G., van Leeuwen, T.G., Faber, D.J.: A literature review and novel theoretical approach on the optical propertiesof whole blood. Lasers Med. Sci. **29**(2), 453–479 (2013). http://dx.doi.org/10.1007/s10103-013-1446-7
4. Bro, R., Jong, S.D.: A fast non-negativity-constrained least squares algorithm. J. Chemometr. **11**(5), 393–401 (1997)
5. Clancy, N.T., Arya, S., Stoyanov, D., Singh, M., Hanna, G.B., Elson, D.S.: Intraoperative measurement of bowel oxygen saturation using a multispectral imaging laparoscope. Biomed. Opt. Express **6**(10), 4179 (2015)
6. Clancy, N.T., Saso, S., Stoyanov, D., Sauvage, V., Corless, D.J., Boyd, M., Noakes, D.E., Thum, M.Y., Ghaem-Maghami, S., Smith, J.R., Elson, D.S.: Multispectral imaging of organ viability during uterine transplantation surgery. In: Advanced Biomedical and Clinical Diagnostic Systems XII. SPIE-The International Society for Optical Engineering, February 2014. http://dx.doi.org/10.1117/12.2040518
7. Clancy, N.T., Stoyanov, D., James, D.R.C., Marco, A.D., Sauvage, V., Clark, J., Yang, G.Z., Elson, D.S.: Multispectral image alignment using a three channel endoscope in vivo during minimally invasive surgery. Biomed. Opt. Express **3**(10), 2567–2578 (2012). http://www.opticsinfobase.org/boe/abstract.cfm?URI=boe-3-10-2567
8. Claridge, E., Hidović-Rowe, D., Taniere, P., Ismail, T.: Quantifying mucosal blood volume fraction from multispectral images of the colon. In: Medical Imaging, p 65110C. International Society for Optics and Photonics (2007)
9. Darzi, A., Mackay, S.: Recent advances in minimal access surgery. Br. Med. J. **324**(7328), 31 (2002)
10. Du, X., Allan, M., Dore, A., Ourselin, S., Hawkes, D.J., Kelly, D.S.: Combined 2D and 3D tracking of surgical instruments for minimally invasive and robotic-assisted surgery. Int. J. Comput. Assist. Radiol. Surg. **11**(6), 1109–1119 (2015)

11. Dunn, A.K., Devor, A., Dale, A.M., Boas, D.A.: Spatial extent of oxygen metabolism and hemodynamic changes during functional activation of the rat somatosensory cortex. NeuroImage **27**(2), 279–290 (2005). http://dx.doi.org/10.1016/j.neuroimage.2005.04.024

12. Fang, Q.: Mesh-based Monte Carlo method using fast ray-tracing in plücker coordinates. Biomed. Opt. Express **1**(1), 165 (2010)

13. Fawzy, Y., Lam, S., Zeng, H.: Rapid multispectral endoscopic imaging system for near real-time mapping of the mucosa blood supply in the lung. Biomed. Opt. Express **6**(8), 2980 (2015)

14. Guazzi, A.R., Villarroel, M., Jorge, J., Daly, J., Frise, M.C., Robbins, P.A., Tarassenko, L.: Non-contact measurement of oxygen saturation with an RGB camera. Biomed. Opt. Express **6**(9), 3320 (2015)

15. Hardeberg, J.Y., Brettel, H., Schmitt, F.J.M.: Spectral characterization of electronic cameras. In: Bares, J. (ed.) Electronic Imaging: Processing, Printing, and Publishing in Color. SPIE-The International Society for Optical Engineering, September 1998. http://dx.doi.org/10.1117/12.324101

16. Nighswander-Rempel, S.P., Shaw, R.A., Mansfield, J.R., Hewko, M., Kupriyanov, V.V., Mantsch, H.H.: Regional variations in myocardial tissue oxygenation mapped by near-infrared spectroscopic imaging. J. Mol. Cell. Cardiol. **34**(9), 1195–1203 (2002)

17. Nishidate, I., Maeda, T., Niizeki, K., Aizu, Y.: Estimation of melanin and hemoglobin using spectral reflectance images reconstructed from a digital RGB image by the Wiener estimation method. Sensors **13**(6), 7902–7915 (2013)

18. Sorg, B.S., Moeller, B.J., Donovan, O., Cao, Y., Dewhirst, M.W.: Hyperspectral imaging of hemoglobin saturation in tumor microvasculature and tumor hypoxia development. J. Biomed. Opt. **10**(4), 044004 (2005)

19. Wirkert, S.J., Clancy, N.T., Stoyanov, D., Arya, S., Hanna, G.B., Schlemmer, H.-P., Sauer, P., Elson, D.S., Maier-Hein, L.: Endoscopic sheffield index for unsupervised in vivo spectral band selection. In: Luo, X., Reich, T., Mirota, D., Soper, T. (eds.) CARE 2014. LNCS, vol. 8899, pp. 110–120. Springer, Heidelberg (2014)

Radiation-Free 3D Navigation and Vascular Reconstruction for Aortic Stent Graft Deployment

Fang Chen, Jia Liu, and Hongen Liao[✉]

Department of Biomedical Engineering, School of Medicine,
Tsinghua University, Beijing, China
liao@tsinghua.edu.cn

Abstract. We propose a radiation-free three dimensional (3D) navigation and vasculature reconstruction method to reduce aortic stent graft deployment time and repeated exposures to high doses of X-ray radiation. 2D intraoperative US images are fused with 3D preoperative magnetic resonance (MR) image to provide intuitive 3D navigation for deployment of the stent-graft in the proposed system. On the other hand, calibrated 2D US images track catheter's tip and construct intraoperative 3D aortic model by combining segmented intravascular ultrasound (IVUS) images. The constructed 3D aortic models can quantitatively assess morphological characteristics of aortic to assist deployment of stent graft. This system was validated by using in vitro cardiac and aorta phantom. The mean target registration error of 2D US-3D MR registration was 2.70 mm and the average tracking error of position of IVUS catheter's tip was 1.12 mm. Accurate contours detection results in IVUS images were acquired. Meanwhile, Hausdorff distances are 0.78 mm and 0.59 mm for outer and inner contours, respectively; Dice coefficients are 90.21 % and 89.96 %. Experiment results demonstrate that our radiation-free navigation and 3D vasculature reconstruction method is promising for deployment of stent graft in vivo studies.

Keywords: Radiation-free 3D navigation · Intravascular ultrasound segmentation · Ultrasound tracking · Registration

1 Introduction

Placement of endovascular stent graft is the most common approach for treatment of acute aorta dissection and aneurysm [1]. In this treatment, a stent graft is inserted into aortic lesions by using a catheter through a dissected femoral artery. For accurate stent graft deployment, there are two critical factors: (1) morphological characteristics information of aorta especially calcification areas for determining the size of stent graft [2]; (2) intuitive relative position information between catheter and three dimensional (3D) cardiac structure for assisting stent graft placement. Stent graft placement is typically guided by fluoroscopic guidance with the use of X-ray contrast. However, fluoroscopic guidance has three distinct disadvantages. First, although fluoroscopy can visualize the catheter excellently, soft tissue structures are not easily visualized. Poor 2Dvisualization of aorta and surrounding anatomy causes incorrect placement of stent.

© Springer International Publishing Switzerland 2016
G. Zheng et al. (Eds.): MIAR 2016, LNCS 9805, pp. 59–71, 2016.
DOI: 10.1007/978-3-319-43775-0_6

Second, 2D X-ray fluoroscopic image can't provide quantitative analysis of the vessel's morphological characteristics [3]. Third, repeated injection of contrast agents influences the health of patient and clinical staff.

To provide intuitive 3D navigation images, Fagan *et al.* proposed a 3D vascular geometry visualization method with rotational angiographic images [4]. Hybrid imaging systems which combined magnetic resonance (MR) and X-ray fluoroscopic images, can realize 3D guidance in endovascular interventions [5]. These methods undoubtedly increase X-ray radiation or bring magnetic compatibility problem. Moreover, electromagnetic (EM) tracking system has been widely used to collect 3D position information of catheter for endovascular guidance [6]. 3D information of catheter is also combined with preoperative images [7]. However, the EM tracking method can't acquire intraoperative movement information of soft tissue and has limitation on accuracy due to the increased size of the EM sensor-attached catheter. Recently, intravascular ultrasound (IVUS) images have been used for in vivo analysis of plaque morphology [8]. IVUS imaging is more accurate to guide stent deployment than conventional angiography including X-ray and MR imaging, because of the relatively higher resolution [9]. The semi-automatic vessel 3D reconstruction method from IVUS video sequences is used to evaluate vessel pathologies [10]. However, this method can only be used for blood vessels with small curvatures and can't acquire catheter position information. A cardiovascular modeling method fusing the IVUS images and EM tracking system is proposed without the utilization of X-ray images [11]. This method provides only 3D model of blood vessel, without 3D structure around target aorta. Real-time 2D echocardiography is commonly used to guide correct stent deployment for aortic dissection because it provides superior diagnostic accuracy than angiography [12], but this method provides only 2D non-intuitive images. In summary, it is still a challenge to develop a navigation method, which provide not only morphological characteristics information of aortic but also 3D guidance image of surrounding soft tissue.

In this paper, we propose novel radiation-free 3D endovascular navigation and vascular reconstruction system for aortic stent grafts deployment. We implement real-time 2D ultrasound (US) image to provide intraoperative information of soft tissue and track catheter. This method can provide 3D navigation image of aorta and surrounding tissue without X-ray radiation by fusing intraoperative 2D US and operative 3D MR images. 3D model reconstruction of aorta is achieved by combining morphological characteristics information obtained from IVUS image with corresponding position of IVUS catheter tip from US image tracking.

2   Materials and Methods

2.1   Configuration of Radiation-Free 3D Navigation and Vascular Reconstruction System

The radiation-free 3D navigation and vascular reconstruction system consists of an US device, a 3D optical tracking system, a computer, and a catheter (Fig. 1). The US system is used to obtain images of the intraoperative surrounding tissue and catheter's tip. The 3D optical tracking system collects the pose of the US probe. In addition, the IVUS scanning probe is inserted into the aorta through a catheter. The collected

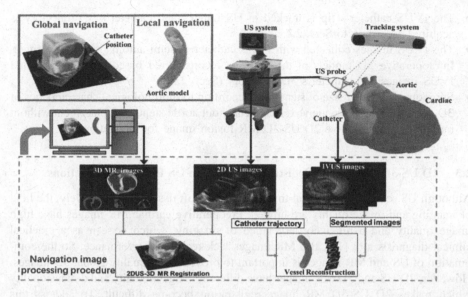

Fig. 1. System configuration of radiation-free 3D navigation and vascular reconstruction.

intraoperative US images, IVUS images and preoperative 3D MR images are combined and processed during image processing procedure. The image processing procedure mainly includes two parts: (1) 2D US-3D MR registration for 3D intuitive image information; (2) construction of 3D aorta model combining segmented IVUS images with catheter's trajectory from US images. Finally, the processed navigation image is displayed to guide aortic stent graft deployment.

2.2 Radiation-Free 3D Navigation and Vascular Reconstruction Workflow

The workflow of the proposed navigation and vascular reconstruction system is divided into two parts: preoperative processing and intraoperative processing.

Preoperative Processing.

- The preoperative high-quality 3D MR images of the cardiac and aorta are collected, which have a large field of view.
- Using the calibrated 3D US probe to collect 3D US image only one time in intraoperative preparatory stage.

Intraoperative Processing. Intraoperatively, the calibrated 2D US probe is implemented to collect real-time 2D US images. The US images contains both anatomical regions relating to the aorta and catheter tip.

- The 2D intraoperative US images are fused with 3D preoperative MR image to acquire intuitive 3D navigation information for stent graft deployment according to registration method in Sect. 2.3.

- The IVUS catheter's tip is tracked in US images and catheter's 3D trajectory is acquired according to Sect. 2.4.
- The IVUS images collected with IVUS catheter is semi-automatically segmented. Intraoperative 3D models of the aortic is reconstructed based on the segmented IVUS images and catheter's 3D trajectory (Sect. 2.5).
- Surgeons decide the size of stent graft according to morphological characteristics of 3D aorta especially plaque voxels and carry out aortic stent graft placement without radiation using intuitive 2D US-3D MR fusion image for navigation.

2.3   2D US-3D MR Image Registration Based on US Probes' Calibrations

Although US scan can obtain real-time imaging of soft tissue intraoperatively, the field of imaging and image quality are limited. Preoperative cardiac MR images have high image quality and a relatively large filed of imaging, which is seen as a practical clinical diagnosis tool [13]. But MR images lack real-time performance. So the combination of US and MR images is important to provide high-quality global 3D images. However, 2D US and 3D MR images have different image modality and dimensionality which makes 2D US-3D MR image registration become difficult. To address this problem, we apply a calibrated 3D US image to simplify traditional rigid 2D US-3D MR registration problem into two easy-achieved steps: 2D-3D US intra-modal registration and 3D US-3D MR intra-dimension registration. In our registration process, rigid registration transformation T_{2DUS}^{3DMR} is calculated by

$$T_{2DUS}^{3DMR} = T_{2DUS}^{3DUS} * T_{3DUS}^{3DMR},$$ (1)

where T_{2DUS}^{3DUS} is transformation between intra-modal 2D and 3D US images, T_{3DUS}^{3DMR} is registration transformation between intra-dimension 3D US and MR images.

In intraoperative preparatory stage, we employ a calibrated 3D US probe to collect 3D US image of the target organ only one time. The collected 3D US image has same dimension as MR image. And 3D US-3D MR preoperative registration is done manually using custom software (3D slicer) to acquire T_{3DUS}^{3DMR}.

In addition, crucial 2D-3D US intra-modal registration T_{2DUS}^{3DUS} is achieved automatically by firstly using the 2D and 3D US probes' calibration results to get a near-optimal start value $\dot{T}_{2DUS}^{3DUS}$ and then doing intensity-based local registration adjustment to acquire final transformation T_{2DUS}^{3DUS}.

Firstly, the near-optimal start value of registration transformation $\dot{T}_{2DUS}^{3DUS}$ can be automatically calculated by

$$\dot{T}_{2DUS}^{3DUS} = T_{2DUS}^{TS} * (T_{3DUS}^{TS})^{-1}$$ (2)

Here

(i) $T_{2DUS}^{TS} = T_{2DPR}^{TS} * T_{2DUS}^{2DPR}$, where T_{2DUS}^{2DPR} is 2D probe's calibration result (transformation between 2D US image coordinate and 2D US probe (2D PR) coordinate); T_{2DPR}^{TS} transform from 2D probe coordinate (2D PR) to tracking system coordinate (TS) and it is recorded by external tracking system;

(ii) $T^{TS}_{3DUS} = T^{TS}_{3DPR} * T^{3DPR}_{3DUS}$, where T^{3DPR}_{3DUS} is 3D probe's calibration result (transformation between 3D US image coordinate and 3D US probe coordinate (3D PR)); T^{TS}_{3DPR} is transformation between 3D probe sensor coordinate (3D PR) to TS coordinate. T^{TS}_{3DPR} is updated according to the pose of the 3D probe sensor and recorded by tracking system.

Secondly, with the acquired near-optimal start value of transformation $\hat{T}^{3DUS}_{2DUS}$, fast automatic intensity-based local registration adjustment is then employed for accurate registration. In local registration adjustment, we utilize mutual information (MI) as similarity metric. We use gradient ascent optimizer to find optimum value of MI metric and final rigid transformation T^{3DUS}_{2DUS}.

During our registration process, to solve used calibrations results of 2D and 3D US probes (T^{2DPR}_{2DUS} and T^{3DPR}_{3DUS}), we design an applicative phantom (length: 26 cm, width: 12 cm, height: 28 cm) (Fig. 2). While performing calibration of 2D US probe, we use N-wire calibration phantom [14] with three N-wires (two types of N-wires) resembled on each layer (Fig. 2(a), (b)). By adding a wire to N-wire shape, we create an IXI-wire shape. For 3D US probe's calibration, we utilize an IXI-wire calibration phantom [15] with four IXI-wires (two types of IXI-wires) on four layers (Fig. 2(c), (d)). More detailed descriptions about calibration and registration procedure can be found in [16].

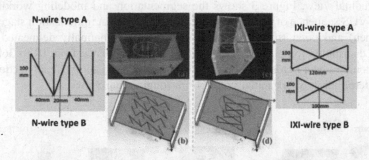

Fig. 2. Calibration phantoms; (a) real N-wire phantom; (b) CAD model of N-wire phantom; (c) real IXI-wire phantom;(d) CAD model of IXI-wire phantom.

2.4 Catheter Tip Tracking for Acquirement of 3D Trajectory

We use real-time 2D US images to collect intraoperative structural information including heart chambers and aorta, and simultaneously track the IVUS catheter's tip with US images. The catheter could be scanned in consecutive cross-sections with tracked US imaging. We apply a normalized correlation coefficient based template matching method to track the catheter tip in collected US images. Template matching algorithm is widely used for location of the signal and target object [17]. In 2D US images, the vessel's cross section is chosen as the region of interest (ROI) to be tracked. To identify the matching area, we try to find the maximum of matching metric which is defined as normalized correlation coefficient, by sliding the template image on the 2D

US images. The template size is set as 40 pixels × 40 pixels according to the size of the blood vessels in US images. Considering the amount of target movement between two adjacent frames, the ratio of template's size to search area's size is 5:1. By normalized correlation coefficient based template matching method, the cross-section of vessel is localized in each US image. Since the intensity of the catheter in US image is much higher than that of most of the speckle in the images, the position of IVUS's catheter can be easily acquired by using a threshold (the threshold value is set at 220 on 256 step scale). After thresholding, a morphological opening operation is performed to remove any spurious points. The tip of IVUS catheter is located in the last US image frame where the catheter can be detected. With 2D US probe's calibration result, the position of the IVUS catheter's tip under 2D US image coordinate can be transformed to the tracking system coordinates by using transform T_{2DUS}^{TS} between 2D US image coordinate and tracking system. Once acquiring real-time positions of IVUS catheter's tip, the 3D trajectory of catheter is constructed.

2.5   IVUS Segmentation for 3D Aortic Reconstruction

3D aortic model can be reconstructed with segmented IVUS sequence and IVUS catheter trajectory. To achieve IVUS sequence segmentation, we apply a segmentation method which uses the information of IVUS sequence's dual views: the cross-sectional and longitudinal view. Figure 3 shows the segmentation and modeling workflow for collected IVUS sequence of the aorta with vascular plaque. In initialization stage, initial inner (lumen) and outer (media-adventitia) contours are manually delineated on six uniformly distributed longitudinal views of the IVUS sequence from 0° to 360°. The initial contours in every cross-section of IVUS sequence are automatically acquired by a linear interpolation of six initial points from longitudinal views.

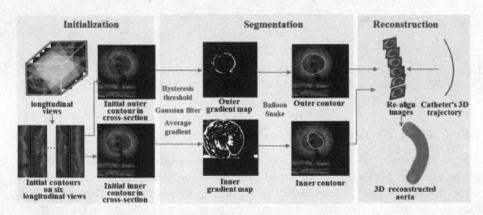

Fig. 3. The workflow of IVUS image segmentation and 3D vessel reconstruction.

In segmentation stage, the balloon snake model [18] is implemented to acquire final inner and outer borders guided by modified gradient maps. Deformable balloon snake model of contour detection applying gradient information as input is heavily susceptible to image artifacts. So preprocessing is required to achieve gradient map with low noise for accurate detection. Firstly, we use the average gradient defined by Plissiti *et al.* [19] instead of standard gradient (difference between adjacent pixels) to avoid sharp changes in gradient and acquire expected smooth contour. Then, hysteresis thresholding and Gaussian filter are used to reduce unwanted gradient information in gradient map. The Gaussian filter is applied to reduce noise while maintaining edges and the hysteresis thresholding is utilized to remove extreme values unlikely to be involved in the detection of contours. The outer gradient map is modified with a hysteresis threshold, primarily to eliminate low gradients associated with the inner contour, and secondarily to eliminate high gradients associated with the catheter "shadow" artifact. For inner gradient map, it is modified with a hysteresis threshold, primarily to eliminate the gradients associated with the outer contour. And inner gradient map is further convolved with a radial Gaussian kernel centered at the average center of the initial inner contour to lower the effects of gradients far from the likely location of the inner contour. Finally, with acquired initial contours and gradient maps, we apply balloon snake to obtain borders in each frame with smoothness maintained.

In the reconstruction stage, with the use of automatic pullback device, constant pullback speed is assumed. Thus segmented IVUS frames can be realigned automatically at equidistant intervals on the acquired 3D catheter trajectory. For the distribution angles for the IVUS frames, image planes are positioned perpendicular to the catheter trajectory. After determining spatial location of each segmented IVUS image, 3D aortic model is reconstructed and is written as VTK file format. The final 3D aortic model is rendered in 3D Slicer.

3   Experiment and Results

The experiment platform was shown in Fig. 4. The 2D US images were collected by using US system (iU22 xMATRIX, Philips) with a 2D linear array probe (VL13-5, Philips). And 3D US image of the cardiac and aortic was collected just one time with 3D phased array probe (S5-1, Philips). Additionally, we used an optical tracking

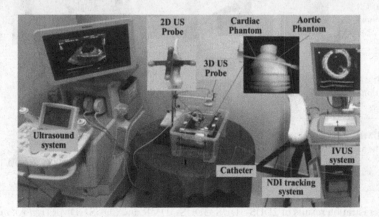

Fig. 4. The aortic and cardiac phantom experiment platform.

system (Polaris, Northern Digital Inc) to track US probes. The IVUS images were collected by using Boston Scientific Galaxy 2 system with a 40 MHz Atlantis SR IVUS probe at a pull-back speed of 0.5 mm per second. The simulated experiment used a MR compatible multi-modality heart phantom (SHELLEY Medical, USA), which contained left ventricular (LV) and right ventricular (RV) and an aortic phantom covered on it. Preoperative 3D MR images were collected with a MR scanner (Philips Achieva 3.0T TX) whose size was $480 \times 480 \times 300$ voxels with resolution 0.4871 mm 0.4871 mm and slice thickness 1.6000 mm. The size of the 2D US images was 600×800 pixels with resolution 0.2382 mm $\times$ 0.2382 mm. IVUS images were 8-bits, 512×512 with in-frame resolution 0.0175 mm $\times$ 0.0175 mm.

3.1   Results of Probes' Calibration and 2DUS-3DMR Registration

2D and 3D Probes' Calibration. Calibration reproducibility (CR) error measured repeatability of a proposed probe calibration method when performed on a new set of images [14]. CR was the Euclidian distance between two calibration transformations (T_{US}^{PRi} and T_{US}^{PRj}) of the same US image point P^{US}. CR error was usually calculated by

$$E^{CR} = \underset{i,j}{mean}\left\{ \left\| T_{US}^{PRi} * P^{US} - T_{US}^{PRj} * P^{US} \right\| \right\} \tag{3}$$

During the evaluations of 2D and 3D probes' calibration, we both performed 8 calibration trials and used 10 images per trial, 80 datasets in total. The acquired CR error of 2D calibration was 0.61 mm and CR error of 3D calibration is 1.42 mm.

2DUS-3DMR Image Registration. Figure 5 showed the registration results of 2DUS-3DUS images, 3DUS-3DMR images and 2DUS-3DMR images during

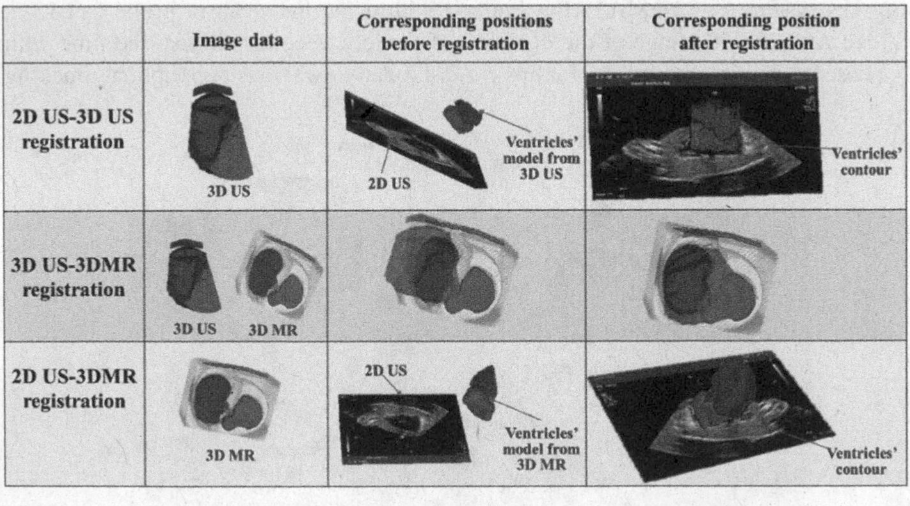

	Image data	Corresponding positions before registration	Corresponding position after registration
2D US-3D US registration	3D US	2D US, Ventricles' model from 3D US	Ventricles' contour
3D US-3DMR registration	3D US 3D MR		
2D US-3DMR registration	3D MR	2D US, Ventricles' model from 3D MR	Ventricles' contour

Fig. 5. Registration results of 2DUS-3DUS, 3DUS-3DMR and 2DUS-3DMR *(red volume is left ventricular model; blue volume is right ventricular model).* (Color figure online)

registration process (see Fig. 5). The ventricle model from 3D US image was registered to corresponding ventricle's contour in 2D US images (see first row in Fig. 5), which verified the 2D-3D US registration based on US probes' calibration. The contours of the ventricle in 2D US and 3D MR images after registration achieved a good agreement (see third row in Fig. 5), which qualitatively demonstrated the proposed 2D US-3D MR image registration method was effective. In addition, 2D US-3D MR registration accuracy was further quantitatively evaluated by calculating the target registration error (TRE). 10 ventricle contour points in 2D US and corresponding ventricle contour points 3D MR model were manually delineated by expert surgeon to serve as fiducial marks. And TRE was defined as average Euclidean distance of these corresponding contour points. The registration result of 2D US and 3D MR image with a mean TRE of 2.70 mm (range 1.05 mm–3.67 mm) was acquired. On phantom experiment, our registration speed was about 11 s per frame in Matlab 2014 platform, which can be speeded up specifically by implementing the algorithm on C++ platform.

3.2 IVUS Segmentation and Catheter Tracking

IVUS Image Segmentation. The performance of the proposed IVUS segmentation method was evaluated using 200 IVUS images obtained from 5 sequences. These five IVUS sequences included one IVUS sequence of aorta phantom and four IVUS sequences of real patients. These sequences were collected by an IVUS expert from Navy PLA General Hospital. The detected inner and outer contours by proposed segmentation method were compared with manual segmentations by the anonymous IVUS expert to evaluate algorithm's accuracy. Figure 6 depicted our automatic segmentation examples of IVUS images along with manual segmentation. In addition, the performance of the segmentation method was quantified by using Hausdorff distance [20] and Dice index [21]. Table 1 provided the comparison results of our proposed

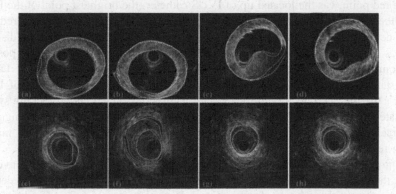

Fig. 6. Segmented contours of IVUS images ((a)–(d): IVUS images of vessel phantom; (e)–(h): IVUS images of real patients); yellow and green contours denote the outer and inner contours respectively. *(dotted lines denote detected contours by manual segmentation and full lines denote detected contours by proposed segmentation method, respectively).* (Color figure online)

Table 1. The segmentation results comparison between proposed method and manual tracing.

Similarity and distance measurements	Outer contour		Inner contour	
	Mean	SD	Mean	SD
Hausdorff distance ·	0.78 mm	0.24 mm	0.59 mm	0.31 mm
Dice index	90.21 %	7.53 %	89.96 %	5.91 %

segmentation method and manual delineation. The mean Hausdorff distance and Dice index between automatic and manual segmentations were 0.59 mm and 89.96 % for inner contour detection. The Hausdorff distance and Dice index were 0.78 mm and 90.2 % for outer contour detection. The results validated that the proposed IVUS segmentation method was effective for detecting outer and inner contours.

IVUS Catheter Tracking and Catheter's 3D Trajectory Reconstruction. During the experiment, we inserted the IVUS catheter into aortic of the heart phantom and collected 2D US images to track the IVUS catheter. Catheter tracking result was shown in Fig. 7.

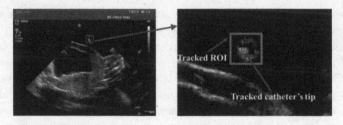

Fig. 7. Tracking results of IVUS catheter's tip. (Color figure online)

As shown in Fig. 7, the red box represents the tracked ROI (vessel's cross section). And the red point was the located tip of IVUS catheter (the brightest point of the ROI). During the experiments, we tracked catheter's tip in 100 US images and compared with manual delineative tip in each image to calculate tracking error. The tracking distance error was defined as the Euclidean distance between the manual delineative position and automatically tracked position. The acquired average tracking error was 1.12 mm with a standard deviation of 0.49 mm. After acquiring real time positions of IVUS catheter's tip, the 3D trajectory of the catheter was reconstructed under tracking system coordinate (Fig. 8). Figure 8 showed the 3D trajectory of the catheter by using automatic tracking results of catheter tip along with 3D catheter trajectory by manual tracking results.

The proposed radiation-free 3D navigation and vascular reconstruction system could provide the surgeon with hybrid navigation information for aortic stent graft deployment. There were three kinds of navigation information (see Fig. 9): (1) Global navigation. In global navigation, 3D MR cardiac structural image is registered with real time US images to provide an updated view of the surrounding tissue. And 3D position information of inserted catheter is overlaid on this 3D image; (2) Local navigation. In

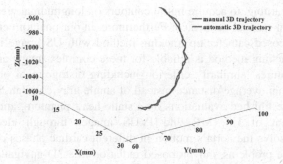

Fig. 8. 3D trajectory of the catheter in tracking system coordinate.

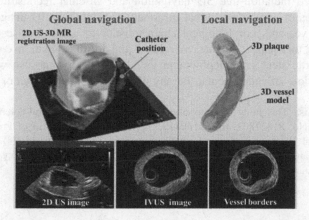

Fig. 9. Navigation information of radiation-free 3D navigation system.

local navigation, real intraoperative 3D model of aorta is reconstructed to provide morphological characteristics information of calcification; (3) Typical 2D views including 2D US images and segmented 2D IVUS images with the detected lumen and media-adventitia border.

4 Discussions and Conclusion

This paper presents a radiation-free 3D navigation and vascular reconstruction method for aortic stent graft deployment with the combination of IVUS, US and MR images. The proposed method can provide not only 3D real-time navigation images of cardiac and surrounding tissue, but also quantitative morphological characteristics of vessel to assist stent graft deployment without X-ray radiation. We have evaluated the proposed method on a realistic cardiac phantom experiment and the results validated the feasibility of the radiation-free 3D navigation method for guiding aortic stent graft deployment.

Our IVUS segmentation method is semi-automatic. In the future, to make segmentation method fully automatic, we will use automatic pixel classification method such as machine learning, to acquire initial contours on longitudinal views of the IVUS sequence instead of manual delineated. Furthermore, in our phantom environment, the reality of our proposed catheter tip tracking method with US image is validated. To ensure that our tracking method is reliable for more complex image artifacts, we will combine more features' similarity criterion including histogram of oriented gradient feature and gray min average distance instead of single gray correlation coefficient. In our study, we have finished evaluations on a static heart phantom, and we will apply temporal alignment of US, MR and IVUS images through electrocardiograph (ECG) signals to solve the aorta's motion in different cardiac phases of beating heart. After solving these problems, our proposed radiation-free 3D navigation method will be used near-automatically to guide the aortic stent graft deployment on animal pig experiment.

The proposed radiation-free 3D navigation and vascular reconstruction method achieves the idea of combining global information of intuitive 3D images with local information of vessels' morphological characteristics to guide precise endovascular intervention. In this paper, the idea of global and local navigation combination is validated in aortic stent graft deployment guidance, and it may also work in other clinical applications of endovascular therapy like catheter intervention of oral cancers.

Acknowledgments. This study was supported in part by National Natural Science Foundation of China (Grant No. 81427803, 61361160417, 81271735), Grant-in-Aid of Project 985, and Beijing Municipal Science & Technology Commission (Z151100003915079). The Authors would like to thank Mr. Yigang Qiu from Department of Cardiology, Navy PLA General Hospital for assistance in acquiring IVUS data for this study.

References

1. Dake, M.D., Kato, N., Mitchell, R.S., et al.: Endovascular stent–graft placement for the treatment of acute aortic dissection. New. Engl. J. Med. **340**(20), 1546–1552 (1999)
2. Timmins, L.H., Meyer, C.A., Moreno, M.R., et al.: Effects of stent design and atherosclerotic plaque composition on arterial wall biomechanics. J. Endovasc. Ther. **15** (6), 643–654 (2008)
3. Vykoukal, D., Chinnadurai, P., Davies, M.G.: Cardiovascular imaging, navigation and intervention: hybrid imaging and therapeutics. In: Garbey, M., Bass, B.L., Berceli, S., Collet, C., Cerveri, P. (eds.) Computational Surgery and Dual Training, pp. 125–148. Springer, New York (2014)
4. Fagan, T., Kay, J., Carroll, J., et al.: 3-D guidance of complex pulmonary artery stent placement using reconstructed rotational angiography with live overlay. Cathet. Cardio. Interv. **79**(3), 414–421 (2012)
5. Rhode, K.S., Sermesant, M., Brogan, D., et al.: A system for real-time XMR guided cardiovascular intervention. IEEE Trans. Med. Imaging **24**(11), 1428–1440 (2005)
6. Abi-Jaoudeh, N., Glossop, N., Dake, M., et al.: Electromagnetic navigation for thoracic aortic stent-graft deployment: a pilot study in swine. J. Vasc. Interv. Radiol. **21**(6), 888–895 (2010)

7. De Lambert, A., Esneault, S., Lucas, A., et al.: Electromagnetic tracking for registration and navigation in endovascular aneurysm repair: a phantom study. Eur. J. Vasc. Endovasc. **43** (6), 684–689 (2012)
8. Nishimura, R.A., Edwards, W.D., et al.: Intravascular ultrasound imaging: in vitro validation and pathologic correlation. Am. Coil. Cardiol. **16**, 145–154 (1990)
9. Brodoefel, H., Burgstahler, C., et al.: Accuracy of dual-source CT in the characterisation of non-calcified plaque: use of a colour-coded analysis compared with virtual histology intravascular ultrasound. Br. J. Radiol. **82**, 805–812 (2009)
10. Sanz-Requena, R., Moratal, D., García-Sánchez, D.R., et al.: Automatic segmentation and 3D reconstruction of intravascular ultrasound images for a fast preliminar evaluation of vessel pathologies. Comput. Med. Imag. Graph **31**(2), 71–80 (2007)
11. Shi, C., Kojima, M., Tercero, C., et al.: Intravascular modeling and navigation for stent graft installation based on data fusion between intravascular ultrasound and electromagnetic tracking sensor. In: 2012 IEEE International Symposium on Micro-NanoMechatronics and Human Science (MHS), pp. 229–234 (2012)
12. Franke, A., Kuhl, H.P., et al.: Quantitative analysis of the morphology of secundum-type atrial septal defects and their dynamic change using transesophageal three-dimensional echocardiography. Circulation **96**, II323–II327 (1997)
13. Finn, J.P., Nael, K., Deshpande, V., et al.: Cardiac MR imaging: state of the technology 1. Radiology **241**(2), 338–354 (2006)
14. Lindseth, F., Tangen, G.A., Langø, T., et al.: Probe calibration for freehand 3-D ultrasound. Ultrasound Med. Biol. **29**(11), 1607–1623 (2003)
15. Bergmeir, C., Seitel, M., Frank, C., et al.: Comparing calibration approaches for 3D ultrasound probes. Int. J. Comput. Assist. Radiol. Surg. **4**(2), 203–213 (2009)
16. Chen, F., Liao, R., Liao, H.: Fast registration of intraoperative ultrasound and preoperative MR images based on calibrations of 2D and 3D ultrasound probes. In: Jaffray, D.A. (ed.) World Congress on Medical Physics and Biomedical Engineering, pp. 220–223. Springer, Toronto (2015)
17. Lewis, J.P.: Fast template matching. In: Vision Interface, pp. 15–19 (1995)
18. Kass, M., Witkin, A., Terzopoulos, D.: Snakes: active contour models. Int. J. Comput. Vis. **1** (4), 321–331 (1988)
19. Plissiti, M.E., Fotiadis, D.I., Michalis, L.K., et al.: An automated method for lumen and media-adventitia border detection in a sequence of IVUS frames. IEEE Trans. Inf. Technol. Biomed. **8**(2), 131–141 (2004)
20. Dice, L.R.: Measures of the amount of ecologic association between species. Ecology **26**(3), 297–302 (1945)
21. Huttenlocher, D.P., Klanderman, G.A., Rucklidge, W.J.: Comparing images using the Hausdorff distance. IEEE Trans. Pattern. Anal. Mach. Intell. **15**(9), 850–863 (1993)

Electromagnetic Guided In-Situ Laser Fenestration of Endovascular Stent-Graft: Endovascular Tools Sensorization Strategy and Preliminary Laser Testing

Sara Condino[1(✉)], Roberta Piazza[1,2], Filippo Micheletti[3],
Francesca Rossi[3], Roberto Pini[3], Raffaella Berchiolli[2], Aldo Alberti[4],
Vincenzo Ferrari[1,5], and Mauro Ferrari[1,2]

[1] EndoCAS Center, Department of Translational Research and of New Surgical
and Medical Technologies, University of Pisa, Pisa, Italy
{sara.condino,roberta.piazza,
ferrari.vincenzo}@endocas.org,
mauro.ferrari@med.unipi.it
[2] Unit of Vascular Surgery of the Department of Translational Research
and of New Surgical and Medical Technologies, University of Pisa, Pisa, Italy
{raffaella.berchiolli,mauro.ferrari}@med.unipi.it
[3] Italian National Research Council (CNR),
Institute of Applied Physics, Florence, Italy
{f.micheletti,f.rossi}@ifac.cnr.it
[4] Department of Translational Research and of New Surgical and Medical
Technologies, University of Pisa, Pisa, Italy
a.albertimd@gmail.com
[5] Department of Information Engineering, University of Pisa, Pisa, Italy

Abstract. The in-situ endograft fenestration, a possible surgical option for the minimally invasive treatment of aneurysms with unfavorable anatomy, is today limited by difficulties in targeting the fenestration site and by the lack of a safe method to perforate the graft. In this work we suggest the use of: a 3D electromagnetic (EM) navigator, to accurately guide the endovascular instruments to the target, and a laser system, to selectively perforate the graft. More particularly we propose to integrate a laser fiber into a sensorized guidewire and we describe an EM sensorization strategy to accurately guide the laser tool. Finally we preliminary explore different laser irradiation conditions to achieve a successful endograft fenestration and we verify that the heating generated by the laser doesn't damage the EM coils.

1 Introduction

Endovascular abdominal aortic aneurysms (AAA) repair (EVAR) involves the minimally invasive implantation of a stent-graft within the aorta to exclude the aneurysm from the circulation thus preventing its rupture.

The feasibility of EVAR is highly dependent on the aorta morphology [1–3]: the presence of one/both renal arteries emerging from the aneurysm is the absolute limit for

© Springer International Publishing Switzerland 2016
G. Zheng et al. (Eds.): MIAR 2016, LNCS 9805, pp. 72–83, 2016.
DOI: 10.1007/978-3-319-43775-0_7

the implantation of a standard stent-graft [4]. This limit can be overcomed by using custom-made grafts with fenestrations or branches to preserve flow to the involved aortic branches [5, 6]. However, fenestrated grafting is technically challenging and time consuming, since graft positioning requires a precise alignment of fenestrations with the target vessels [7]. Customized solutions are also very expensive and not available for acute syndromes. All these reasons have led operators to test technical alternatives [8] such as the percutaneous in-situ graft fenestration [9, 10], which involves the careful creation of holes in the stent-graft after its deployment.

The reliability of this procedure is today principally limited by the difficulties in guiding the endovascular tools to the proper fenestration site: the endograft deployment temporarily blocks the flow of contrast medium into the aorta branches, thus the targeting of renal ostia cannot be supported by angiography. Other major issues to be addressed for the successful in-situ graft fenestration are: mechanical support and stability during fenestration, selective perforation of the graft material to safeguard the arterial wall, long term stability of the fenestrated component.

In this work we propose an innovative electromagnetic (EM) guided fenestration system based on laser technology.

In previous studies [11–13] we provided proof-of-concept of the accuracy (1.2 ± 0.3 mm) and efficacy of a 3D EM navigator to guide endovascular procedures,

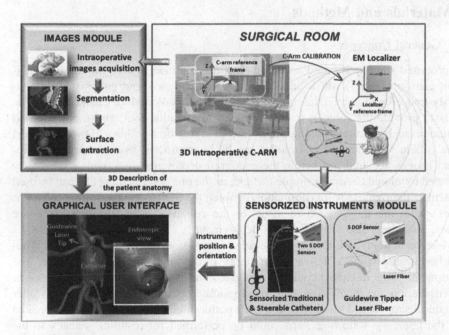

Fig. 1. Schematic representation of the navigation system architecture which include: an Image Module, implemented using the EndoCAS Segmentation Pipeline [11], which generates an accurate 3D model of the patient vasculature starting from intraoperative 3DRA images; a Sensorized Instruments Module with endovascular tools for the fenestration procedure; a Graphical User Interface which displays the position of the endovascular tools inside the 3D model of the patient anatomy.

allowing avoidance of the need for real-time fluoroscopy and angiography, thus reducing X-ray exposure and contrast medium injection. The accuracy obtained can be considered sufficient to cannulate most of the abdominal aorta visceral branches which, in adults, have a mean diameter two times greater than the system maximum error (i.e. Right Renal Artery 5.2 ± 1.3 mm, Left Renal Arteries 5.1 ± 1.0 mm) [14]. Ultrasound images can be exploited as intraoperative information to perform a deformable registration and/or to update 3D static patient-specific models [15].

As regard the endograft perforation, literature works [16–20] have identified laser fenestration as a safe and promising procedure, even if so far no dedicated solutions exist to selectively fenestrate the graft material without damaging the arterial wall. Existing clinical research studies indeed are based on the use of laser atherectomy catheters, designed specifically for the atherosclerotic plaque vaporization, as a surrogate solution to perforate the graft material.

In this paper we propose innovative navigation concepts and EM sensorization strategies for an accurate targeting of the fenestration site and guidance of the laser tool. Finally, we preliminarily test different laser settings to perforate the graft material in presence of human blood and we verify that the heating generated by the laser doesn't damage the EM coils.

2 Materials and Methods

2.1 General Concepts

The proposed strategy is based on the integration of a laser system into an EM navigation platform (Fig. 1) which includes sensorized catheters and guidewires simultaneously tracked with the NDI Aurora (Northern Digital, Waterloo, Canada) [11]. The aim is to provide the surgeon with a selective fenestration tool whose position and orientation can be accurately tracked and showed in real-time within a 3D virtual model of the patient vasculature. Such model can be reconstructed from volumetric radiological images acquired just before the endograft deployment, e.g. with a previously calibrated rotational C-Arm (a simple method, as the one described in [11], can be used to calculate the rigid static transformation between the 3DRA and the Aurora reference frames), allowing the surgeon to visualize the collateral arteries during the entire surgical procedure, also after endograft deployment.

More particularly, the idea is to use a guidewire laser fiber (a laser fiber incorporated into a guidewire) to deliver laser energy to the graft material at the target fenestration site. This laser tool could be navigated and positioned in correspondence to the fenestration site thanks to a sensorized guiding catheter designed ad-hoc to offer mechanical support and stability during graft perforation. Once a hole has been created with the laser, the following steps could be performed for restoring patency to the occluded renal arteries:

- Advancement of the guidewire tipped laser fiber through the newly created fabric hole into renal arteries;
- Withdrawal of the guiding catheter maintaining the guidewire tipped laser fiber in place;

- Using of the guidewire tipped laser fiber as a rail for advancing a cutting balloon dilatation device (as suggested in [21]) or an ad-hoc designed laser catheter to enlarge the fabric hole;
- Deployment of a stent approximately one-quarter into the endograft lumen and three-quarters into the renal artery.

The following paragraph details a sensorization strategy allowing for the real-time tracking of the involved endovascular tools.

2.2 Sensorized Tools

Sensorized Guidewire Laser Fiber. Laser fibers used in current laser therapy procedures are glass optical fibers coaxially surrounded by protective plastic jacket or coating. In general, laser fibers are transparent to fluoroscopy, moreover they have a relatively small diameter and a sharp distal end which can cause arterial punctures/damages while the fiber is being advanced up a tortuous vascular path [22].

In order to deal with guidance issues and to facilitate an atraumatic advancement of the fiber through the patient vasculature the laser fiber can be integrated, together with an EM sensor coil, into a guidewire (Fig. 2). The guidewire could be formed of a metal microtube and could have a diameter of about 0.035 in., a standard diameter for endovascular guidewires used in the clinical practice.

In this work a first prototype of a sensorized guidewire laser fiber was developed by using:

- A tailored nitinol helical hollow strand (suitable for endovascular application) from Fort Wayne Metals (Fort Wayne, Indiana, USA) 0.035 in. in diameter and 180 cm long;
- A 0.22 Numerical Aperture (NA), high power multimode fiber from Thorlabs, Inc. (Newton, New Jersey, USA) 260 ± 6 µm in diameter;
- A 5 degrees of freedom (DOF) EM sensor coil from NDI Aurora, 0.3 mm in diameter and 13 mm long.

Figure 2 illustrates the inner structure of the guidewire laser fiber.

The EM sensor coil at the microtube tip offers the user the possibility to track in real-time the position of the laser fiber end. At this aim methods described in [11] can be employed to calibrate the guidewire sensor and to manually refine the calibration. The selected laser fiber has a double-clad fiber construction (TECS hard coating over fluoride-doped silica cladding) for an improved bending performance: the short-term bend radius, the minimum radius allowed during use and handling, is 12 mm. This parameter is very important for our particular application. Considering that for creating a clean circular fenestration the laser fiber should be ideally oriented at a 90° angle to the endograft [20], and that the sensor coil should not be bent during the procedure, the fiber short-term bend radius should satisfy the following relation (Fig. 3):

$$R_{bent} < D_{endo} - L_{coil} \tag{1}$$

Where:
R_{bent} is the fiber short-term bend radius
D_{endo} is the endograft main body diameter
L_{coil} is the EM coil length

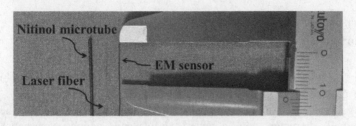

Fig. 2. Components of the guidewire laser fiber.

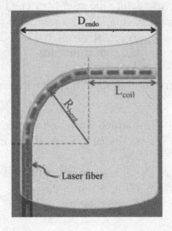

Fig. 3. Schematic representation of a sensorized catheter inside an endograft to evaluate the relation among the fiber short-term bend radius, the endograft main body diameter and the EM coil length. A yellow dotted line shows the position of the sensorized guidewire laser fiber. (Color figure online)

Sensorized Catheters. At least two 5 degrees of freedom (DOF) EM sensors are needed to properly navigate an endovascular catheter allowing the surgeon to visualize in real-time the catheter tip position and the curvature of its distal part without the need for live fluoroscopy [11, 12].

In our particular application, there are no particular limitations on catheter maximum size (the profile of currently available components of endograft delivery systems indeed ranges from 11 to 27 F in outer diameter [23]) and solutions including more than two sensors can be designed.

Figure 4 illustrates a convenient configuration to precisely calculate the catheter tip position and orientation and to derive the catheter distal part curvature by using three 5 DOF EM coils. In this configuration sensor 1 and 2 are positioned according to the method proposed in [11], and sensor 3 is additionally integrated into the catheter to improve the tip localization accuracy.

Figure 4 illustrates the local coordinate system of each Aurora sensor which, by default, has the origin in the coil center and the z-axis along the coil length.

Sensor data can be elaborated to:

- Calculate position $(\vec{o}_t)$ and orientation $(\hat{x}_t, \hat{y}_t, \hat{z}_t)$ of the catheter tip.
- Infer the deformation of the catheter distal part (the tract between sensor 1 and sensor 2).

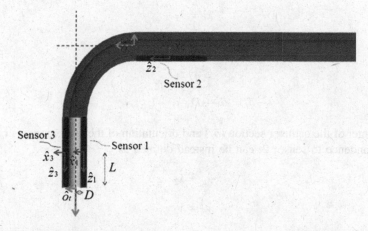

Fig. 4. Possible configuration of sensors. Sensor 1 and sensor 3 are arranged parallel each other at the catheter tip, and sensor 2 is inserted into the same accessory lumen of sensor 1.

To derive these information a calibration procedure is needed. The core of this procedure is the definition of the x and y axes of each sensor i: this is because for 5 DOF sensors the rotation around the coil axis is undetermined and consequently the x and y axes are not fixed.

A possible calibration procedure is described in [11]. This procedure is based on Eqs. 2 and 3 and on the assumption that sensor 1 and sensor 2 (and thus their z axes) lie in the same plane (or at least in two parallel planes).

$$\hat{y}_1 = \hat{y}_2 = \frac{\hat{z}_1 \times \hat{z}_2}{|\hat{z}_1 \times \hat{z}_2|} \qquad (2)$$

$$\hat{x}_i = \hat{z}_i \times \hat{y}_i \qquad (3)$$

This assumption can fall due torsions and bending of the catheter during endovascular navigation. For this reason a more trustful solution can be adopted to accurately derive the catheter tip position and orientation. More particularly, sensor 3 can be added as shown in Fig. 4 in a fixed position and orientation (which do not change during catheter manipulation) relative to sensor 1. Thus, a very simple solution to define the $\hat{x}_i$ and $\hat{y}_i$ axis is:

$$\hat{y}_1 = \frac{\hat{z}_1 \times \frac{\vec{o}_3 - \vec{o}_1}{|\vec{o}_3 - \vec{o}_1|}}{\left|\hat{z}_1 \times \frac{\vec{o}_3 - \vec{o}_1}{|\vec{o}_3 - \vec{o}_1|}\right|} \tag{4}$$

$$\hat{x}_1 = \hat{z}_1 \times \hat{y}_1 \tag{5}$$

Consequently the position and orientation of the catheter tip can be calculated as follows:

$$\hat{x}_t = \hat{x}_1 \tag{6}$$

$$\hat{y}_t = \hat{y}_1 \tag{7}$$

$$\hat{z}_t = \hat{z}_1 \tag{8}$$

$$\vec{o}_t = \vec{o}_1 + D \cdot \hat{x}_1 + L \cdot \hat{z}_t \tag{9}$$

The center of the catheter section ($\vec{o}_c$) and orientation of the catheter axis ($\hat{x}_c, \hat{y}_c, \hat{z}_c$) in correspondence to sensor 2, can be instead defined as:

$$\hat{x}_c = \hat{x}_2 \tag{10}$$

$$\hat{y}_c = \hat{y}_2 \tag{11}$$

$$\hat{z}_c = \hat{z}_2 \tag{12}$$

$$\vec{o}_c = \vec{o}_2 + D \cdot \hat{x}_2 \tag{13}$$

The deformation of the catheter distal part can be finally estimated by using Bezier curves [11], a trustful method providing the advantage of high shape reconstruction accuracy [24] and which can be successfully use to infer the deformation of tubular structures [25–27].

An alternative sensorization strategy could be based on a unique 6 DOF EM coil for the catheter tip and a 5 DOF EM coil to infer the catheter curvature. This strategy is intrinsically more accurate since it doesn't require a calibration procedure to calculate the catheter tip orientation, however the first one should be preferred for mechanical consideration: at the present time the minimum diameter of 6 DOF sensor is more than two times than that of 5 DOF EM coils (0.8 mm versus 0.3 mm) and it would more largely affect the catheter tip mechanical properties.

3 Experimental Design

Preliminary in-vitro test were performed in order to:

- To test different laser settings to perforate the graft material in presence of human blood;
- To verify whether or not the EM sensor can be damaged by the heating generated by the laser.

The first stage of the experiment consisted in testing different laser irradiation condition by controlling laser power, irradiation time, beam source-polyester fabric distance.

A sample of stent-graft polyester fabric was fixed to an ad-hoc build support grid and placed into a plastic container filled with 33 ml of human blood. The polyester fabric was standard woven Dacron from COOK (Bjaereskov, Denmark); blood was obtained from a hematologically healthy adult donor by venipuncture.

As showed in Fig. 5, the polyester fabric was immersed to a depth of 5 mm below the surface of the blood sample.

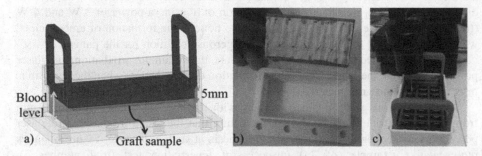

Fig. 5. Experimental setup for laser irradiation test: (a) schematic representation of the support grid for the stent-graft polyester fabric and the plastic container; the illustration shows the position of the graft sample and the blood level; (b) graft sample fixed on the lower surface of the support grid (red), (c) complete experimental setup: the fiber tip, secured on a holder of the micropositioner, can be positioned at different distances from the graft sample. The grid is used as a reference to distinguish between trials with different irradiation conditions. (Color figure online)

A 0.22 Numerical Aperture (NA), high power multimode fiber from Thorlabs, Inc. (Newton, New Jersey, USA) 260 ± 6 μm in diameter, was connected to a diode laser system (SMARTY A800, DEKA) with a 810 nm wavelength and a maximum power of 10 W. The fiber tip was placed on a 3 axis micropositioner allowing the user to precisely regulate the distance between the fiber tip and the graft. The tested irradiation conditions and distances are listed in Table 1.

After irradiation was performed, the fabric sample was washed with physiologic solution and observed under an optical microscope to verify whether or not the laser had fenestrated the tissue and thus to identify the best irradiation conditions.

Then, to verify whether or not the EM sensor can be damaged during laser activation, a final irradiation test was performed using the prototype of sensorized guidewire laser fiber. The sensorized guidewire, connected to the Aurora NDI System Control Unit, was opportunely placed on the 3 axis micropositioner positioning its tip at the desired distance from the stent-graft fabric. Irradiation parameters, as well as the distance between the guidewire tip and the graft, were defined by selecting among all the successful tested conditions the worst case in terms of generated heating. The static position of the guidewire was measured before and after laser activation to evaluate if the heating generated by the laser damages the EM sensor (i.e. by deforming the coil) and thus compromises the sensor measurements. 100 samples were collected and the mean position (distance from the aurora emitter), standard deviation and span (maximum distance – minimum distance) were calculated for each experiment and compared with each other. At the end of the experiment the fabric sample was washed with physiologic solution and observed under optical microscope.

4   Results and Conclusions

Results of the fenestration test are summarized in Table 1. As for trials with an irradiation time of 0.9 s, we obtained a fenestration only using a power of 3 W and 4 W (trial 2 and 3). However during these trials we noticed the formation of emboli/clots, which in the clinical scenario represent a dangerous condition for the patient.

Among the tested conditions, 0.5 s/3 W are the minimum irradiation time/laser power to perforate the fabric without the formation of emboli/clots when the laser tip is in contact with the graft material.

No fenestrations were obtained in trials with the laser tip at a distance of 3 mm from the fabric (trial numbers 16–19), indicating that the tested irradiation time/laser powers are not enough to perforate the prosthesis at such a distance. Figure 6 shows representative examples of: (a) unsuccessful fenestration test (trial number 5), (b) successful fenestration test (trial number 15). Irradiation conditions of trial 7 (power = 4 W, irradiation time = 0.5 s, distance = 0 mm) were selected to test the sensorized guidewire laser fiber. Figure 7 shows the results of this test confirming that, as expected, the graft was properly perforated.

As demonstrated by results summarized in Table 2, the EM sensor was not damaged during the laser activation, indeed no significant difference can be observed between sensor data acquired before and after irradiation. To conclude, this paper presents the main technical concepts for the electromagnetic guided in-situ laser fenestration of endovascular stent-graft, an interesting surgical option for the minimally invasive treatment of aneurysms with unfavorable anatomy.

This procedure can potentially make EVAR available to a greater number of patients, also to those in need of emergency surgery. In this work, we describe the main endovascular tools and surgical steps to perform the procedure, and we propose a sensorization strategy to accurately and effectively guide the targeting of the fenestration site. Preliminary in-vitro results show that a successful fenestration can be achieved without comprising the EM coils used for the endovascular tool tracking. Further extensive studies are needed to identify the best laser irradiation conditions,

Table 1. Results of fenestration test under different irradiation condition. An "X" in the last column indicates that the laser has fenestrated the fabric while a "-" indicates that the current irradiation parameter didn't allow a proper perforation of the material

Trial number	Irradiation time [s]	Power [W]	Distance from the fabric [mm]	Fenestration
1	0.9	2	0	-
2	0.9	3	0	X
3	0.9	4	0	X
4	0.5	2	0	-
5	0.5	2.5	0	-
6	0.5	3	0	X
7	0.5	4	0	X
8	0.5	2	1	-
9	0.5	2.5	1	X
10	0.5	3	1	-
11	0.5	4	1	X
12	0.5	2	2	-
13	0.5	2.5	2	-
14	0.5	3	2	-
15	0.5	4	2	X
16	0.5	2	3	-
17	0.5	2.5	3	-
18	0.5	3	3	-
19	0.5	4	3	-

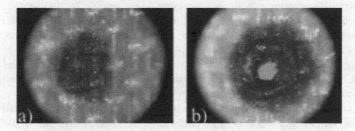

Fig. 6. Optical microscope images: (a) trial number 5, (b) trial number 15.

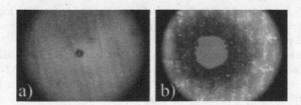

Fig. 7. Optical microscope images of the final irradiation test using the prototype of sensorized guidewire laser fiber.

Table 2. Evaluation of the static position of the guidewire before and after laser activation. The mean position, standard deviation and span of 100 measurements were reported.

	Mean position [mm]	Standard deviation [mm]	Span [mm]
Before laser activation	286.34	0.10	0.47
After laser activation	286.31	0.08	0.38

including human aorta samples in the experimental set-up to verify that the laser can selectively perforate the graft material without damaging the biological tissue.

Acknowledgments. This research has been supported by the scientific project "Electromagnetic guided in-situ laser fenestration of endovascular endoprosthesis" funded by the Italian Ministry of Health and Regione Toscana through the call "Ricerca Finalizzata 2011–2012".

References

1. Dillavou, E.D., Muluk, S.C., Rhee, R.Y., Tzeng, E., Woody, J.D., Gupta, N., Makaroun, M. S.: Does hostile neck anatomy preclude successful endovascular aortic aneurysm repair? J. Vasc. Surg. **38**, 657–663 (2003)
2. Choke, E., Munneke, G., Morgan, R., Belli, A.M., Loftus, I., McFarland, R., Loosemore, T., Thompson, M.M.: Outcomes of endovascular abdominal aortic aneurysm repair in patients with hostile neck anatomy. Cardiovasc. Intervent. Radiol. **29**, 975–980 (2006)
3. Cameron, J.L., Cameron, A.M.: Current Surgical Therapy. Elsevier Health Sciences, Amsterdam (2013)
4. Bertoni, H.G., Girela, G., Peirano, M., Leguizamón, J.H., Ludueña, S., Barone, H.: Endovascular exclusion of an abdominal aortic aneurysm with a fenestrated balloon-expandable stent-graft. Revista argentina de cardiología **76**, 403–406 (2008)
5. Verhoeven, E.L., Zeebregts, C.J., Kapma, M.R., Tielliu, I.F., Prins, T.R., van den Dungen, J. J.: Fenestrated and branched endovascular techniques for thoraco-abdominal aneurysm repair. J Cardiovasc. Surg. (Torino) **46**, 131–140 (2005)
6. Greenberg, R.K., Qureshi, M.: Fenestrated and branched devices in the pipeline. J. Vasc. Surg. **52**, 15S–21S (2010). Official publication, the Society for Vascular Surgery [and] International Society for Cardiovascular Surgery, North American Chapter
7. Health Quality Ontario: Fenestrated endovascular grafts for the repair of juxtarenal aortic aneurysms: an evidence-based analysis. Ont. Health Technol. Assess. Ser. **9**, 1–51 (2009)
8. Oderich, G.S., Ricotta 2nd, J.J.: Modified fenestrated stent grafts: device design, modifications, implantation, and current applications. Perspect. Vasc. Surg. Endovasc. Ther. **21**, 157–167 (2009)
9. McWilliams, R.G., Fearn, S.J., Harris, P.L., Hartley, D., Semmens, J.B., Lawrence-Brown, M.M.: Retrograde fenestration of endoluminal grafts from target vessels: feasibility, technique, and potential usage. J. Endovasc. Ther. **10**, 946–952 (2003)
10. Riga, C.V., Bicknell, C.D., Wallace, D., Hamady, M., Cheshire, N.: Robot-assisted antegrade in-situ fenestrated stent grafting. Cardiovasc. Intervent. Radiol. **32**, 522–524 (2009)
11. Condino, S., Ferrari, V., Freschi, C., Alberti, A., Berchiolli, R., Mosca, F., Ferrari, M.: Electromagnetic navigation platform for endovascular surgery: how to develop sensorized catheters and guidewires. Int. J. Med. Robot. + Comput. Assist. Surg. MRCAS **8**, 300–310 (2012)

12. Condino, S., Calabro, E.M., Alberti, A., Parrini, S., Cioni, R., Berchiolli, R.N., Gesi, M., Ferrari, V., Ferrari, M.: Simultaneous tracking of catheters and guidewires: comparison to standard fluoroscopic guidance for arterial cannulation. Eur. J. Vasc. Endovasc. Surg. Off. J. Eur. Soc. Vasc. Surg. **47**, 53–60 (2014)
13. Turini, G., Condino, S., Postorino, M., Ferrari, V., Ferrari, M.: Improving endovascular intraoperative navigation with real-time skeleton-based deformation of virtual vascular structures. In: De Paolis, T.L., Mongelli, A. (eds.) AVR 2016. LNCS, vol. 9769, pp. 82–91. Springer International Publishing, Switzerland (2016)
14. Pennington, N., Soames, R.W.: The anterior visceral branches of the abdominal aorta and their relationship to the renal arteries. Surg. Radiol. Anat. **27**, 395–403 (2005)
15. Zhang, L., Parrini, S., Freschi, C., Ferrari, V., Condino, S., Ferrari, M., Caramella, D.: 3D ultrasound centerline tracking of abdominal vessels for endovascular navigation. Int. J. Comput. Assist. Radiol. Surg. **9**, 127–135 (2014)
16. Murphy, E.H., Dimaio, J.M., Dean, W., Jessen, M.E., Arko, F.R.: Endovascular repair of acute traumatic thoracic aortic transection with laser-assisted in-situ fenestration of a stent-graft covering the left subclavian artery. J. Endovasc. Ther. **16**, 457–463 (2009). An official Journal of the International Society of Endovascular Specialists
17. Ahanchi, S.S., Almaroof, B.H., Stout, C.L., Panneton, J.M.: In situ laser fenestration and stenting during TEVAR: a new approach to subclavian artery revascularization. J. Vasc. Surg. **53**, 552–553 (2011)
18. Ahanchi, S.S., Almaroof, B., Stout, C.L., Panneton, J.M.: In situ laser fenestration for revascularization of the left subclavian artery during emergent thoracic endovascular aortic repair. J. Endovasc. Ther. **19**, 226–230 (2012). An official Journal of the International Society of Endovascular Specialists
19. Redlinger Jr., R.E., Ahanchi, S.S., Panneton, J.M.: In situ laser fenestration during emergent thoracic endovascular aortic repair is an effective method for left subclavian artery revascularization. J. Vasc. Surg. **58**, 1171–1177 (2013)
20. Topaz, O.: Lasers in Cardiovascular Interventions. Springer, London (2015)
21. Saari, P., Manninen, H.: Fenestration of aortic stent grafts-in vitro tests using various device combinations. J. Vasc. Interv. Radiol. **22**, 89–94 (2011)
22. Zinn, K., Welch, J., Root, H.: Guidewire tipped laser fiber. Google Patents (2009)
23. Arslan, B., Turba, U.C., Sabri, S., Angle, J.F., Matsumoto, A.H.: Current status of percutaneous endografting. Semin. Intervent. Radiol. **26**, 67–73 (2009)
24. Song, S., Li, Z., Yu, H.Y., Ren, H.L.: Electromagnetic positioning for tip tracking and shape sensing of flexible robots. IEEE Sens. J. **15**, 4565–4575 (2015)
25. Maria Viglialoro, R., Condino, S., Gesi, M., Ferrari, M., Ferrari, V.: Augmented reality simulator for laparoscopic cholecystectomy training. In: De Paolis, L.T., Mongelli, A. (eds.) AVR 2014. LNCS, vol. 8853, pp. 428–433. Springer, Heidelberg (2014)
26. Ferrari, V., Viglialoro, R.M., Nicoli, P., Cutolo, F., Condino, S., Carbone, M., Siesto, M., Ferrari, M.: Augmented reality visualization of deformable tubular structures for surgical simulation. Int. J. Med. Robot. Comput. Assist. Surg. **12**, 231–240 (2016)
27. Viglialoro, R., Condino, S., Gesi, M., Ferrari, M., Ferrari, V., Freschi, C., Cutolo, F.: AR visualization of ``Synthetic Calot's Triangle'' for training in cholecystectomy. In: 12th IASTED International Conference on Biomedical Engineering, BioMed 2016 (2016)

A Cost-Effective Navigation System for Peri-acetabular Osteotomy Surgery

Silvio Pflugi[1(✉)], Rakesh Vasireddy[1], Li Liu[1], Timo M. Ecker[2], Till Lerch[2], Klaus Siebenrock[2], and Guoyan Zheng[1]

[1] Institute for Surgical Technology and Biomechanics,
University of Bern, Bern, Switzerland
{silvio.pflugi,guoyan.zheng}@istb.unibe.ch
[2] Department of Orthopedic Surgery, Inselspital,
University of Bern, Bern, Switzerland

Abstract. *Purpose.* To develop and evaluate a low-cost, surgical navigation solution for periacetabular osteotomy (PAO) surgery.

Methods. A commercially available low-cost miniature computer is used together with a camera board (Raspberry Pi 2 Model B, Camera Module PiNoir) to track planar markers (Aruco markers). The overall setup of the tracking unit is small enough to be attached directly to the patient's pelvis. The patient's pelvis is registered by estimating the pose of a planar marker which is attached to an anterior pelvic plane (APP) digitization device. Next, one marker is attached to the acetabular fragment and the initial orientation of the fragment is recorded. The estimated orientation of the fragment is transmitted to the host computer for visualization.

Results. A plastic bone study (eight hip joints) was performed to validate the proposed system. The comparison with a previously developed optical tracking-based system showed no statistical significant difference between measurements obtained from the two systems. In all eight hip joints the mean absolute difference was below 2° for both anteversion and inclination and a very strong correlation was observed.

Conclusions. We show that with our proof-of-principle system, we are able to compute the acetabular orientation accurately.

1 Introduction

Periacetabular osteotomy (PAO) surgery is a type of hip preservation surgery which works by reorienting the acetabular fragment in order to improve femoral head coverage. Several cuts are necessary to separate the acetabular fragment from the rest of the pelvis, leaving the soft tissue unharmed. The separated fragment can then be slowly rotated (due to soft tissue constraints) to the desired new orientation. The desired fragment orientation can be planned pre-operatively, however, the goal of computer assisted surgery (CAS) is to validate if the planned reorientation is achieved intra-operatively. Surgical navigation for PAO has been done before [6,7,10,11]. It has been shown that the use of CAS systems improve accuracy [8,15,21], nevertheless, CAS systems are not yet

© Springer International Publishing Switzerland 2016
G. Zheng et al. (Eds.): MIAR 2016, LNCS 9805, pp. 84–95, 2016.
DOI: 10.1007/978-3-319-43775-0_8

widely used in clinical routine, which can be attributed to certain deficiencies of current navigation techniques. More specifically, the current gold-standard is optical tracking where two cameras track reflective spheres in space. Optical tracking-based systems suffer from the line-of-sight problem and are generally very expensive [5]. Many alternatives were proposed to overcome these drawbacks. Hybrid systems [2,3,5,12,19] combining two or more tracking technologies to overcome each other's drawbacks are usually very expensive and have increased complexity. Other well-known tracking technologies such as electromagnetic tracking [25] or inertial sensor-based tracking [1,16–18,24] still lack the accuracy and show difficulties in magnetic field distorted environments [1,16]. In this paper, we propose a low-cost system solely based on a monocular camera. It tracks planar markers known from augmented reality applications [4]. Our contribution is to put the monocular camera directly on the patient's pelvis to eliminate the line of sight impediment. We use a miniature computer board (Raspberry Pi 2 Model B, Raspberry Pi Foundation, UK) together with a camera module (PiNoir, Raspberry Pi Foundation, UK) to estimate the pose of the marker attached to the acetabular fragment. Patient registration is based on a previously developed system by directly measuring the orientation of the anterior pelvic plane (APP) [17]. The small working volume together with the usage of a regular camera module allows us to use well established image processing and marker tracking techniques. Augmented reality using planar markers was previously introduced for other surgical interventions [14,20,22]. Compared to previously reported work, we directly attach the marker and the monocular camera to the patient's bone, this frees up space in the operating room compared to the usually large installments necessary when using optical tracking-based navigation systems.

2   Materials and Methods

2.1   System Components

The system is divided into two parts: (A) The credit card-sized single-board computer (Raspberry Pi 2 Model B, Raspberry Pi Foundation, UK) with the monocular camera module (Pi NoIR, Raspberry Pi Foundation, UK) which is attached to the patient's pelvis and is responsible for position tracking and (B) the host computer which visualizes the current orientation of the acetabular fragment (Fig. 1). The surgeon can control the workflow and settings directly from the host computer. Communication between the Raspberry Pi and the host computer is done using a local area network (LAN) connection using the transmission control protocol (TCP). The Raspberry Pi is connected using an Ethernet cable, however, the final system is planned to have a wireless connection based on the same communication protocol and an additional battery pack to remove any cabling.

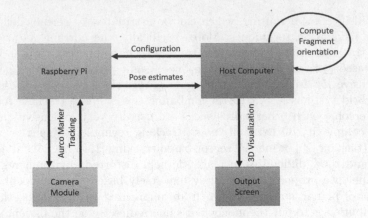

Fig. 1. Red: The Raspberry Pi tracks the Aruco marker using the PiNoir camera module. The pose estimates are then sent to the host computer. Blue: The host computer uses the pose estimates to compute the acetabular orientation and updates the 3D visualization on the screen. (Color figure online)

2.2 Marker Tracking

The camera module is first calibrated using OpenCVs calibration framework. This must be done once for the PiNoir camera, the results including distortion parameters are stored. Once the host computer successfully connected to the Raspberry Pi, the marker tracking starts in a separate thread. During normal operation, the camera module provides grayscale images which are processed to detect planar Aruco markers [4] (see Fig. 2). The detection is implemented in C/C++ using OpenCV (Version 3.1) for all image processing tasks and the marker size was set to 25 mm. The 25 mm were determined empirically and offer a good tradeoff between size and detection accuracy. Simple thresholding is performed first and contours are detected. Contours are filtered by approximating each contour by a polygon and rejecting all contours which cannot be represented by four individual points (rectangle). The final marker candidates are rectified and evaluated whether they represent an Aruco marker [4] or not (Fig. 2). Once the marker is identified, the pose of the marker in the camera's coordinate system is estimated. Two pose estimation algorithms were tested: OpenCVs pose estimation and the robust pose estimation algorithm proposed by Schweighofer and Pinz [23]. The robust pose estimation by Schweighofer et al. showed slightly more stable results with the drawback of being slower (approx. 4 Hz compared to 8 Hz). For our experiments, we decided to use [23] since we think that for our purpose, update rate is less important than accuracy. To reduce outliers, an empirically chosen reprojection error threshold was set to 2 pixels to reject pose estimates with high reprojection error. Additionally, a linear Kalman filter was implemented to improve stability [9]. Pose estimates consist of a 3-by-3 rotation matrix and a 3-by-1 translation vector. The employed Kalman filter was designed to have a state vector x with 18 states:

$$x = \left(x, y, z, \dot{x}, \dot{y}, \dot{z}, \ddot{x}, \ddot{y}, \ddot{z}, \gamma, \theta, \phi, \dot{\gamma}, \dot{\theta}, \dot{\phi}, \ddot{\gamma}, \ddot{\theta}, \ddot{\phi}\right)^T \tag{1}$$

The positional data (x, y, z) and their first and second derivatives make up the first 9 states. The rotation matrix is converted to Euler angles (γ, θ, ϕ) and together with their first and second derivatives make up the second part of the state vector.

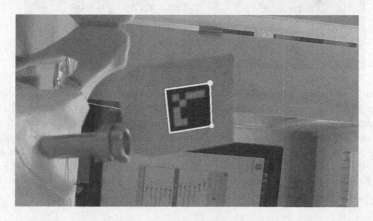

Fig. 2. A screen shot of a detected Aruco marker which is attached to the acetabular fragment as seen by the camera. The white lines are projected back on to the image based on the estimated pose.

2.3 Host Computer Application

A patient-specific computer model is necessary for visualization. This is acquired from segmented computed-tomography (CT) data (using AMIRA, Visage Imaging, San Diego, USA). Next, five landmarks are picked, they include the right and left anterior superior iliac spines and the right and left pubic tubercles. These landmarks define the anterior pelvic plane (APP) which is later used for registration. The fifth landmark is the femur head center which is estimated by fitting a sphere to the femoral head and selecting the sphere center as the femur head center. Furthermore, the acetabular cup plane normal is necessary to compute acetabular orientation (inclination and anteversion). The cup plane normal is computed using a previously developed PAO planning system [11]. The system first automatically detects the acetabular rim points and then fits a plane to these points to get the plane normal. Once all this data is collected, a TCP connection can be established with the Raspberry Pi. The host application as it appears to the surgeon during reorientation is shown in Fig. 3.

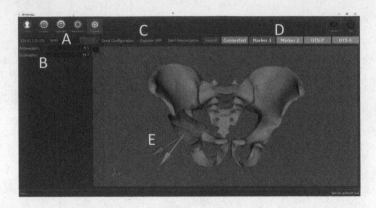

Fig. 3. Host computer application during reorientation: (A) Connection details to establish a TCP connection to the Raspberry Pi (address and port number) (B) The updated anteversion and inclination values (C) Buttons to control the workflow, first the configuration details are sent to the Raspberry Pi, these include marker size, Aruca marker ID and threshold value (D) Labels indicating the current state and if markers are visible (here for our system and for the optical tracking that is running for comparison) (E) The original acetabular cup plane normal (red arrow) is shown together with the updated cup plane normal (green). (Color figure online)

2.4   Anatomy Registration

Patient model registration is done using a special device which was previously developed for APP registration using an inertial measurement unit (IMU) [17] (see Fig. 4). This device has three pillars which are positioned over the right and left iliac spines and on one pubic tubercle. The pillars are of equal length and align the device's top plate with the APP. The estimated pose of the attached marker represents the orientation of the patient's APP in the camera coordinate system. The computer model can then be transformed in a way that its APP (known from the previously picked landmarks) has the same orientation as the patient's APP. Several pose estimates are recorded and averaged to improve robustness of the registration process.

2.5   Reorientation Setup

Before starting the reorientation, the Raspberry Pi is placed on the pelvis with the camera facing towards the fragment. The Aruco marker is attached to the fragment so that it is visible in the camera's view (see Fig. 5).

The reorientation is initiated by sending a command to the Raspberry Pi to get the initial pose estimates of the marker attached to the fragment. Using this pose estimate (represented as a rotation matrix), the starting orientation (anteversion/inclination) is computed according to [13]. From this point on forward, the orientation of the fragment is updated ($\approx$4 Hz) as the surgeon moves the fragment (see Fig. 3). At every time point t_k, the difference in rotation to

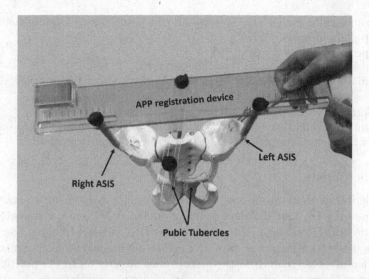

Fig. 4. The previously developed APP registration device. The three pillars with equal length are placed on the right and left anterior iliac spine and one of the two pubic tubercles. The top plate is aligned with the anterior pelvic plane.

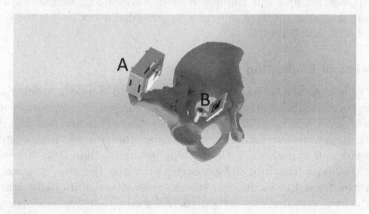

Fig. 5. The current setup: (A) The tracking unit consisting of the Raspberry Pi with the monocular camera is placed directly on the pelvis facing towards the acetabular fragment. (B) The Aruco marker is attached to the fragment.

the previous time point t_{k-1} is computed. The updated rotation matrix is sent to the host computer where the acetabular orientation values and the fragment model are updated. The pose estimate's translation part is not considered in this work. The overall procedure is outlined below.

- Pre-operative
  - Acquire 3D patient-specific model of the pelvis and proximal femur.
  - Pick all landmarks on the pelvis/femur.

○ Automatically detect the acetabular rim points and compute acetabular cup plane normal.
- Intra-operative
  ○ Establish a connection to the Raspberry Pi.
  ○ Send configuration details including Aruco marker ID, marker size and threshold value.
  ○ Perform APP registration.
  ○ Mount Aruco marker to the fragment and initialize re-orientation state.
  ○ Start re-orientation process until target orientation is reached.

2.6   Experiments

The validation of the system was performed using a plastic bone study using 8 hip joints (4L, 4R, four different pelvis models). A CT scan was acquired for each plastic bone. A commercial software (AMIRA, Visage Imaging, SanDiego, USA) was used to segment the data and create 3D models of the pelvis and the proximal femur. A surgeon drew the osteotomies directly on to the plastic bones. The fragments were cut using a coping saw. A previously developed navigation system using an optical tracking camera (Polaris, NDI Canada) was used to get ground truth measurements [11]. The two navigation techniques were merged into one application and ran simultaneously. Anteversion, inclination and the intermediate fragment rotation matrix were recorded every 3 s for the proposed system and the ground truth.

2.7   Statistical Evaluation

Wilcoxon rank-sum test and correlation was used to compare anteversion and inclination values to the optical tracking-based system. We hypothesized that the measurements performed with the proposed systems are **not** significantly different than the measurements acquired using the ground truth system. We will reject the null hypothesis if the p value is smaller than 0.05. Secondly, we compared the mean absolute difference between the the two systems, again, we treat anteversion and inclination values separately. Additionally, correlation between the two systems was computed. All evaluation was performed using Matlab (Mathworks, Natick, MA, USA).

The recorded rotation matrix (fragment orientation) was also compared to the ground truth system as it better represents the accuracy since anteversion and inclination are projected 2D angles. To compare the rotation matrices, we converted them to quaternion representation. q_{rpi} represents the quaternion measured with our system, q_{ots} is the quaternion computed by converting the rotation matrix measured by the optical tracking-based system. For any two unit quaternions, Eq. 2 holds.

$$0 \le abs(dot(q_{rpi}, q_{ots})) \le 1 \tag{2}$$

If two unit quaternions represent the same rotation, then $abs(dot(q_{rpi}, q_{ots})) = 1$. This relationship is used as a metric to compare the rotation matrices stemming from the two systems.

3   Results

Tables 1 and 2 show the results for all eight hip joints. The results show for all eight hips that we have a strong correlation (>0.9) and that the measurements from both systems are **not** significantly different from each other ($p > 0.05$). The mean absolute difference between the two systems is always below $2.0°$.

Table 1. Quantitative results for anteversion. The mean absolute difference for all eight hip joints was below two degrees. No significant difference ($p < 0.05$) was found for all hip joints.

Pelvis	Mean abs	Max abs	Correlation	p val
1R	1.36	6.6	0.9908	0.2113
1L	1.71	5.5	0.9652	0.6847
2R	1.46	4.1	0.9953	0.1730
2L	0.45	2.5	0.9971	0.6982
3R	1.01	4.8	0.9950	0.9402
3L	1.11	3.1	0.9967	0.4029
4R	0.92	6.7	0.9960	0.8261
4L	1.07	3.1	0.9973	0.4436

Table 2. Quantitative results for inclination. The mean absolute difference for all eight hip joints was below two degrees. No significant difference ($p > 0.05$) was found for all hip joints.

Pelvis	Mean abs	Max abs	Correlation	p val
1R	1.31	4.9	0.9921	0.2469
1L	1.26	3.8	0.9968	0.3108
2R	0.49	2.3	0.9944	0.7571
2L	0.48	6.4	0.9965	0.9430
3R	0.93	3.8	0.9932	0.4266
3L	1.36	3.6	0.9928	0.2970
4R	0.82	6.7	0.9968	0.6524
4L	1.11	3.7	0.9927	0.9606

The comparison of the rotation matrices also show a tight correlation between the two systems. The mean quaternion dot product over all measurements is 0.9998 ± 0.0002). Figures 6 and 7 show qualitative results for anteversion and inclination for one hip joint (3R).

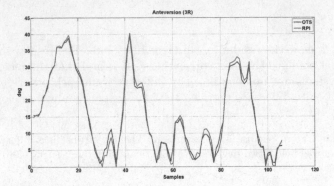

Fig. 6. Anteversion comparison between optical tracking-based system (blue) and our proposed monocular camera-based system (red) for on hip joint (3R). (Color figure online)

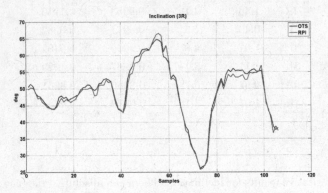

Fig. 7. Inclination comparison between optical tracking-based system (blue) and our proposed monocular camera-based system (red) for on hip joint (3R). (Color figure online)

4   Discussion

In this work we proposed and evaluated a low-cost system for PAO. The prototype uses a monocular camera running on a miniature computer (Raspberry Pi). The Raspberry Pi is directly attached to the patient's pelvis and tracks a planar marker (Aruco marker [4]) fixed to the acetabular fragment (see Fig. 2). The system was compared to the current gold standard, optical tracking. The results have shown a strong correlation between the two systems. This proof-of-principle prototype demonstrates the applicability of a miniature system which is directly attached to the patient, decreasing the risk of interrupting the line of sight that is necessary for camera-based tracking systems.

We have not manufactured special clamps and holders, this will be part of future work. In this work, the Aruco marker was simply fixed on top of the dynamic reference base used by the optical tracking system. The results indicate an error which is in average always below two degrees. However, a maximum difference of up to 6.7° was recorded. This big error is not necessarily from wrong pose estimates but from errors during APP registration. The APP registration device was taken from previous work and was not specifically designed to be used with the proposed system. The Aruco marker was attached to the top plate which caused it to be mostly visible at the image boarder, resulting in a reduced detection accuracy. Detection accuracy is also depending on marker size and distance to the camera. The distance to the camera varies during reorientation. An additional factor that influences detection accuracy is the camera's focus. No auto-focus is used and depending on the current orientation, it might well be possible that the marker is slightly out of focus (see Fig. 2).

The proposed system successfully reduces the line of sight impediment known from optical tracking-based navigation systems. The small working volume established by directly placing the monocular camera on to the patient increases convenience and removes the need for large equipment in the operating room. Additionally, we believe that the smaller size together with the low cost, our system is a first step towards a miniaturized and cost-effective navigation system that offers higher convenience to the surgeon.

5   Conclusion

We successfully demonstrated the feasibility of our low-cost system which reduces the line of sight problem and still is able to accurately estimate the acetabular orientation. Future work will focus on developing specialized tools and fixation devices and on miniaturizing the system even more (e.g. using microcontrollers). Furthermore we will further develop a prototype without any additional cables (e.g. use a battery and wireless technology). The possibility of using additional sensors (such as inertial measurement units) will also be evaluated.

Acknowledgements. The authors would like to thank Thomas Wyss, Tobia Brusa, Urs Rohrer and the team from the machine shop for the valuable support in conducting this prototype.

References

1. Behrens, A., Grimm, J.: Inertial navigation system for bladder endoscopy. In: 2011 Annual International Conference of the IEEE Engineering in Medicine and Biology Society, pp. 5376–5379 (2011)
2. Beller, S., Eulenstein, S.: Upgrade of an optical navigation system with a permanent electromagnetic position control. J. Hepatobiliary Pancreat. Surg. **16**(2), 165–170 (2009)
3. Claasen, G., Martin, P., Picard, F.: High-bandwidth low-latency tracking using optical and inertial sensors. In: 2011 5th International Conference on Automation, Robotics and Applications (ICARA), pp. 366–371 (2011)

4. Garrido-Jurado, S., Munoz-Salinas, R., Madrid-Cuevas, F.J., Marin-Jimenez, M.J.: Automatic generation and detection of highly reliable fiducial markers under occlusion. Pattern Recogn. **47**(6), 2280–2292 (2014)

5. Haid, M., Kamil, M., Chobtrong, T., Guenes, E.: Machine-vision-based and inertial-sensor-supported navigation system for minimal invasive surgery. In: AMA Conferences 2013 - Sensor 2013 (2013)

6. Hsieh, P., Chang, Y., Shih, C.: Image-guided periacetabular osteotomy: computer-assisted navigation compared with the conventional technique: a randomized study of 36 patients followed for 2. Acta Orthop. **77**, 591–597 (2006)

7. Jaeger, M., Westhoff, B., Wild, A., Krauspe, R.: Computer-assisted periacetabular triple osteotomy for treatment of dysplasia of the hip. Zeitschrift fuer Orthopaedie und Ihre Grenzgebiete **142**(1), 51–59 (2004)

8. Jolles, B., Genoud, P., Hoffmeyer, P.: Computer-assisted cup placement techniques in total hip arthroplasty improve accuracy of placement. Clin. Orthop. Relat. Res. **426**, 174–179 (2004)

9. Kalman, R.: A new approach to linear filtering and prediction problems. J. Fluids Eng. **82**, 35–45 (1960)

10. Langlotz, F., Stucki, M.: The first twelve cases of computer assisted periacetabular osteotomy. Comput. Aided Surg. **2**(6), 317–326 (1997)

11. Liu, L., Ecker, T., Schumann, S., Siebenrock, K., Nolte, L., Zheng, G.: Computer assisted planning and navigation of periacetabular osteotomy with range of motion optimization. In: Golland, P., Hata, N., Barillot, C., Hornegger, J., Howe, R. (eds.) MICCAI 2014, Part II. LNCS, vol. 8674, pp. 643–650. Springer, Heidelberg (2014)

12. Mahfouz, M., Kuhn, M.: Integration of UWB and wireless pressure mapping in surgical navigation. IEEE Trans. Microw. Theor. Tech. **57**(10), 2550–2564 (2009)

13. Murray, D.: The definition and measurement of acetabular orientation. J. Bone Joint Surg. Br. **75**, 228–232 (1993)

14. Nicolau, S.A., Pennec, X., Soler, L., Ayache, N.: A complete augmented reality guidance system for liver punctures: first clinical evaluation. In: Duncan, J.S., Gerig, G. (eds.) MICCAI 2005. LNCS, vol. 3749, pp. 539–547. Springer, Heidelberg (2005)

15. Nogler, M., Kessler, O., Prassl, A.: Reduced variability of acetabular cup positioning with use of an imageless navigation system. Clin. Orthop. Relat. Res. **426**, 159–163 (2004)

16. O'Donovan, K., Kamnik, R.: An inertial and magnetic sensor based technique for joint angle measurement. J. Biomech. **40**, 2604–2611 (2007)

17. Pflugi, S., Liu, L., Ecker, T., Cullmann, J., Siebenrock, K., Zheng, G.: A cost-effective surgical navigation solution for periacetabular osteotomy (PAO) surgery. Int J CARS. doi:10.1007/s11548-015-1267-1

18. Ren, H., Kazanzides, P.: Investigation of attitude tracking using an integrated inertial and magnetic navigation system for hand-held surgical instruments. IEEE/ASME Trans. Mechatron. **17**(2), 210–217 (2012)

19. Ren, H., Rank, D., Merdes, M.: Multisensor data fusion in an integrated tracking system for endoscopic surgery. IEEE Trans. Inf. Technol. Biomed. **16**(1), 106–111 (2012)

20. Rhienmora, P., Gajananan, K.: Augmented reality haptics system for dental surgical skills training. In: Proceedings of the 17th ACM Symposium on Virtual Reality Software and Technology, pp. 97–98 (2010)

21. Ryan, J., Jamali, A., Bargar, W.: Accuracy of computer navigation for acetabular component placement in THA. Clin. Orthop. Relat. Res. **468**(1), 169–177 (2010)

22. Sauer, F., Khamene, A., Vogt, S.: An augmented reality navigation system with a single-camera tracker: system design and needle biopsy phantom trial. In: Dohi, T., Kikinis, R. (eds.) MICCAI 2002, Part II. LNCS, vol. 2489, pp. 116–124. Springer, Heidelberg (2002)
23. Schweighofer, G., Pinz, A.: Robust pose estimation from a planar target. IEEE Trans. Pattern Anal. Mach. Intell. **28**(12), 2024–2030 (2006)
24. Walti, J., Jost, G., Cattin, P.: A new cost-effective approach to pedicular screw placement. Augment. Environ. Comput. Assist. Interv. **8678**, 90–97 (2014)
25. Zhang, H., Banovac, F., Lin, R.: Electromagnetic tracking for abdominal interventions in computer aided surgery. Comput. Aided Surg. **11**(3), 127–136 (2006)

Motion-Based Technical Skills Assessment in Transoesophageal Echocardiography

Evangelos B. Mazomenos[1(✉)], Francisco Vasconcelos[1], Jeremy Smelt[2],
Henry Prescott[4], Marjan Jahangiri[2], Bruce Martin[3], Andrew Smith[3],
Susan Wright[2], and Danail Stoyanov[1]

[1] Centre for Medical Image Computing, University College London, London, UK
e.mazomenos@ucl.ac.uk
[2] St George's University Hospitals, NHS Foundation Trust, London, UK
[3] St Bartholomew's Hospitals, NHS Foundation Trust, London, UK
[4] Glassworks Ltd, London, UK

Abstract. This paper presents a novel approach for evaluating technical skills in Transoesophageal Echocardiography (TEE). Our core assumption is that operational competency can be objectively expressed by specific motion-based measures. TEE experiments were carried out with an augmented reality simulation platform involving both novice trainees and expert radiologists. Probe motion data were collected and used to formulate various kinematic parameters. Subsequent analysis showed that statistically significant differences exist among the two groups for the majority of the metrics investigated. Experts exhibited lower completion times and higher average velocity and acceleration, attributed to their refined ability for efficient and economical probe manipulation. In addition, their navigation pattern is characterised by increased smoothness and fluidity, evaluated through the measures of dimensionless jerk and spectral arc length. Utilised as inputs to well-known clustering algorithms, the derived metrics are capable of discriminating experience levels with high accuracy (>84 %).

Keywords: Skill assessment · Motion analysis · Transoesophageal echocardiography

1 Introduction

Transoesophageal echocardiography (TEE) is carried out by imaging the heart with an ultrasound (US) transducer, attached to the tip of a flexible endoscope (probe), navigated through the oesophagus proximally to the heart. TEE provides clear and detailed imaging of the four chambers and the valves, enabling accurate cardiovascular diagnosis and monitoring. As a minimally-invasive (MI), image-guided procedure, TEE requires complex psychomotor skills and a high

© Springer International Publishing Switzerland 2016
G. Zheng et al. (Eds.): MIAR 2016, LNCS 9805, pp. 96–103, 2016.
DOI: 10.1007/978-3-319-43775-0_9

level of coordination. Professional accreditation organisations routinely publish guidelines and recommendations on training practices and the cognitive and technical skills required for performing TEE [3,9]. In summary, TEE practitioners must demonstrate proficiency in: (a) navigating the US probe safely through the oesophagus; (b) adjusting the scanning plane so as to obtain the necessary imaging views; (c) accurately evaluating the heart's functionality and recognising abnormal conditions. Essentially, (a) and (b) pertain to technical manipulation skills while (c) to medical knowledge and understanding of pathologies.

In order for new interventionalists to develop the necessary technical skills, specific and constructive assessment/feedback is necessary. However, the current gold standard of surgical evaluation through expert supervision and manual assessment is inefficient, laborious and with limited standardisation. As a result, alternative directions for training and assessment ought to be explored. Breakthroughs in computing enabled the development of virtual reality (VR) systems that simulate the operational environment with high fidelity. They provide a platform for trainees to hone primarily their dexterous skills in an environment that poses no patient risk, without the need for direct supervision. To fully compliment surgical training, VR simulators must incorporate detailed performance feedback that will assist users to refine their skills. So far these systems are restricted in providing generic metrics without benchmarking, that are generally considered as surrogate markers of surgical competency [6,8].

Motion analysis as a tool to evaluate competency is currently unexplored in the field of TEE. Motivated by studies in MI procedures (e.g. laparoscopic, endovascular) that have reported a strong correlation between tool kinematics and surgical ability [5,7,10], we hypothesised that by analysing the motion pattern of the tip of the TEE probe (that carries the US transducer) and deriving representative metrics, surgical skills can be objectively evaluated. Thus far, basic probe kinematics have only been used to measure the improvement of trainees during training/teaching with simulators, but not for TEE skills assessment [4,11]. This work differs from such studies, which chiefly employ qualitative manual evaluation [2,11]. Intuitively, differences are expected between experts and novices, but the features to best represent these are not established. Our main objective is to identify the motion metrics that can effectively characterise and assess TEE surgical experience. This is crucial towards automated assessment and has not been reported for TEE.

We employed a high-fidelity TEE simulator, equipped with a probe with the same manoeuvrability as standard probes, in experiments with both expert and novice practitioners. The motion of the probe was captured with the simulator's software. A set of kinematic features was derived, introducing previously unexplored smoothness measures as we expect this feature to be indicative of the skill level. We then investigated their correlation with experience and found that the majority of the formulated metrics show statistical significance. Ultimately, the derived features were used as inputs to clustering algorithms yielding high accuracy (>84 %) in classifying the participants according to their experience group.

2   Methods

2.1   HeartWorks VR Simulator

The HeartWorks TEE simulator (Inventive Medical, Ltd, London, UK) was used as the experimentation platform. This system, illustrated in Fig. 1a involves an upper-torso mannequin with a mouth opening to emulate probe insertion. The HeartWorks probe has similar shape, dimensions and articulation capabilities (flexion, rotation, angulation), as standard TEE probes. Dedicated VR software generates a high-fidelity 3D rendering (Fig. 1b) of a beating human heart simulating cardiovascular activity (normal and abnormal). An ultrasound detector in the mannequin detects the position and orientation of the US plane which is then used to generate the 2D US image (Fig. 1c) from the heart model. Both the 2D US image and the 3D animation of the heart with the inserted probe are illustrated in the simulator's monitor. This allows the user to associate the obtained US image with the anatomical position of the probe. By visualising only the US screen the overall experience of the HeartWorks simulator is similar to an actual TEE system in the operating theatre, as it was the case in our experimentation.

Similar to standard multi-plane TEE probes the HeartWorks probe is capable of five movements, visualised in Fig. 2. Firstly, moving the probe up and down (advancement/withdrawal) in the oesophagus. The probe can be also twisted to the right (clockwise from the operators prospective at the head) or left (counterclockwise) at the full range of $\pm180°$. Control knobs enable anteflexion (flex anteriorly) and retroflexion (flex posteriorly) as well as lateral flexion (flex left

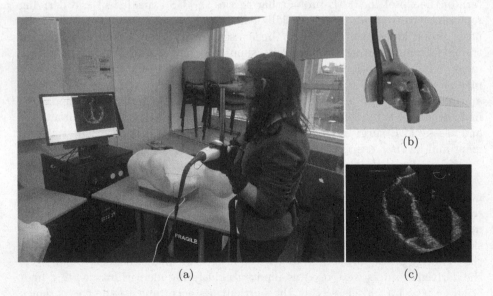

(a)   (b)

                                                            (c)

Fig. 1. (a) A volunteer operating the HeartWorks simulator; (b) 3D rendering of the heart model, the probe and US scanning field; (c) the simulated US image

and right) at the range of ±90°. Finally the US transducer on the tip can be rotated within the range of 0° (horizontal plane) to 180°, using buttons on the probe's handle.

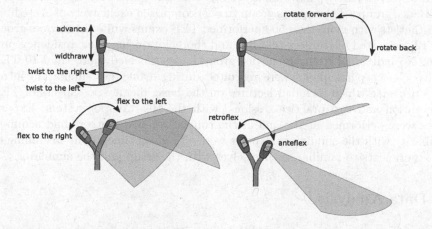

Fig. 2. The HeartWorks TEE probe movements: (upper-left) advancement/withdrawal and twist, (lower-left) flexion, (upper-right) US transducer rotation, (lower-right) anteflecion/retroflexion

2.2 Designed Study

For our assessment study, an experiment was designed where the participant was asked to obtain 10 image planes in a specific sequence with the simulator. These 10 cross-sectional views, listed in Table 1, are a subset of the 20 suggested views, designated by various organisations, as essential for a comprehensive cardiovascular evaluation during a TEE exam [3]. In the experiments, the participant

Table 1. Sequence of the 10 US image planes used in the study

Sequence	US image view
1	Mid-Esophageal 4-Chamber (centered at tricuspid valve) - ME4C (TV)
2	Mid-Esophageal 2-Chamber - ME2C
3	Mid-Esophageal Aortic Valve Short-Axis - ME AV SAX
4	Transgastric Mid-Short-Axis - TG mid SAX
5	Mid-Esophageal Right Ventricle inflow-outflow - ME RV inflow-outflow
6	Mid-Esophageal Aortic Valve Long-Axis - ME AV LAX
7	Transgastric 2-Chamber - TG2C
8	Mid-Esophageal 4-Chamber (centered at left ventricle) ME4C (LV)
9	Deep Transgastric Long-Axis - dTG LAX
10	Mid-Esophageal Mitral Commissural - ME MV commissural

operated the US probe while a supervisor (expert anaesthetist) provided support by guiding the participant through the views sequence and operating the HeartWorks software.

A total of 19 participants volunteered for this study and were divided into two experience groups. The experts group (n = 7) comprised exclusively of accredited anaesthetists with more than 500 performed TEE exams while the novices group (n = 12) consisted of trainees (cardiac and thoracic) during their residency program. No individual from the novice group had performed more than 10 TEE exams. Novice participants were recruited during a one-day simulation introduction course which included lectures on the basic diagnostic aspects of TEE intervention and two practice sessions, with the HeartWorks system. Experiments were performed at the end of the course, when volunteers had acquired familiarity with the simulator. Experts were also given time at the beginning of the experiments to familiarise themselves with the setup and the simulator.

3   Data Analysis

Data are logged in a timestamped datafile with the values of the probe articulation parameters (depth of insertion, ante/retro flexion, lateral flexion, twist and transducer angulation). These are controlled directly by the operator. The software-generated 6DoF (3D position and orientation) of the probe's tip, used for positioning the probe in the 3D scene based on the user's handling, are also included. Figure 3 illustrates representative examples of the depth and resulting probe trajectory, obtained from an expert and a novice volunteer. The differences are obvious with the expert demonstrating superior dexterity skills, resulting in smoother and fluid probe manipulation. Moreover the novice's erratic movement is dangerous for causing oesophageal perforation or trauma. The total procedure time (T_t) was extracted from the timestamp values. From the depth $(d(t))$ which is the main translation parameter we calculated the total path length (pl) travelled by the tip, the average velocity (v_d) and acceleration (a_d) as well as two measures of smoothness. The dimensionless jerk (j_d), a jerk metric independent of duration and amplitude and the spectral arc length (η_{sal}) a recently proposed, also dimensionless metric, found to be consistent and robust in measuring movement smoothness [1]. Considering the 1D parameter of depth, the two smoothness metrics are defined as:

$$j_d = \left(0.5 \int_{t_i}^{t_e} \dddot{d(t)}^2 dt \right) \cdot \frac{T_t^5}{p^2} \qquad \eta_{sal} = -\int_0^{\omega_c} \sqrt{\left(\frac{1}{\omega_c} \right)^2 + \left(\frac{\|dV_d(\omega)\|}{d\omega} \right)^2} \, d\omega$$

where $\|V_d(\omega)\|$ is the amplitude normalised Fourier magnitude spectrum of the speed and ω_c is the upper frequency limit of the movement spectrum. This was set to $\omega_c = 40\pi$ rad/s or 20 Hz considering the spectrum of human hand movement. From the rotational parameters of the probe, the average values of twist (tw) and flexion (fl), were calculated and included in our analysis.

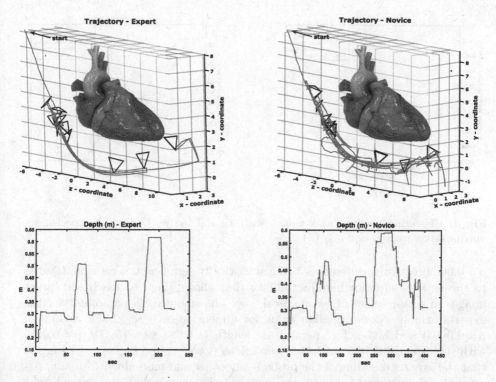

Fig. 3. Probe tip trajectories (top), coordinates are in 3D scene units (i.e. scaled meters), with position and orientation of US scanning fields (black triangles) in the 10 captured views; and depth (bottom) for an expert (left) and a novice (right). The smoothness and fluidity of the expert operator is evident compared to the novice.

The obtained data were compared with the nonparametric Mann-Whitney U test with the difference considered significant for p-value <0.05. The median and p-values for each parameters are listed in Table 2. We observe that experts complete the test faster (226.2 s vs 439.9 s, p = 0.0007) and demonstrate higher velocity (0.009 m/s vs 0.007 m/s, p = 0.0004) and acceleration (0.304 m/s vs 0.240 m/s,

Table 2. Median values and p-values of the calculated features

Parameter	Novices	Experts	p-value (MW)
T_t - Total time (sec)	439.9	226.2	0.0007
pl - Depth path length (m)	2.838	2.509	0.482
v_d - Average depth velocity (m/s)	0.007	0.009	0.0004
a_d - Average depth acceleration (m/s^2)	0.240	0.304	0.009
j_d - Depth dimensionless jerk	15.938	2.353	0.0004
η_{sal} - Depth spectral arc length	−15.478	−6.684	0.028
tw - Average twist (deg)	18.832	11.906	0.0004
fl - Average flexion (deg)	6.748	5.619	1

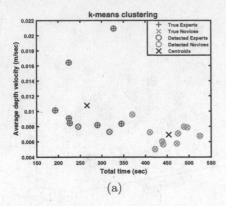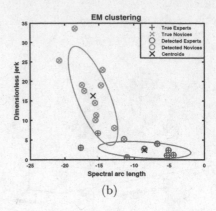

          (a)   (b)

Fig. 4. Clustering results; (a) k-means with T_t and v_d (89.47 %); (b) expectation-maximisation with j_d and η_{sal} (84.21 %)

$p = 0.0009$) with the differences being statistically significant. This is attributed to the experts superior handling ability that allows them to reach the target images in a more efficient, economical way. The smoothness parameters of the experts exhibit a lower median value for dimensionless jerk (2.353 vs 15.938, $p = 0.0004$) and higher for spectral arc length (-6.684 vs -15.478, $p = 0.028$) with significant differences. Both observations (lower j_d and higher η_{sal}) suggest that the experts handling of the probe is smoother and more fluent. Finally, significant difference was found for the average twist exercised on the probe by the two groups. The rest of the rotation parameters (flexion, lateral flexion and scanning field rotation) did not show statistical significance. This is because these are used to adjust the US scanning field at a specific orientation once the tip has reached the desired position, but users do not alter them during probe navigation (advance/withdrawal and twist) resulting in them having a static pattern. Also their nominal value in the 10 views, is roughly known from practice, thus the lack of variation across users.

To further evaluate the ability of the derived kinematic parameters to discriminate the level of experience, we conducted experiments with established unsupervised learning methods. Figure 4 illustrates two clustering examples; (a) k-means clustering using the total time and average depth velocity resulting in 89.47 % (17/19) classification accuracy; and (b) expectation - maximisation (EM) with the two smoothness features which yields a 84.21 % (16/19) accuracy.

4   Conclusions

This paper presented an investigation on the applicability of motion-based metrics for TEE skill evaluation. A cohort of 19 participants, comprising of novice and expert practitioners performed experiments, acquiring 10 standard TEE views, on the HeartWorks VR simulator. Statistical analysis revealed significant differences ($p < 0.05$) in motion-based metrics that represent economy and efficiency (procedure time, average speed, average acceleration) as well as motion smoothness and fluidity (dimensionless jerk, spectral arc length). We run clustering experiments with the derived feature set and participants were classified to their respective group with high accuracy ($>84\%$). We thus conclude that the kinematic analysis of the TEE probe presents high potential for the development of objective skill assessment methods in TEE. Future work will focus on integrating information about tool-tissue interaction (force exercised by probe's tip) and from the image analysis of the acquired TEE views. Ultimately, we aim to develop an automated performance score that correlates well with manual assessment. Such a system, can be integrated into the HeartWorks software providing detailed self-assessment and further facilitating the development of dexterous skills with VR simulation training.

References

1. Balasubramanian, S., Melendez-Calderon, A., Burdet, E.: A robust and sensitive metric for quantifying movement smoothness. IEEE Trans. Biomed. Eng. **59**(8), 2126–2136 (2012)
2. Charron, C., Prat, G., Caille, V., et al.: Validation of a skills assessment scoring system for transesophageal echocardiographic monitoring of hemodynamics. Intensive Care Med. **33**(10), 1712–1718 (2007)
3. Hahn, R.T., Abraham, T., Adams, M.S., et al.: Guidelines for performing a comprehensive transesophageal echocardiographic examination: recommendations from the American Society of Echocardiography and the Society of Cardiovascular Anesthesiologists. J. Am. Soc. Echocardiogr. **26**(9), 921–964 (2013)
4. Matyal, R., Montealegre-Gallegos, M., Mitchell, J.D., et al.: Manual skill acquisition during transesophageal echocardiography simulator training of cardiology fellows: a kinematic assessment. J. Cardiothorac. Vasc. Anesth. **29**(6), 1504–1510 (2015)
5. Mazomenos, E.B., Chang, P.L., Rippel, R.A., et al.: Catheter manipulation analysis for objective performance and technical skills assessment in transcatheter aortic valve implantation. Int. J. Comput. Assist. Radiol. Surg. **11**(6), 1121–1131 (2016)
6. Mitchell, E.L., Arora, S., Moneta, G.L., et al.: A systematic review of assessment of skill acquisition and operative competency in vascular surgical training. J. Vasc. Surg. **59**(5), 1440–1455 (2014)
7. Moorthy, K., Munz, Y., Sarker, S.K., Darzi, A.: Objective assessment of technical skills in surgery. Brit. Med. J. **327**(7422), 1032–1037 (2003)
8. Neequaye, S.K., Aggarwal, R., Van Herzeele, I., et al.: Endovascular skills training and assessment. J. Vasc. Surg. **46**(5), 1055–1064 (2007)
9. Quinones, M.A., Douglas, P.S., Foster, E., et al.: ACC/AHA clinical competence statement on echocardiography: a report of the American College of Cardiology/American Heart Association/American College of Physicians-American Society of Internal Medicine Task Force on Clinical Competence. J. Am. Coll. Cardiol. **41**(4), 687–708 (2003)
10. Rolls, A.E., Riga, C.V., Bicknell, C.D., et al.: A pilot study of video-motion analysis in endovascular surgery: development of real-time discriminatory skill metrics. Eur. J. Vasc. Endovasc. Surg. **45**(5), 509–515 (2013)
11. Sohmer, B., Hudson, C., Hudson, J., et al.: Transesophageal echocardiography simulation is an effective tool in teaching psychomotor skills to novice echocardiographers. Can. J. Anaesth. **61**(3), 235–241 (2014)

Advanced Design System for Infantile Cranium Shape Model Growth Prediction

Kamal Shahim[1]([✉]), Mauricio Reyes[1], Ruben Simon[2], Philipp Jürgens[3],
and Christoph Blecher[2]

[1] Institute for Surgical Technology and Biomechanics,
University of Bern, Bern, Switzerland
kamal.shahim@istb.unibe.ch
[2] Cranioform AG, Alpnach, Switzerland
[3] Department of Cranio-Maxillofacial Surgery, Faculty of Medicine,
University of Basel, Basel, Switzerland

Abstract. We present a longitudinal statistical shape/volumetric model of the cranium of infants and use it as prior information to support the design of cranial shape correction helmets. In addition, a logical approach based on natural brain growth is considered to derive necessary formulation to calculate the required treatment duration. The respective morphological analysis and statistical model will be integrated into the current haptic-based design pipeline of a company to produce an effective computer-assisted design system.

Keywords: Infants · Cranium · Longitudinal statistical shape model · Volume growth

1 Introduction

Infantile cranium is vulnerable to deformation due to the lack of rigidity mostly up to the fourth or fifth month of life. The brain may start developing abnormal shape due to the limited head mobility and external forces acting on the head. Hence, the skull grows normally but in asymmetric manner. Therapy focus on constraining the baby cranium by providing a helmet which should be worn for several months. The treatment may take from eight weeks to eight months, depending on the child's age of the child and the degree of asymmetry and depends on the cause, the age of the child and the severity of the head deformity. It consists in patient specific treatments, meaning surgeon defines manually for each baby the normal region and outlines volumetrically the correction for the asymmetric cranial shape and constructs a helmet based on medical specifications where head growth is not restricted. To our knowledge, there is no algorithm available to provide surgeons with statistical information of infantile cranium growth and indeed the treatment duration for which baby should wear the helmet. Due to the lack of information on the statistical shape model of infant cranium, several checkups normally are carried out and correction to the helmet might be necessary. For the sake of illustration, the extra volumes are

© Springer International Publishing Switzerland 2016
G. Zheng et al. (Eds.): MIAR 2016, LNCS 9805, pp. 104–113, 2016.
DOI: 10.1007/978-3-319-43775-0_10

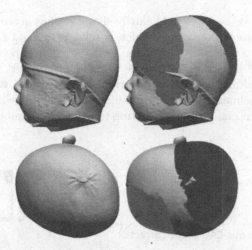

Fig. 1. During the shape correction process, the surgeons add manually extra volumes to the scanned model in order to correct the asymmetrical shape of the skull and fabricate the patient specific helmet.

shown in Fig. 1 where two volumes are added to the front and back side in order to correct the asymmetry of skull.

In this paper, we present an advanced setup which integrates the statistical shape model of infantile cranium by creating a longitudinal volume model of the cranium of infants generated from large number of scans. The shape model can be used as prior information to support the design of cranial shape correction helmets. In addition, we generate the logical approach based on natural brain growth to derive necessary formulation to calculate the required treatment duration. With such improvement, surgeons are able to assess head growth and the expected treatment duration and how much correction volume is needed in the regions based on the statistical information. They can either mark the extra volume needed and our algorithm provides the treatment duration or the model predicts directly both the correction and treatment time. This model will be integrated into the current haptic-based design pipeline of a company active in this domain to produce an effective computer-assisted design system.

2   Current and Proposed Design System

Current helmet design work flow is schematically described in Fig. 2. First of all, a 3D scanning of the baby's head is needed to obtain a shape representation of the initial state of the cranium. Then, this three-dimensional representation is used within in a special CAD program to perform shape corrections and the ideal individual shape is established. This step is sensitive to the operators experience, being crucial in understanding cranial shape growth in infants, and translating this knowledge into a patient-specific scenario. In addition, this step requires estimation of the expected healthy shape at that given time. Due to the complexity of this shape prediction, which is related to head's shape, deformity locations, missing volume and baby's age, every predicted healthy shape needs to be inspected and if necessary corrected by surgeon expert in the area. This introduces a constraining factor in the current helmet design workflow. Figure 2 shows the current helmet design and manufacturing workflow. Text in red indicates inspection from main expert, affecting the effective number of helmets that can be produced.

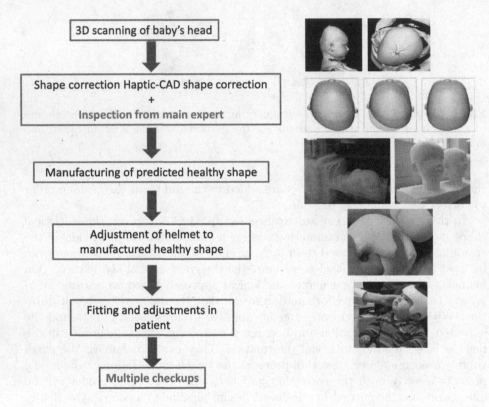

Fig. 2. Schematic of current helmet design and manufacturing workflow.

Due to the manual correction involved in the current design system, multiple check-ups (approximately five visits) of the patient to the treating doctor are needed to perform corrections or, in some cases, manufacturing of a new corrected helmet. As a third step, the resulting CAD model is manufactured using a CNC grinding machine, yielding a patient-specific model on which the helmet is fitted and tunned to (fourth step). At last, a fifth step involves fitting and adjustments to the baby's head. After this first visit, several checkups (about five), are conducted to perform adjustments, and if necessary manufacturing of a new corrected helmet. From these steps, the sought strategy is to reduce the time for the design phase and the number of check-ups. In order to achieve the planned goals, the following improvements are made to the current design system, based on the clinical cases form different centers, an insight analysis of morphology and volume changes are performed. These improvements are introduced into the current design system, based on the clinical cases from different centers. Then, we construct longitudinal statistical shape model of infant cranium in Statismo format [1]. At then end, for evaluation purposes, cranial shape from sparse temporal surface information are reconstructed using specific morphing algorithms. The rationale underpinning the use of a statistical shape model is to support the complex decision making process of designing a healthy (or corrected) patient-specific cranial shape while taking into account growth patterns of the baby's head. The following subsections describe in detail the construction of such statistical model and how it is planned to be used within the helmet design workflow.

3   Data Cohort and Morphological Measurements

The input data used to build the statistical shape model consists on a set of surface scans collected over the years. About 360 clinical cases (cad corrected or healthy shape), plus 700 scans were collected from different centers and used for further analysis such as elementary morphological measurements and data statistics. The correspondence was made between models and age of the baby and their scanning time. The number of scans is higher as the surgeon normally monitors and controls the brain growth development in several visits. Each surface scan contains the complete head of the baby, face and part of the neck and shoulder (see example in Fig. 1). Therefore the first step is to select the surface areas that only include cranial information. To this end, user-driven selection of surface landmarks were performed for each case in order to mark the cranium section in each baby's head. Given the birth information, the resulting meshes were annotated along with the age of the baby. The pipeline was made semi-automatic using computer tools in order to gain timing in different tasks such as cropping the region of interest covering the full baby crani. Open source library Visualization toolkit [3] was employed for cropping the region of interest and rigid landmark alignment. Figures 3 and 4 present the statistics on the available clinical cases used to create the model.

The age of the babies being scanned ranges from 4 to 20 months of age and is concentrated in the lower range, as the corrections are mostly performed during the first months of development. The approximate frequency of the scans per age bin (bin width corresponding to 1 month) is about 20 to 100 scans (babies with 4–8 months old). The feasibility of building a comprehensive longitudinal model relies also on how well the sample is representative of the population. This in turns depends on the temporal granularity of the shape variability; the more cases per age (or age bin) we have at our disposal, the more variability is captured at the specific time points. Based on these figures we estimate to have an appropriate sampled population.

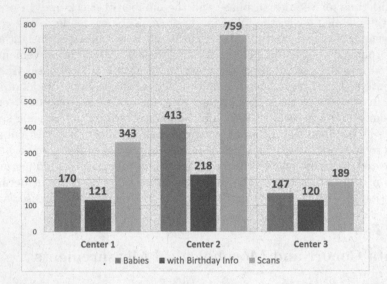

Fig. 3. Number of scans and cad correction models received from different centers (Color figure online).

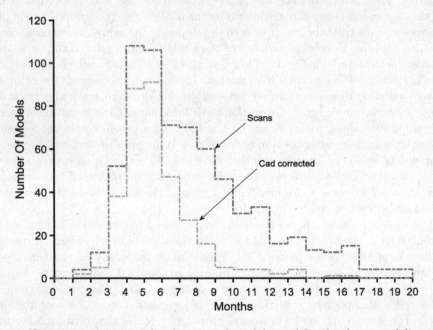

Fig. 4. Histogram of scans and cad corrected models used for the shape modeling and further volumetric analysis.

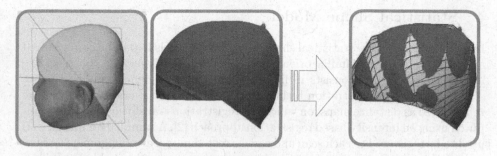

Fig. 5. Each scan and cad corrected model were cropped, co-aligned. A template surface mesh is registered to each cropped mesh using Deformetrica software [2].

To assess the volumetric growth (which is independent of the helmet effect) both scans and cad corrected shapes were used to create volume growth chart. Both scans and cad corrected models are manually landmark annotated, followed by mesh cropping to eliminate regions that are not to be modeled (see Fig. 5). For each aligned configuration of baby cranium, we calculated the volume of both scanned models and card corrections. The confidence interval for the resulting volume arranged per birthday time was obtained using Matlab software [5]. The appropriate equations from the fitted graph to scans and cad correction data is helpful to determine the approximate timing needed for extra volume for correction phase. Due to the confidential requirement, the resulting equation and chart for cad corrected volume growth are not presented (Fig. 6).

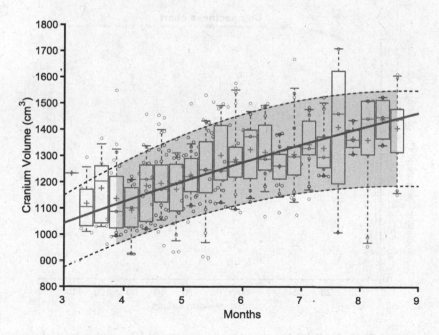

Fig. 6. Confidence interval for volumes of scanned models.

4   Statistical Shape Model

In order to develop the statistical shape model, the models had to be co-registered and aligned to have a similar orientation and reference frame. To construct the model, the procedure consists in finding point-correspondences among subject scans by means of registration techniques. To this end, the cranial surfaces are represented as distance maps, on which the registration transformation were computed using an intensity based registration approach [2]. A sampled temple mesh is used to be registered to each scan and cad corrected model after alignment. As the temporal information among subjects is not homogeneous (i.e. babies age varies on scanning) and the number of scans per subject is low and not consistent among subjects, the resulting data set is regarded as a time series. The longitudinal model

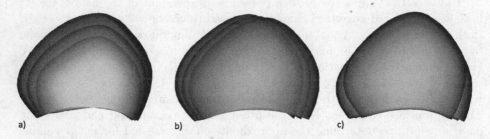

Fig. 7. Shape models variation are shown for three major eigenvalue (mean and −3 and +3 standard deviations)

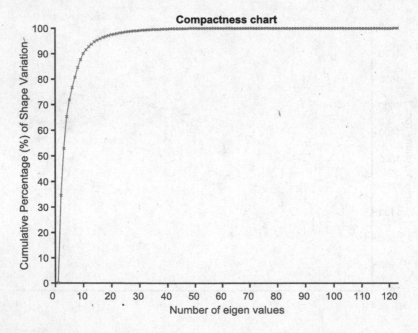

Fig. 8. Compactness chart for the shape model generated from cad corrected models.

will be built based on the recovered healthy shape for each baby, which is performed for each case using a CAD software. After point-correspondences were defined, the library Statismo was employed to encode temporal information and generate the statistical shape model of cranium growth [1]. Using the Statismo library, we were able to produce shape model and its variation shown as level of compactness presented in Figs. 7 and 8. The resulting model (available in hdf5 format) allow us to derive instances of cranial shape at a given age of development, and use the model for shape prediction from sparse information, which is described in detailed in evaluation step.

5   Cross-Validation

To evaluate the accuracy of the estimated cranial shape, a cross-evaluation analysis was performed. To perform shape prediction for a given unhealthy cranium condition, we employed the concept of model fitting into a given observation. 50 cases were randomly selected to evaluate the ability of the model to predict the shape of cranial shapes that were not employed during model construction. The evaluation process is shown schematically in Fig. 9 and includes the following steps:

1. Selection of healthy/unhealthy regions: The sparse information on which the model is fitted to can be interactively selected using brushing tools available in in-house software. This selection allows the system to differentiate between what is considered healthy from unhealthy shape information. To this end, selected regions shown in green color in Fig. 9(a), is considered as healthy therefore our statistical model should be constrained to the these regions during the morphing process.
2. Shape prediction and surface merging: The model is then fitted to the healthy cranial shape in a two-step approach, consisting of pose and shape estimation. Through this process the most plausible complete cranial shape can be estimated. A mean model driven from the statistical model developed in the previous section is generated and is aligned to the patient coordinate reference using semi-automatic model initialization. The mean model is shown in white color and the resulting fitted model is shown in green closer in Fig. 9(b). The fitting process employs the plausible deformation which is constrained to the healthy region. Through a class available in Statismo library, a mean model can be deformed to pass through the constrained region.
3. Model comparison and distance error evaluation: In this part, the fitted result is compared to the cad corrected model designed by the surgeon. The corresponding point-point distance analysis was performed using a software which enables manual selection of landmarks and mesh-to-mesh distance comparison [4]. A distance error is measured per corresponding point in the fitted cranium and is given in millimeters. The resulting mean and absolute mean error distribution are as a boxplot for all 50 cases in Fig. 10.
4. Possibility for further correction: As the last step (not considered in evaluation process), we compared the fitted result to the unhealthy cranium. In this step, surgeons can further modify the final fitted result if necessary.

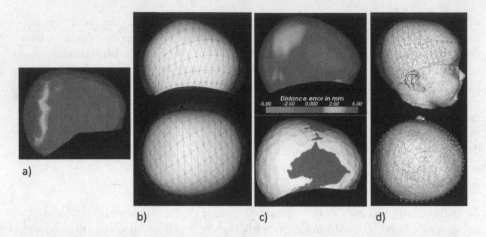

Fig. 9. Evaluation procedure carried out for 50 cases. (a) Detection of healthy/ unhealthy regions (b) Shape prediction and surface merging (c) Model comparison and distance error evaluation (d) Possibility for further correction (Color figure online).

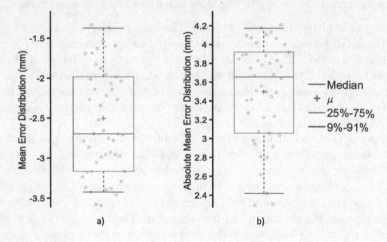

Fig. 10. Mean (a) and absolute mean (b) error distribution chart for predicted cases (Color figure online).

6   Conclusion

In this paper, we presented an advanced system for infant design system which enable surgeons to predict the duration of treatment based on the amount of added volume and indeed a possible shape correction of unhealthy baby cranium. The evaluation of the model was performed using a cross-evaluation n-leave-out procedure with quantitative metrics being the surface prediction error. With such improvement, we are not only able to define how fast but also which head region is growing, and when the therapy can be expected to conclude. The results will be updated in relation to requirements based on current practice considering expected functional and security error margins used in helmet manufacturing.

Acknowledgment. This work was funded by the Swiss Commission for Technology and Innovation (CTI) project number: 16226.3 PFLS-LS.

References

1. Lüthi, M., Blanc, R., Albrecht, T., Gass, T., Goksel, O., Büchler, P., Kistler, M., Bousleiman, H., Reyes, M., Cattin, P., Vetter, T.: Statismo - a framework for PCA based statistical models (2012). University of Basel
2. Stanley, D., Marcel, P., Nicolas, C., Julie, R.K., Sarang, J., Guido, G., Alain, T.: Morphometry of anatomical shape complexes with dense deformations and sparse parameters. NeuroImage **101**, 35–49 (2014)
3. Visualization Toolkit. http://www.vtk.org/
4. Kim, H., Jürgens, P., Weber, S., Nolte, L.P., Reyes, M.: A new soft-tissue simulation strategy for cranio-maxillofacial surgery using facial muscle template model. Prog. Biophys. Mol. Biol. **103**(2), 284–291 (2010)
5. Matlab software. http://www.mathworks.com/

Augmented Reality and Virtual Reality

Interactive Mixed Reality for Muscle Structure and Function Learning

Meng Ma[1,2(✉)], Philipp Jutzi[1], Felix Bork[1],
Ina Seelbach[3], Anna Maria von der Heide[3], Nassir Navab[1,4],
and Pascal Fallavollita[1]

[1] Technische Universität München, Munich, Germany
meng@in.tum.de
[2] National University of Defense Technology, Changsha, China
[3] Chirurgischen Klinik und Poliklinik - Innenstadt, LMU, Munich, Germany
[4] Johns Hopkins University, Baltimore, MD, USA

Abstract. Understanding the structure and function of the muscular system is important in many different medical scenarios, such as student and patient education, muscle training, and rehabilitation of patients with kinetic problems. The structure and function of muscles are difficult to learn as muscle movement is imperceptible using the traditional methods. In this paper, an interactive mixed reality system is proposed for facilitating the learning of the muscles of the upper extremities. The proposed system consists of two main components: an AR view, overlaying the virtual model of the arm on top of the video stream, and a VR view, providing a more detailed understanding of the muscles. The mixed reality view helps the user to mentally map the behaviour of muscles to his/her own body during different movements. A user study including twenty students was performed by a questionnaire framework. The results indicate that our system is useful for learning the structure and function of the muscle and can be a valuable supplement to established muscle learning paradigms.

Keywords: Muscle learning · Augmented reality · Mixed reality · Anatomy learning · User interface · Kinect

1 Introduction

Muscle learning is an important topic in many scenarios, e.g. medical education, patient education, and rehabilitation. The muscular system of the human body is composed of many different types of muscles, enabling the movement of bones and consequently different motions. Quite a few muscles are used during walking or running, but also during very delicate movements such as suturing or cutting during surgery. For all those tasks, multiple muscles are stimulated and dynamically work together in antagonistic pairs to perform the motion. Due

---

M. Ma, P. Jutzi, and F. Bork—These three authors have contributed equally to this work.

© Springer International Publishing Switzerland 2016
G. Zheng et al. (Eds.): MIAR 2016, LNCS 9805, pp. 117–128, 2016.
DOI: 10.1007/978-3-319-43775-0_11

to these interrelations, how the muscular system works is quite a complex topic to learn. Traditional methods for learning the structure and function of muscles include textbooks, 3D models, and cadaver studies [14]. Inherently, these methods cannot reflect the dynamic nature of muscle movements and are therefore not optimal. Animated anatomy videos [1] and web-based learning platforms have been developed as a potential solution in the past, such as Zygote[1]. However, these contents are pre-generated and therefore do not correspond to the motion of the user, and there is the intricacy of mental mapping during the learning procedure. McMenamin [15] proposed an artistic solution by painting muscles and other structures onto the skin of medical students and got predominantly positive feedback. However, this methodology requires anatomical knowledge of the painter and is associated with high efforts and inconveniences for the anatomical models. With the recent advances in Mixed Reality (MR), an *in-situ* visualization of muscles can also be achieved in a computerized fashion. Augmented Reality (AR) in particular can be used to project virtual anatomical information onto the user's body.

1.1 Related Work

The General Medical Council recently proposed standards for effective teaching and learning of medical students [9]. They stated that: "...medical schools should take advantage of new technologies" to deliver teaching." Many commercially available systems use Virtual Reality (VR) for medical education and psychomotor skills training [3,12]. These systems have indeed proven to be valid and useful. Augmented reality research has matured to a level that its applications can now be found in both mobile and non-mobile devices [2] and research on AR has also demonstrated its usefulness for increasing student motivation in the learning process [5,8]. By combining computer models of anatomical structures with custom software we can showcase to students new ways of interacting with anatomy that could not be achieved during cadaveric dissections or in static images and diagrams for increasing their learning satisfaction [2,10,16].

Augmented reality systems for visualization of anatomy have been shown before. Davis et al. [7] presented a system that augmented a 3D model of anatomical airways onto a patient phantom using a head mounted display (HMD). Juan et al. [11] created a system that used a HMD to visualize human anatomy onto a phantom, and this system allowed students to open the abdomen of the phantom and visualize different organs on the phantom. The AR view provides real-time manipulation of these visualizations and direct feedback to students. An AR system for patient-doctor communication has recently been presented [18]. This system used a hand-held projector to project anatomy onto the skin of the patient. Several AR systems have already been developed specifically for anatomy education [4,6,19]. Blum et al. [4,17] described 'Mirracle' which was an AR system that can be used for undergraduate anatomy education. The set-up of that system is as follows: the trainee stands in front of a TV screen that has a camera and the Kinect attached to it. The camera image of the trainee is flipped

---

[1] www.zygotebody.com.

horizontally and is shown on the TV screen, mimicking a mirror function. Part of an anonymous patient CT dataset is augmented on the user's body and shown on the TV screen. This creates the illusion that the trainee can look inside their body. In addition, Ma et al. proposed a personalized augmented reality system to improve the accuracy of the AR view for anatomy learning [13,16].

1.2 Contribution

In this paper, we present an interactive mixed reality system for learning the structure and function of the muscles associated with an upper extremity. We propose a muscle model developed in consultation with medical experts, which reflects the physiology of real human muscles. An AR view is generated by over-laying the virtual model of the arm on top of the video stream of an RGB-D sensor, which is displayed in a mirror-like way on a large TV screen. In addition, our system includes a purely VR view, which can be controlled by the user in order to obtain the details of the interrelations between muscles during certain movements. All the movements of the virtual model correspond to the user's real motions. Our mixed reality system provides an interactive feedback which facilitates the mental mapping compared to traditional learning modalities. A user study including twenty anatomy students was performed during evaluation. Results indicate that the proposed system is useful for learning the structure and function of the muscle and it can offer a valuable supplement to established muscle learning paradigms.

2   Materials and Methods

A realistic muscle model is at the heart of our interactive muscle learning system and is therefore described in detail in the following subsection. Furthermore, we illustrate our system design, which allows the user to observe the muscle model from different viewpoints to learn the structure and motion function and provides a flexible learning experience.

2.1   Muscle Model

Based on discussions with our medical partners (three experienced orthopedic surgeons), we developed a muscle model that reflects the physiology of a real muscle to a great extent. A human muscle has at least two attachment points to a bone, the origin (or anchor), and the insertion. The former connects the muscle to an immovable bone, the latter to a movable bone. The contraction of a muscle is then characterized by the insertion moving towards the origin. Muscles of the arm, that are responsible for the movements *flexion*, *extension*, *pronation*, and *supination* were included, as seen in Table 1. The *musculus coracobrachialis* is added to this collection according to our medical partners' suggestion, although it does not contribute to the motions mentioned above. Each of those muscles has two virtual attachment points to the respective bones.

Table 1. The selected motions of one arm and the corresponding main muscles

Motion	Muscles
Flexion	M.biceps brachii, M.brachialis
Extension	M.triceps brachii, M.anconeus
Pronation	M.pronator teres, M.pronator quadratus
Supination	M.supinator

In our interactive learning system, virtual bone models of the arm and the shoulder were obtained from an anatomical model of a human male body from ANATOMIUM 3D[2]. Their virtual muscle models, however, did not resemble their real counterparts closely enough. Therefore, they were custom modeled from a cylindrical base mesh and created using polygonal modeling techniques and subdivision algorithms according to images from the Sobotta Atlas of Human Anatomy in Autodesk 3ds Max[3]. Only the *musculus supinator* and the *musculus pronator quadratus* are modeled from a flat box, due to their shape. Appropriate textures were designed to provide a realistic visual effect. Figure 1 illustrates a virtual arm for all four arm movements and their associated muscles.

To improve realism even further, the muscle model should deform when the user performs a certain arm motion. The muscles' animation for contraction and expansion was achieved in 3DS MAX via stretchy bones, which automatically contract or expand if their length is changed. To enable this animation of the virtual arm model, the bones are weighted to different armatures that consist of one control object. The ulna and radius are weighted to separate control objects to behave correctly when the hand is rotated. To deform the muscles, the vertices of each model are weighted to several control objects, which can be transformed easily according to the bones (see Fig. 2). The vertices follow the transformation of each related object to a certain percentage, which is determined by their weighting.

2.2   System Design

Hardware Setup. Our interactive mixed reality muscle learning system is comprised of only two main hardware components, namely a display device and an RGB-D sensor placed on the top of the former. In our setup, a 42″ screen and the Microsoft Kinect v2 were employed. In order to correctly position the virtual arm model, the skeleton tracking data provided by the Microsoft Kinect SDK is used. Joint positional and rotational information is acquired in each frame and used to update the model accordingly.

---

[2] http://www.anatomium.com/.
[3] http://www.autodesk.com/products/3ds-max/overview.

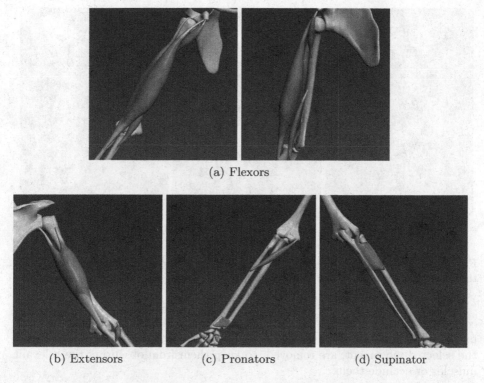

(a) Flexors

(b) Extensors   (c) Pronators   (d) Supinator

Fig. 1. Muscle models. Each picture shows the muscles involved in each motion.

Mixed Reality View. The proposed system employs the color camera to create a mirror-like AR effect for the user, and all the non-physical visual feedback is generated based on the user's skeleton and personal information via rendering the corresponding medical information. This AR view shows the color image from the Kinect with the augmented virtual arm, and it helps the user to map all the activities of the bones and muscles onto their own arm. The details of the muscle are very important, so a virtual view is introduced to present a close-up view of the arm model to show the attachment points and the spatial relationship (see Fig. 4). The VR view is also synchronized with the real arm motion, and it concentrates on the upper or lower arm, showing the details of the muscle structure and function. To preserve the connection between the user and the virtual arm, the AR-view is shown on the left side of the screen after the system finishes calibration (see Fig. 3).

There are several solutions to place the virtual camera. One is that the camera rotates around a special object and generates the virtual view from different angles. The cameras are attached to a rotating helper object to create an orbiting movement around the arms. The close-up views are implemented with additional cameras and copies of the arm model. By putting these copies into separate layers it is ensured that these cameras only render their respective objects. The first

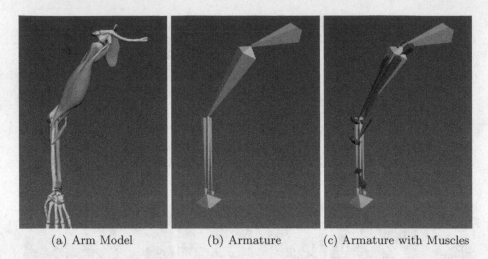

(a) Arm Model   (b) Armature   (c) Armature with Muscles

Fig. 2. Muscle deformation model. The bones are weighted to different armatures and the vertices of each model are weighted to several control objects in the armetures.

copy takes part in just the flexion and extension, while the second one participates in the pronation and supination. The muscles, which are not responsible for the selected movement, are removed, to keep them from obscuring the relevant muscles or occlude them.

2.3   Learning Functions

Self-Control Virtual View. A self-control virtual camera is introduced and its position and rotation can be controlled by the user. When the user's right hand is placed close to the left arm, the self-control camera model is triggered (see Fig. 3). The camera moves to the position of the hand and tries to focus on the desired area by calculating the closest point on the arm and rotating towards it. This point is computed in the user-controlled arm's local coordinate system and transformed into that of the arm currently observed (see Fig. 5). Hence, the user can naturally move the virtual camera to focus on different objects from different view angles. This function introduces more friendly interaction for muscle learning.

Interactive Learning. Two learning models are designed, 'muscle-oriented', the muscle is displayed one by one, and 'motion-oriented', the user performs the target motions and only the muscles related the current motion is shown. A configuring class is defined, including methods to control the muscles' visibility, the highlighting of working muscles and of anchor points, and the labels that display the muscles' names and function. Highlighting it determines the angle between the upper and lower arm, as well as the rotation of the hand, relative to the frame before. This information is used to determine which motion is

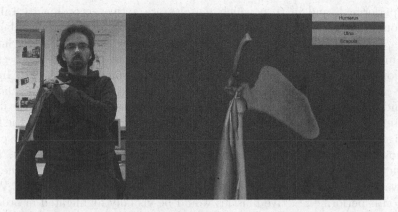

Fig. 3. Framework design. There is an AR-view and a VR view. The current learning function is "Self-control virtual view", which can be triggered when the user's right hand is placed close to the left arm. The virtual camera is controlled by the user's right hand.

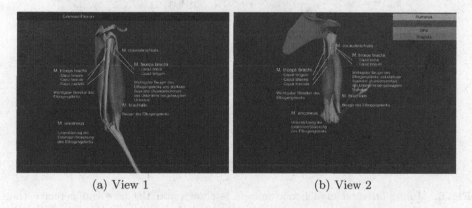

(a) View 1   (b) View 2

Fig. 4. Virtual camera concentrating on flexion and extension. (Color figure online)

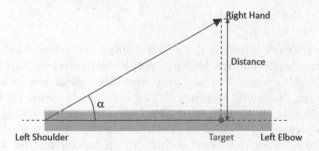

Fig. 5. The camera moves to the position of the hand and tries to focus on the desired area by calculating the closest point on the arm and rotating towards it.

being performed, and in turn which muscles are active according to Table 1. Additional functions are created to toggle the visibility of all muscle-labels to the user interface and control the visibility of muscles by type (see Fig. 4). Similar to the muscles, the bones are controlled by a configuring class. These determine the color-coding of the bones and expose this functionality to the UI. In the muscle oriented model, one or more muscles are shown successively and the AR view and virtual view of the muscle is generated. The user can perceive the detail of the muscle, the start and end point and the spatial relationship with the bone (see Fig. 6). In the motion oriented model, users are asked to perform special arm movements and only the muscle involved is highlighted (see Fig. 4b). Then the functions of the muscle are learned. During the learning procedure, the user can always move the arm and see the muscle state and shape deformation. When a motion is performed, active muscles would be visually highlighted in order to make them more prominent.

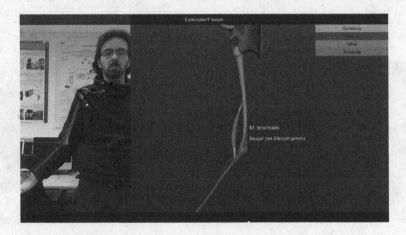

Fig. 6. Muscle oriented model: one muscle is shown and the user can perceive the detail of the muscle, the start and end points, and the spatial relationship with the bone. (Color figure online)

Learning Sequence. Based on the mixed reality view, the system can generate a lot of learning material. We prefer a simple user interface and let the user focus on the learning instead on how to control this system. Hence, we introduce another function, "Learning Sequence". The sequence of events for the learning session is predefined via a configuring file. This is an easily editable text format with values separated by semicolons. Each line in this file contains the data for one event. The data for one event consists of an integer for the duration and the camera mode, boolean values to enable or disable the color-coding for the bones, the muscles' labels and highlighting of their anchor points, and a bitmask that determines the muscles visibility. An optional group of values can be used to display text at the desired position of the screen. This file is opened and read line after line by a simple parser at the start of the program, and the data is stored in an array of event structures. The sequence is played using a coroutine that takes one entry from the event-array and uses its values to set the relevant parameters and waits for the specified time before triggering the next event, until it reaches the end of the array. Simple functions can control the running sequence by stopping and restarting the coroutine or by modifying the array-index to skip or replay events.

3   Evaluation and Results

In order to evaluate the potential of our mixed reality muscle learning system, a user study was designed together with our medical partners. Every participant went through a previously developed *learning sequence*, which is described in more detail in the following subsection. After successful completion of the learning sequence, participants were asked to fill out a questionnaire focusing on the system's suitability for acquiring knowledge about the structure and function of muscles.

3.1   User Study Design

Study Procedure. At the heart of our user study is a predefined learning sequence, which every participant has to go through. In the beginning, the user is presented with an AR view exclusively showing the bones of the arm identified by different colors. After that, it switches to the VR view and introduces the muscles responsible for *flexion* and *extension* individually. Furthermore, each muscle is annotated with a label displaying its name and additional information about its function (see Fig. 4). After the muscles contributing to each motion have been introduced, they are shown together to give the user the opportunity to review. This process is then repeated for *pronation* and *supination*. The whole sequence runs for approximately ten minutes.

Participants. Twenty first year anatomy students without muscle education, having an average age of 22 ± 4.7 years, were included in this user study. The gender distribution was 6 male and 14 female.

Questionnaire Design. A questionnaire with twelve questions was designed based on three hypotheses that were subject to investigation during our experiments:

H1: The system increases the user's motivation to learn the muscular system.
H2: The information provided by our system is easy to comprehend.
H3: The system is suitable for transferring knowledge about the structure and
    function of muscles.

After the learning sequence, participants were asked to assess the proposed system by responding to the following 12 questions:

Q1-The program increases my motivation to study.
Q2-It is fun to study with this system.
Q3-It increases my attention while studying.
Q4-The information is acceptable.
Q5-It promotes "active" studying.
Q6-It helps me to study on my own.
Q7-It provides important knowledge about the muscle.
Q8-It presents the muscle in a well arranged fashion.
Q9-It supports memorizing knowledge.
Q10-It helps to study the anatomy of the arm.
Q11-It increases my understanding of different movements of the arm.
Q12-It supports learning the function of muscles during certain motions.

Responses to questions were based on a four point Likert Scale: (1) *strongly disagree*, (2) *disagree*, (3) *agree*, and (4) *strongly agree*. Questions Q1-Q2 were used to investigate H1, questions Q3-Q9 for H2, and questions Q10-Q11 for H3 respectively.

3.2   Results

Frequencies and average Likert value of responses for all the twelve questions are given in Table 2. The results show that the overall feedback on the system is very positive. It motivates participants to learn and provides a fun and interactive experience. It provides the desired information in an easily understandable fashion and is suitable for acquiring knowledge about the structure and function of muscles of the arm. Regarding the ability of the system to make people study on their own, opinions of the participants varied quiet a lot. Results from Q11–Q12 indicate, that the most difficult and important aspect of muscle learning, the interrelations of muscles during certain motions, could be successfully achieved.

Table 2. Likert scale value of the questionnaire.

Frequencies	Q1	Q2	Q3	Q4	Q5	Q6	Q7	Q8	Q9	Q10	Q11	Q12
Strongly agree(4)	6	9	4	11	12	5	6	8	6	7	11	9
Agree(3)	10	6	9	6	5	7	12	8	8	10	6	10
Disagree(2)	3	4	7	3	2	6	1	2	5	3	2	1
Strongly disagree(1)	1	1	0	0	1	2	1	2	1	0	1	0
Average (Value)	3.05	3.15	2.85	3.5	3.4	2.75	3.15	3.1	2.95	3.2	3.35	3.4

4   Discussion and Conclusion

Based on our discussion with anatomy students we found that they really liked the AR visualization on their own bodies. However, as results of Q3 and Q6 indicate, they were not used to the natural user interface and gestures required for interaction. We note here that the anatomy students are more used to textbook learning paradigms instead of human-computer interaction ones. A learning curve was necessary for them to appease initial frustrations they had when first using our system. Most students who tried the application viewed it as an interesting and engaging source of information. The possibility of viewing the arm from every direction offered them a new insight that they could not get from static images. The students confirm the effectiveness of acquiring knowledge with an AR-program. However, this application is limited by necessity, so the textbook still constitutes a more universal resource and it can function as a useful supplement. In the future, we plan to extend the system to incorporate muscles of the entire body. A larger scale user study could be performed to evaluate the interactive mixed reality system for the muscle learning in different scenarios with user groups of varying education background.

It is very difficult to create a perfect AR view, which includes ideal scale factors for virtual information, accurate tracking for the overlay and excellent rendering for natural perception. In the proposed system, Kinect automatically does the calibration procedure when a user is well detected, and the raw skeleton information from Kinect SDK is directly employed to scale and transform the medical model onto the user's body. The accuracy of the AR view is limited by the tracking technologies, but interactive registration [13] can be used to improve the performance later.

In this paper, we proposed an interactive mixed reality system for learning the structure and function of muscles of the upper extremities. A custom designed muscle model is employed, which was developed with medical experts to mirror the physiology of real human muscles. An AR view was developed where the movements of the user correspond to the movements of the virtual arm, facilitating the mental mapping in comparison to traditional muscle learning modalities. A VR view for acquiring more details about the muscles responsible for certain arm movements with a self-controlled virtual camera is another major component of the system. A user study was conducted, which demonstrated that participants dominantly award the system with the potential to be a valuable alternative to traditional methods for learning the structure and function of the muscle. We believe our system offers the alternative to transform the way the muscular system is learned in many different application areas, including student and patient education, rehabilitation, and fitness training.

References

1. Azer, S.A.: Can "YouTube" help students in learning surface anatomy? Surg. Radiol. Anat. **34**(5), 465–468 (2012)

2. Bacca, J., Baldiris, S., Fabregat, R., Graf, S.: Augmented reality trends in education: a systematic review of research and applications. Educ. Technol. Soc. **17**(4), 133–149 (2014)
3. Basdogan, C., Sedef, M., Harders, M., Wesarg, S.: VR-based simulators for training in minimally invasive surgery. IEEE Comput. Graph. Appl. **27**(2), 54–66 (2007)
4. Blum, T., Kleeberger, V., Bichlmeier, C., Navab, N.: Mirracle: an augmented reality magic mirror system for anatomy education. In: Proceedings of the IEEE Virtual Reality, pp. 115–116, March 2012
5. Chang, K.E., Chang, C.T., Hou, H.T., Sung, Y.T., Chao, H.L., Lee, C.M.: Development and behavioral pattern analysis of a mobile guide system with augmented reality for painting appreciation instruction in an art museum. Comput. Educ. **71**, 185–197 (2014, 2015)
6. Chien, C.H., Chen, C.H., Jeng, T.S.: An interactive augmented reality system for learning anatomy structure. In: Proceedings of the International Multi Conference Engineers and Computer Scientists I (2010)
7. Davis, L., Hamza-Lup, F.G., Daly, J., Ha, Y., Frolich, S., Meyer, C., Martin, G., Norfleet, J., Lin, K.C., Imielinska, C., Rolland, J.P.: Application of augmented reality to visualizing anatomical airways. Proc. SPIE **4711**, 400–405 (2002)
8. Di Serio, Á., Ibáñez, M.B., Kloos, C.D.: Impact of an augmented reality system on students' motivation for a visual art course. Comput. Educ. **68**, 585–596 (2013)
9. General Medical Council: Tomorrow's Doctors - Outcomes and standards for undergraduate medical education. No. 1, UK: General Medical Council, Manchester (2009)
10. Johnson, L., Adams Becker, S., Estrada, V., Freeman, A.: The NMC Horizon Report: 2015 Higher Education Edition. The New Media Consortium, Austin (2015)
11. Juan, C., Beatrice, F., Cano, J.: An augmented reality system for learning the interior of the human body. In: Proceedings of the 8th IEEE International Conference on Advanced Learning Technologies ICALT 2008, pp. 186–188 (2008)
12. Lu, J., Pan, Z., Lin, H., Zhang, M., Shi, J.: Virtual learning environment for medical education based on VRML and VTK. Comput. Graph. **29**(2), 283–288 (2005)
13. Ma, M., Fallavollita, P., Seelbach, I., Heide, A.M.V.D., Euler, E., Waschke, J., et al.: Personalized augmented reality for anatomy education. Clin. Anat. **29**(4), 446–453 (2015)
14. McHanwell, S.: Atlas of anatomy. J. Anat. **217**(1), 83–83 (2010)
15. McMenamin, P.G.: Body painting as a tool in clinical anatomy teaching. Anat. Sci. Educ. **1**(4), 139–144 (2008)
16. Meng, M., Fallavollita, P., Blum, T., Eck, U., Sandor, C., Weidert, S., Waschke, J., Navab, N.: Kinect for interactive AR anatomy learning. In: 2013 IEEE International Symposium on Mixed and Augmented Reality, ISMAR 2013, Adelaide, Australia, pp. 277–278, October 2013
17. Navab, N., Blum, T., Wang, L., Okur, A., Wendler, T.: First deployments of augmented reality in operating rooms. Comput. (Long. Beach. Calif) **45**(7), 48–55 (2012)
18. Ni, T., Karlson, A.K., Wigdor, D.: AnatOnMe. In: Proceedings of 2011 Annual Conference on Human Factors in Computing Systems, CHI 2011, p. 3333 (2011)
19. Thomas, R.G., John, N.W., Delieu, J.M.: Augmented reality for anatomical education. J. Vis. Commun. Med. **33**(1), 6–15 (2010)

Visualization Techniques for Augmented Reality in Endoscopic Surgery

Rong Wang[1,2(✉)], Zheng Geng[1], Zhaoxing Zhang[1], and Renjing Pei[1,2]

[1] Institute of Automation, Chinese Academy of Sciences, Beijing, China
wangrong2013@ia.ac.cn
[2] University of Chinese Academy of Sciences, Beijing, China

Abstract. Augmented reality (AR) is widely used in minimally invasive surgery (MIS), since it enhances the surgeon's perception of spatial relationship by overlaying the invisible structures on the endoscopic images. Depth perception is the key problem in AR visualization. In this paper, we present a video-based AR system for aiding MIS of removing a tumor inside a kidney. We explore several different AR visualization techniques. They are transparent overlay, virtual window, random-dot mask and the ghosting method. We also introduce the depth-aware ghosting method to further enhance the depth perception of virtual structure which has complex spatial geometry. Both simulated and in vivo experiments were carried out to evaluate these AR visualization techniques. The experimental results demonstrate the feasibility of our AR system and AR visualization techniques. Finally, we conclude the characteristics of these AR visualization techniques.

Keywords: Visualization · Augmented reality · Depth perception · Minimally invasive surgery

1 Introduction

Augmented reality (AR) becomes popular in medical applications where minimally invasive surgery (MIS) is becoming common in practice [1,2]. In MIS, video images of the surgical scene recorded by an endoscopic camera are presented to surgeons through a display monitor to guide their operation maneuvers. Although MIS has many benefits for patients, such as small wound size and shorter recovery time, it presents significant challenges to surgeons since the targets (e.g. tumor or vessels) are usually located behind the visible surface. AR techniques can be used to enhance the surgeon's perception of 3D spatial relationship by combining the virtual structures and the endoscopic image in visualization. AR visualization can guide surgeons during the surgery, hence promising to reduce surgical time and increase surgical precision.

Augmented reality has been applied to kidney surgery [3–6]. An entire AR system usually includes tracking, registration, reconstruction and visualization. However, at present time, AR visualization techniques for MIS have not received sufficient attention in the previous publications, and have a lot of room for

© Springer International Publishing Switzerland 2016
G. Zheng et al. (Eds.): MIAR 2016, LNCS 9805, pp. 129–138, 2016.
DOI: 10.1007/978-3-319-43775-0_12

improvement. Depth perception, which means to obtain the correct spatial relationship between the virtual and the real structures, is the main issue in AR visualization. For more knowledge about medical AR visualization, please refer to [7,8].

To the best of our knowledge, only [9,10] explored different visualization techniques in medical AR. Therefore, medical AR visualization is worth further exploring and it is the focus of this paper.

General AR visualization can be classified into (1) the video-based method; (2) the see-through method; and (3) the projection-based method [8]. Considering the characteristics of MIS where only a small incision is available, the video-based method is more suitable than others. Although many visualization strategies are proposed in general video-based AR, transparent overlay is most widely used in medical AR [3,4,6] due to its simplicity. However, it easily results in a common problem that the virtual structure seems to be located above the real surface rather than below it [11]. Virtual window [12] is an alternative way to observe virtual structure occluded by the real surface. However, it partly covers the real surface which weakens the user's perception of the real scene. Random-dot mask [13] is then proposed to achieve the minimal destruction of the real surface. This method creates a feeling of observing the virtual structure through many small holes on the real surface. The ghosting method [14] is another popular visualization strategy. It assigns different transparency for each pixel by analyzing the importance of the camera image. However, according to these publications, random-dot mask and the ghosting method are rarely applied to medical applications.

In this paper, we apply different visualization techniques (modes) to our medical AR system to evaluate their characteristics. The modes we developed and tested in our AR platform include: (1) transparent overlay; (2) virtual window; (3) random-dot mask; and (4) the ghosting method. We choose these modes because they are representative and commonly used in general AR. We also introduce the depth-aware ghosting method to further enhance perception of spatial relationship. Our AR system concentrates on the ablation of tumor inside the kidney. We conducted both simulated and in vivo experiments in our study. The visualization modes are presented, evaluated and compared with each other. In the next section, we will briefly introduce the components of our AR system and the implementation of each visualization mode.

2   Methods

In this section, we first introduce the components of our AR system and then the technical approach in each visualization mode.

2.1   Overview of Our AR System

In AR system, the precise position of invisible structures (e.g. tumor or vessels) is required for rendering. Our AR system consists of 4 parts: segmentation, reconstruction, registration and AR visualization, which are illustrated in Fig. 1(a).

In the segmentation part, a series of CT slices was acquired beforehand. The 3D Slicer toolkit [15] was used to obtain segmented surfaces of kidney and tumor, where tumor is the small object inside the kidney. In the reconstruction part, we use 5 captured endoscopic images and adopt the algorithm in [16] to get a reconstructed depth map and point cloud. The reconstructed point cloud of partial kidney is in the camera coordinate which is shown as the blue point cloud in Fig. 1(b). In the registration part, we use the iterative closest point (ICP) algorithm [17] to register CT segmented kidney model to the reconstructed one. After registration, the pose of the CT model with respect to the camera coordinate is identified, which is illustrated in Fig. 1(b). The image for AR visualization is rendered after the acquisition of this explicit spatial relationship.

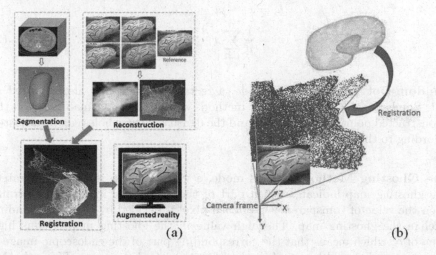

Fig. 1. Overview of our AR system: (a) the components of our AR system; (b) an illustration of the spatial relationship for AR rendering

2.2 Technical Approach of Each Visualization Mode

In this part, we will present the technical implementation of each visualization mode. Assume the original endoscopic image is denoted by $O(x, y)$. The virtual object rendered from the point of view of the camera is $V(x, y)$. The AR view is denoted as $R(x, y)$.

Transparent Overlay. In this mode, the AR view is obtained through Eq. 1. The adjustable transparency parameter α is a user-specified constant.

$$R = O \cdot \alpha + V \cdot (1 - \alpha) \tag{1}$$

Virtual Window. In this mode, we need the reconstructed point cloud of the viewing object on which a window is created. This provides a feeling of getting a view of the inside of the object. A user should define a rectangular framework of the virtual window at first. In order to generate the sense of reality, the window wall is also created after the definition of the window normal. In our method, the window normal is defined by the average of the point normals in the specified rectangular area. A normal for a vertex x_1 is calculated as the eigenvector of S with the smallest eigenvalue. S is the covariance matrix of all the neighboring vertices $x_i(i = 1, \ldots, n)$ around x_1 and is computed in Eq. 2. The wall and the background are decorated with some textures in order to further generate the sense of reality.

$$S = YY^T$$
$$Y = (y_1, y_2, \ldots, y_n)^T$$
$$y_i = x_i - m$$
$$m = \frac{1}{n} \sum_{i=1}^{n} x_i \qquad (2)$$

Random-Dot Mask. In this mode, a rectangular region is also required at first. Similar to the virtual window method, we create many small holes on the reconstructed point cloud. The size and the density of these holes can be adjusted according to the user's preference.

The Ghosting Method. In this mode, a ghosting map is firstly generated. The ghosting map indicates which part of the endoscopic image is important. Then the value of transparency α of each pixel is decided by the corresponding pixel in the ghosting map. The high value in the ghosting map assigns high value of α, which means that the corresponding part of the endoscopic image is important and should be less disturbed by the virtual structure. Then, the AR view is obtained through Eq. 3.

$$R = O \cdot \alpha(x, y) + V \cdot (1 - \alpha(x, y)) \qquad (3)$$

The ghosting map in our system is obtained by analyzing the endoscopic image. Inspired by [14], the analysis includes edge detection, color differences and local contrast. Edges are seen as important parts of the original image. Color difference is computed in Eq. 4 from the global point of view, where $\overline{O}$ is the mean color of the entire image. Local contrast is computed in Eq. 5. We define a region around a pixel (x, y). The pixels in the region are $O_i(i = 1, \ldots, m)$, where m is the number of these pixels and $\overline{O}_m$ is the mean color in this region. All the above color computation is calculated in the CIELAB color space, since it conforms with human color perception. The pixel is considered to be important in the camera image and assigned to 1 in the ghosting map if it satisfies one of the following conditions: (1) It belongs to the detected edges; (2) Its color difference is larger than a pre-defined threshold; (3) Its local contrast is larger than another threshold. The final ghosting map is a binary map. Figure 2 shows the process to generate the ghosting map.

$$Color(x, y) = \|O(x, y) - \overline{O}\| \tag{4}$$

$$Contrast(x, y) = \sqrt{\frac{\sum_{i=1}^{m}(O_i - \overline{O}_m)^2}{m}} \tag{5}$$

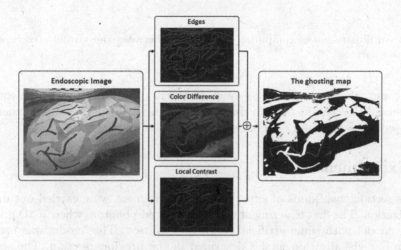

Fig. 2. The process of generating the ghosting map

The Depth-Aware Ghosting Method. This mode is our improvement based on the original ghosting method [14]. In the ghosting method, the virtual objects can be correctly perceived to be behind the visible surface rather than floating over it. This is because the method considers the saliency of the endoscopic image. However, depth information between the virtual structure and the real surface is not presented in it. This information is important when the virtual structure has complex spatial geometry. Therefore, we integrate the distance between the virtual structure and the visible surface in the final AR view [18] after adopting the ghosting method. This process is illustrated in Fig. 3. First, a ray connecting a viewer and a vertex v_i of the virtual object is created. Then, a vertex o_i of the visible surface which is closest to the ray is picked. The distance is computed between v_i and o_i and it is used to modulate the transparency obtained in the ghosting method. In the above process, surface models of the virtual structure and the visible surface need to be acquired which is not difficult in our study. Both CT segmented surface and the reconstructed surface can be used.

In our study, the virtual objects can be divided into simple and complex categories. AR visualization of simple virtual structure like tumor can be achieved in transparent overlay, virtual window, random-dot mask and the ghosting method. Because some complex structures like vessels are usually wide spread, completely observing them through a small window is not possible. In these cases, transparent overlay and the ghosting method are more suitable. We also adopt the

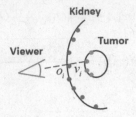

Fig. 3. An illustration of computing the distance between the virtual structure and the visible surface

depth-aware ghosting method to them. In the next section, we will present our AR visualization results of both simulated and in vivo experiments. Further, we will discuss the pros and cons of each visualization mode.

3   Experiments

In this section, two kinds of experimental environment were carried out in AR visualization. The first experiment used a simulated phantom where a 3D printed kidney model with some artificial textures was used. This model was used to explain our visualization modes described in the previous section. The second was a in vivo experiment with a real pig's kidney. The real operation scene is shown in Fig. 4. The augmented tumor or vessels are illustrative and do not reflect the real situation. Our paper focuses on the effect of AR visualization rather than the entire AR system. In both experiments, only AR visualization is evaluated and the accuracy of segmentation, reconstruction and registration is not discussed.

AR visualization results of simulated experiment are shown in Fig. 5. The in vivo results are presented in Fig. 6. These results indicate that AR visualization can provide useful navigation and vital structures targeting during a surgery.

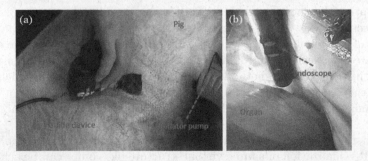

Fig. 4. The operation scene for in vivo experiment: (a) the external scene of the operation. The guide device is used to control the orientation of the endoscope through magnet and the inflator pump is used to pump air into the pig's abdomen to provide enough space for the movement of the endoscope; (b) the internal scene of the operation

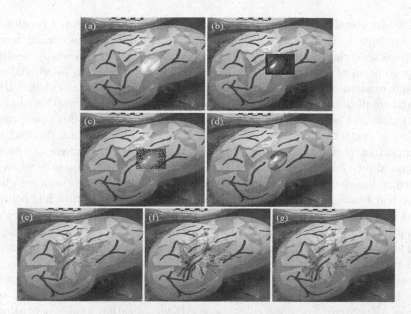

Fig. 5. AR visualization results of simulated experiment: (a)–(d) visualization of the tumor by transparent overlay, virtual window, random-dot mask and the ghosting method; (e)–(g) visualization of the vessels by transparent overlay, the ghosting method and the depth-aware ghosting method

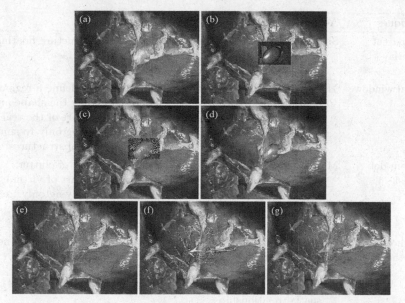

Fig. 6. AR visualization results of in vivo experiment: (a)–(d) Visualization of the tumor by transparent overlay, virtual window, random-dot mask and the ghosting method; (e)–(g) Visualization of the vessels by transparent overlay, the ghosting method and the depth-aware ghosting method

Different visualization modes are analyzed from these presented results. We asked students from our lab for their opinions on the AR visualization modes. Transparent overlay does not consider occlusion cues and can easily result in false perception of spatial relationship [11]. As for visualization by virtual window and random-dot mask, correct occlusion relationship is provided. Virtual wall and small holes can be seen as visual cues to cause the sensation that the virtual structure is behind the real surface. However, random-dot mask causes a feeling of clutter and has a bad user experience. The ghosting method uses the important region of the endoscopic image to create the sense of the correct spatial relationship. However, this method has poor performance when the endoscopic image does not have sufficient features [13]. The depth-aware ghosting method has improved performance when the virtual structure has complex spatial geometry. Comparing its results with the ones in the ghosting method, the depth information of the furcations of the vessels are clearer in the depth-aware ghosting method. We can tell which furcations are in the front and which are in the back from the depth-aware ghosting method. We conclude the pros and cons of these AR visualization modes in Table 1. As all the visualization modes have shortcomings as well as advantages, we can combine all those modes into our AR system. Surgeons can choose AR visualization modes according to their personal preference.

Table 1. Comparison of different AR visualization modes

Techniques	Advantage	Disadvantage
Transparent overlay	Simple to operate; Applying to both simple and complex virtual structures	Causing virtual structure floating over the real surface
Virtual window	Maintaining correct spatial relationship between real and virtual structures	Requiring user to define a region of interest; Missing the shape and color of some part of the real surface; Applying only to simple and small virtual structures
Random-dot mask	Maintaining correct spatial relationship; Solving the problem of real surface removal	Causing the feeling of clutter; Missing some part of virtual structures; Applying only to simple and small virtual structures
The ghosting method	Applying to both simple and complex virtual structures; Maintaining the sense of the correct spatial relationship	Fail when the real image does not have sufficient features; Requiring some image processing techniques
The depth-aware ghosting method	Providing clearer depth information of complex virtual structures	Revealing usefulness only in complex virtual structures

4   Conclusions

In this article, we implement a whole AR system and different AR visualization modes. The AR visualization modes in our system are: Transparent overlay, virtual window, random-dot mask and the ghosting method. We also introduce the depth-aware ghosting method for improved perception of the depth information of the complex virtual structures.

These visualization modes are tested on both simulated and in vivo experiments. The outcome indicates the feasibility of different visualization modes. We also evaluated and compared these visualization modes. The pros and cons of each visualization mode are summarized in a table.

In our current AR visualization, tumor and vessels are presented separately. In the future, we plan to demonstrate the visualization technique to display tumor and vessels at the same time and consider strategies to reveal the relative relationship between them. The visualization evaluation in this paper is mainly based on qualitative results. A more quantitative assessment from experts will be given in the future. Furthermore, the AR system's accuracy and stability will be evaluated thoroughly. Our ultimate goal is to apply our AR system and AR visualization techniques to real surgery operations.

Acknowledgments. This work has been supported by the National High-tech R&D Program (863 Program) of Institute of Automation, Chinese Academy of Sciences (CASIA), grant 2012AA011903 and 2015AA015905.

References

1. Collins, T., Pizarro, D., Bartoli, A., Canis, M., Bourdel, N.: Computer-assisted laparoscopic myomectomy by augmenting the uterus with pre-operative MRI data. In: ISMAR, pp. 243–248 (2014)
2. Kim, J.-H., Bartoli, A., Collins, T., Hartley, R.: Tracking by detection for interactive image augmentation in laparoscopy. In: Dawant, B.M., Christensen, G.E., Fitzpatrick, J.M., Rueckert, D. (eds.) WBIR 2012. LNCS, vol. 7359, pp. 246–255. Springer, Heidelberg (2012)
3. Schneider, A., Pezold, S., Sauer, A., Ebbing, J., Wyler, S., Rosenthal, R., Cattin, P.C.: Augmented reality assisted laparoscopic partial nephrectomy. In: Golland, P., Hata, N., Barillot, C., Hornegger, J., Howe, R. (eds.) MICCAI 2014, Part II. LNCS, vol. 8674, pp. 357–364. Springer, Heidelberg (2014)
4. Puerto-Souza, G.A., Mariottini, G.L.: Toward Long-term and accurate augmented-reality display for minimally-invasive surgery. In: ICRA, pp. 5384–5389 (2013)
5. Teber, D., Guven, S., Simpfendörfer, T., Baumhauer, M., Güven, E.O., Yencilek, F., Gözen, A.S., Rassweiler, J.: Augmented reality: a new tool to improve surgical accuracy during laparoscopic partial nephrectomy? Preliminary in vitro and in vivo results. Eur. Urol. **56**(2), 332–338 (2009)
6. Su, L.M., Vagvolgyi, B.P., Agarwal, R., Reiley, C.E., Taylor, R.H., Hager, G.D.: Augmented reality during robot-assisted laparoscopic partial nephrectomy: toward real-time 3D-CT to stereoscopic video registration. Urology **73**(4), 896–900 (2009)

7. Kersten-Oertel, M., Jannin, P., Collins, D.L.: The state of the art of visualization in mixed reality image guided surgery. Comput. Med. Imaging Graph. **37**(2), 98–112 (2013)

8. Nicolau, S., Soler, L., Mutter, D., Marescaux, J.: Augmented reality in laparoscopic surgical oncology. Surg. Oncol. **20**(3), 189–201 (2011)

9. Kersten-Oertel, M., Gerard, I., Drouin, S., Mok, K., Sirhan, D., Sinclair, D.S., Collins, D.L.: Augmented reality in neurovascular surgery: feasibility and first uses in the operating room. Int. J. Comput. Assist. Radiol. Surg. **10**(11), 1823–1836 (2015)

10. Sielhorst, T., Bichlmeier, C., Heining, S.M., Navab, N.: Depth perception – a major issue in medical AR: evaluation study by twenty surgeons. In: Larsen, R., Nielsen, M., Sporring, J. (eds.) MICCAI 2006. LNCS, vol. 4190, pp. 364–372. Springer, Heidelberg (2006)

11. Buchmann, V., Nilsen, T., Billinghurst, M.: Interaction with partially transparent hands and objects. In: AUIC, vol. 40, pp. 17–20 (2005)

12. Fuchs, H., Livingston, M.A., Raskar, R., Keller, K., State, A., Crawford, J.R., Rademacher, P., Drake, S.H., Meyer, A.A.: Augmented reality visualization for laparoscopic surgery. In: Wells, W.M., Colchester, A.C.F., Delp, S.L. (eds.) MICCAI 1998. LNCS, vol. 1496, pp. 934–943. Springer, Heidelberg (1998)

13. Otsuki, M., Kuzuoka, H., Milgram, P.: Analysis of depth perception with virtual mask in stereoscopic AR. In: International Conference on Artificial Reality and Telexistence, Eurographics Symposium on Virtual Environments (2015)

14. Zollmann, S., Kalkofen, D., Mendez, E., Reitmay, G.: Image-based ghostings for single layer occlusions in augmented reality. In: ISMAR, pp. 19–26 (2010)

15. 3D Slicer. http://www.slicer.org

16. Newcombe, R.A., Lovegrove, S.J., Davison, A.J.: DTAM: dense tracking and mapping in real-time. In: ICCV, pp. 2320–2327 (2011)

17. Best, P.J., McKay, N.D.: A method for registration of 3-D shapes. IEEE Trans. Pattern Anal. Mach. Intell. **14**(2), 239–256 (1992)

18. Marques, B., Haouchine, N., Plantefeve, R., Cotin, S.: Improving depth perception during surgical augmented reality. In: SIGGRAPH 2015 Posters, p. 24 (2015)

Augmented Reality Imaging for Robot-Assisted Partial Nephrectomy Surgery

Philip Edgcumbe[1], Rohit Singla[2(✉)], Philip Pratt[3], Caitlin Schneider[2],
Christopher Nguan[4], and Robert Rohling[2,5]

[1] MD/PhD Program, University of British Columbia, Vancouver, BC, Canada
edgcumbe@ece.ubc.ca
[2] Electrical and Computer Engineering, University of British Columbia,
Vancouver, BC, Canada
{rsingla, rohling}@ece.ubc.ca
[3] Surgery and Cancer, Faculty of Medicine, Imperial College London,
London, UK
[4] Urologic Sciences, University of British Columbia, Vancouver, BC, Canada
[5] Mechanical Engineering, University of British Columbia, Vancouver,
BC, Canada

Abstract. Laparoscopic partial nephrectomy (LPN) is a standard of care for
small kidney cancer tumours. A successful LPN is the complete excision of the
kidney tumour while preserving as much of the non-cancerous kidney as possible. This is a challenging procedure because the surgeon has a limited field of
view and reduced or no haptic feedback while performing delicate excisions as
fast as possible. This work introduces and evaluates a novel surgical navigation
marker called the Dynamic Augmented Reality Tracker (DART). The DART is
used in a novel intra-operative augmented reality ultrasound navigation system
(ARUNS) for robot-assisted minimally invasive surgery to overcome some of
these challenges. The DART is inserted into a kidney and the DART and
pick-up laparoscopic ultrasound transducer are tracked during an intra-operative
freehand ultrasound scan of the tumour. After ultrasound, the system continues
to track the DART and display the segmented 3D tumour and location of
surgical instruments relative to the tumour throughout the surgery. The ultrasound point reconstruction root mean squared error (RMSE) was 0.9 mm, the
RMSE of tracking the da Vinci surgical instruments was 1.5 mm and the total
system RMSE, which includes ultrasound imaging and da Vinci kinematic
instrument tracking, was 5.1 mm. The system was evaluated by an expert surgeon who used the DART and ARUNS to excise a tumour from a kidney
phantom. This work serves as a preliminary evaluation in anticipation of further
refinement and validation *in vivo*.

Keywords: Augmented reality · Robot-assisted laparoscopic surgery ·
Ultrasound imaging

P. Edgcumbe and R. Singla—These authors are both first authors and have contributed equally to
this work.

G. Zheng et al. (Eds.): MIAR 2016, LNCS 9805, pp. 139–150, 2016.
DOI: 10.1007/978-3-319-43775-0_13

1 Introduction

Minimally invasive surgery (MIS) is growing in popularity for many types of abdominal surgery. Advantages of MIS include smaller incisions, less post-operative pain and shorter recovery times after surgery. However, MIS also has shortcomings such as reduced dexterity, limited haptic feedback, a limited field of view and poor depth perception, particularly with a monocular camera, for the surgeon [1]. This paper proposes the Dynamic Augmented Reality Tracker (DART), a custom-designed surgical navigation marker, to facilitate tumour-centric augmented reality. In particular, the DART is used in an intra-operative augmented reality ultrasound navigation system (ARUNS) that was built to overcome some of the shortcomings of MIS and to maximize the usefulness of laparoscopic ultrasound (LUS) during surgery. Surgeons use LUS as it is a real-time, non-ionizing, low-cost and intra-operative imaging modality. The system is designed for use in partial nephrectomy surgery in order to reduce the positive margin rate, the volume of healthy kidney tissue that is removed, warm ischemia time and total operating time. Maximizing healthy kidney tissue [2] and having a warm ischemia time of less than 30 min [3] results in better retention of kidney function. The purpose of this paper is to present and evaluate the DART and ARUNS in the context of a robot-assisted partial nephrectomy (RAPN) surgery in a laboratory setting.

According to a recent survey of European urologists performing RAPN, the majority use LUS and 86 % expect that augmented reality (AR) during RAPN will be useful in the future [4]. Furthermore, 82 % of surgeons practising endoscopy expect an increase in the use of LUS in the future [5]. However, in most kidney surgeries the ultrasound image is only displayed during the ultrasound scanning stage which occurs after kidney exposure and before the excision of the tumour. Displaying previously acquired ultrasound images requires that the ultrasound images be registered to the surface where the images were taken so that the surgeon sees the images moving with the organ. Tracking the surface of the smooth kidney is difficult [6].

In the context of RAPN, the DART (Fig. 1) is the proposed solution for tracking the local kidney surface and displaying the LUS ultrasound images. The surgeon places the DART in the kidney and performs a freehand ultrasound scan of the kidney and tumour. During this scan, both the DART and LUS are optically tracked. A 3D model of the tumour in the DART coordinate system is generated using optical tracking information and ultrasound segmentation. The positions of the surgical instruments relative to the tumour are displayed to the surgeon as direct AR, in two virtual camera viewpoints, and as a colour-coded warning system that alerts the surgeon if his/her instruments come dangerously close to the tumour. These two orthogonal virtual camera viewpoints, called the top and side views, are displayed to provide the surgeon with a better understanding of the location of the surgical instruments relative to the tumour. Furthermore, a guiding principle in the design of the ARUNS and introduction of virtual camera viewpoints is that surgeons generally dislike direct graphical overlays that obscure the surgical field and prefer simple stylized graphics placed beside the surgical scene [7]. The ARUNS relies on a tumour-centric tracking paradigm where ultrasound, camera, surgical instruments and DART are all related via relative, not absolute, 6-DOF tracking to maximize accuracy of the guidance.

Related work preceded ARUNS. Reviews by Lango et al. [8] and Hughes-Hallett et al. [9] summarize the significant amount of work that has already been done in the field of LUS and image-guided abdominal soft tissue surgery. Noteworthy augmented reality LUS research includes electromagnetically-tracked ultrasound for a kidney phantom model resection [10], optical tracking of the LUS for the first use of registered intra-operative ultrasound overlay in in vivo trans-anal surgery [11] and RAPN [12]. Cheung et al. showed that AR ultrasound shortens planning time [10] and Hughes-Hallett et al. used optically registered LUS to account for intra-operative tissue deformation and displayed freehand 3D reconstruction of the ultrasound image on the operative view [13]. Teber et al. previously developed a real-time AR display of the kidney tumour for the execution phase of LPNs. They employed landmark-based registration of the pre-operative segmented CT and intra-operative field of view and maintained the registration by tracking navigational aids that the surgeon had placed into the kidney [14].

The main novelties here are the invention of the DART, the tumour-centric tracking in the ARUNS, and the virtual camera display of the LUS-generated 3D tumour model and the positions of the surgical instruments relative to the tumour throughout the surgery. The ARUNS is broadly applicable to MIS and, in this first iteration, has been designed for RAPN with the da Vinci S® and Si® surgical systems (Intuitive Surgical, Sunnyvale, CA). The DART and ARUNS were tested through a user study in which an expert surgeon excised a tumour from a phantom model of a kidney tumour.

2   Materials and Methods

The DART (Fig. 1) is designed in Solidworks (Waltham, MA) and 3D printed in stainless steel at a low cost of $26 USD each to enable sterilization by autoclave (Xometry, Gaithersburg, MD). The DART can be inserted via the surgical assistant's

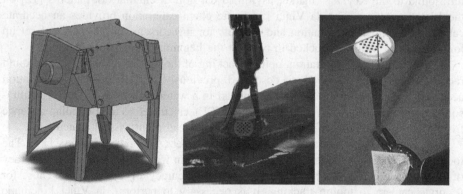

Fig. 1. The DART with repeatable grasp (left); the DART with KeyDot® marker as it is inserted into an ex vivo porcine kidney (centre); and display of modified DART for total system error analysis (right). The red circle is the centre of the pinhead as determined by ultrasound calibration and KeyDot® tracking. The vertex of the yellow cone is the location of the pinhead as determined by da Vinci surgical instrument kinematics. (Color figure online)

12 mm trocar, has a flat surface for placement of the KeyDot® optical marker [12], and can be picked up in a repeatable manner by the da Vinci Pro-Grasp™ [15]. One advantage of the repeatable grasp is that there is a fixed transform from the DART to the surgical instrument. This fixed transform means it is theoretically possible to perform da Vinci kinematic calibration by simply grasping the DART. As well, the DART facilitates a unique tumour-centric tracking system for the ARUNS. The accuracy of the generated tumour model displayed to the surgeon relies on the assumptions that the DART is fixed relative to the tumour and local tissue deformation does not occur. To that end, the DART includes legs with barbed hooks of length 10 mm that are intended to anchor it in a fixed position relative to the tumour.

The LUS transducer is designed for robot-assisted minimally invasive surgeries [15]. It has a 10 MHz 28 mm linear array and it is compatible with the Ultrasonix ultrasound machine (Analogic, Richmond, BC, Canada). The KeyDot® optical markers on the LUS transducer and DART are approved for human use (Key Surgical Inc., Eden Prairie, MN, USA). ITK-Snap [16] and Gmsh [17] are used for ultrasound segmentation and model generation. The user study is performed with the da Vinci Si® (Intuitive Surgical, Sunnyvale, CA), using the Pro-Grasp™ instrument and Monopolar curved scissors.

10–30 mm spherical inclusions at a depth of approximately 20 mm in cylindrical PVC white phantoms with a curved top surface are created using Super Soft Plastic and white colour (M-F Manufacturing, Fort Worth, TX). The phantom's elastic modulus is 15 kPa, which is consistent with the reported elastic modulus for human kidneys [18].

2.1   Calibration and Accuracy Tests

There are several components in the ARUNS system that require calibration. These include the ultrasound tracking and da Vinci kinematic chain. The purpose of the ultrasound calibration is to calculate the transformation from the linear array of the ultrasound to the KeyDot® marker asymmetrical grid of circular dot patterns [12] on the LUS transducer. The da Vinci kinematic chain calibration provides an accurate camera to tooltip transformation and corrects for inaccuracies in the da Vinci set up joint encoders, which are locked in place at the beginning of each operation.

During ultrasound calibration, optical tracking of the KeyDots®, and 3D ultrasound reconstruction are performed as described previously [12]. Ultrasound calibration accuracy is determined by imaging a pinhead in a water bath from 10 different ultrasound poses. The root mean squared error (RMSE), calculated as the Euclidian distance from each pinhead point to the centroid of the pinhead points, is calculated.

The camera is calibrated using the Caltech Camera Calibration toolbox [19]. The tooltip arm is a 12-foot-long, 13-DOF kinematic chain with absolute tracking accuracy of approximately 50 mm and relative tracking accuracy of 1 mm [20]. Thus, for accurate camera to tooltip tracking, it is necessary to perform da Vinci kinematic calibration and register the camera coordinate system to the robot coordinate system. This is achieved via registration of 14 pairs of points, one in the camera coordinate and one in the robot coordinate system. To generate each pair of points the KeyDot® is moved to a unique location and at each location the surgical instrument tip touches the origin of the KeyDot®. In turn, a leave-one-out error for each of the 14 pairs is calculated based on a registration of the other 13 pairs. The RMSE of those 14 errors are reported.

Finally, to characterize the accuracy of the overall system, a modified DART is designed with a flat top and 2.5 mm pinhead (to simulate the tumour centre) rigidly attached exactly 25 mm below the DART surface. A model of the pinhead is generated in the DART coordinate system. Next, the da Vinci surgical instrument is used to pick up the pinhead (Fig. 1). The instrument's location in the DART coordinate system is recorded. The error is calculated as the distance between the pinhead centroid and the surgical instrument. This measure meets the goal of providing user feedback on tool-to-tumour distance. The RMSE of 10 different poses is reported.

2.2 Theory

When using the ARUNS, the surgeon sees the tumour and tooltips via the direct camera feed and via virtual cameras that appear fixed relative to the real camera. The underlying linear algebra that makes this possible is presented in this section.

The abbreviations for the coordinate frames of the ARUNS (Fig. 2) are listed here: Pick-up LUS transducer (P), DART (D), ultrasound image (U), surgical instrument (I), camera (C) and virtual cameras (VC). In the equations in this section, T is a 4×4

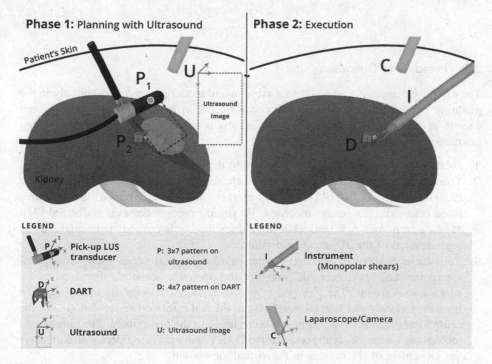

Fig. 2. System configuration with labeled coordinate frames and components for both phases.

transformation matrix, the subscript is the initial coordinate frame, the superscript is the resulting coordinate frame, the subscript of the coordinate frame subscript o indicates the frame at time = 0, and the camera uses the OpenCV coordinate system convention.

The ultrasound images and the locations of the da Vinci surgical instrument tooltips are transformed into the DART coordinate system via Eqs. 1 and 2 respectively:

$$^D T_U = {^D T_C} * {^C T_P} * {^P T_U} \tag{1}$$

$$^D T_I = {^D T_C} * {^C T_I} \tag{2}$$

$^P T_U$ is determined by ultrasound calibration and $^D T_C$ and $^C T_P$ are determined by optical tracking of the KeyDots® on the DART and pick-up LUS transducer respectively. $^C T_I$ is determined via the da Vinci kinematic chain from tooltip to camera.

The transformations from the virtual camera coordinate systems to the initial DART coordinate system, $^{Do} T_{VC}$, are calculated as translational and rotational components. The translations are a pre-set constant that determines the distance between the tumour and virtual cameras. The rotations are pre-set orthogonal rotations around the y and x axes of the camera. When the DART moves, a new transformation from virtual camera to the DART at time t, $^D T_{VC}$, is calculated as follows:

$$^D T_{Do} = {^D T_C} * {^C T_{Co}} * {^{Co} T_{Do}} \tag{3}$$

$$^D T_{VC} = {^D T_{Do}} * {^{Do} T_{VC}} \tag{4}$$

2.3   Principle of Operation

The DART placement, tracked ultrasound scan and model generation occur only in the planning phase. The augmented reality step occurs in both planning (phase 1) and execution (phase 2). The surgeon's console view is shown in Fig. 3. The step-by-step instructions for ARUNS' usage are below:

1. *DART placement*: The DART is placed into the kidney near to the tumour (Fig. 1).
2. *Tracked ultrasound scan:* During the freehand ultrasound scan of the kidney, the LUS transducer and DART KeyDot® markers are optically tracked and synchronised ultrasound images are recorded. 3D volume reconstruction is performed [21].
3. *Model generation:* A 3D model of the kidney tumour is created via manual tumour segmentation of the 3D ultrasound volume.
4. *Augmented reality:* In addition to the regular surgical scene view, orthogonal viewpoints and one direct AR image of the operative scene are displayed to the surgeon in real-time. The viewpoints include rendered tumour and tooltips, shown from the top view and side view, relative to the real camera. The views both face the centroid of the tumour and remain fixed relative to the real camera. The tumour and tooltips are continuously rendered as the DART moves. The rendering also displays the movement of the tumour in the virtual viewpoints.

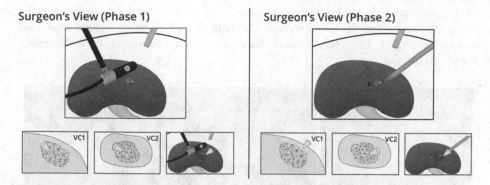

Fig. 3. The surgeon's view during the phases of the surgery. VC1 and VC2 are the orthogonal virtual camera viewpoints for top and side views. Refer to Fig. 2's legend.

5. *Tumour excision*: During the excision of the tumour, if the da Vinci surgical instrument tooltips come within a set threshold distance of the centroid of the tumour the viewpoints flash red to warn the surgeon he/she is approaching the tumour. Last, the DART is removed together with the tumour and surrounding tissue.

2.4   Surgeon User Study

One expert urological surgeon versed in robot-assisted partial nephrectomies participated in the study. The goal of the user study was to evaluate the ARUNS in a simulated RAPN surgery. In the first case, the surgeon was only given the LUS transducer. In the second case, the surgeon was given the LUS transducer and the ARUNS (LUS+ARUNS). The surgeon spent 20 min familiarizing himself with the user interface of the LUS+ARUNS system after which he was given the phantom for resection and the simulated surgery started. The phantoms provided in each case had inclusions that were purposefully unique in shape and location, limiting the surgeon's ability to learn from one case to the other. The AR overlay and orthogonal virtual camera viewpoints are placed at the bottom of the surgeon's screen using TilePro® (Figs. 3 and 4). At the end of the user study, the surgeon answered a questionnaire in which he provided feedback about both cases and both systems. The survey included questions regarding usability and helpfulness of each system.

During the planning phase of both the LUS and LUS+ARUNS cases, the surgeon marked the phantom's surface with the tip of a permanent marker held by the monopolar curved scissors. This simulated the use of electrocautery to mark the kidney surface in surgery. In both the LUS and LUS+ARUNS cases, the surgeon started the execution phase immediately after he finished the planning phase. During the execution phase he used the da Vinci surgical instruments and did not use the LUS.

The LUS+ARUNS tumour model and orthogonal virtual viewpoints were enabled at the start of the planning stage. This was possible because, for this user study, the tumour was scanned and manually segmented prior to the start of the planning phase.

The volume of excised tissue was recorded after subtracting the tissue between the top of the tumour and the tissue surface. The ratio of excised tissue to tumour volume was also recorded. The excised tissue mass was cut into 10 mm slices to determine margin status and size.

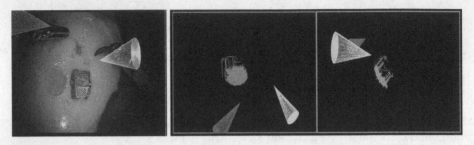

Fig. 4. The direct AR (left) and virtual camera viewpoints (middle and right) that are shown to the surgeon using LUS+ARUNS in addition to his/her normal view. The middle pane is the top-down view and right pane is the side view of the surgical scene.

3 Results

3.1 Calibration and Accuracy Tests

The ultrasound calibration result of the pinhead reconstruction relative accuracy was 0.9 mm. Over the course of capturing the 10 ultrasound images of the pinhead, the ultrasound transducer covered a range of $16 \times 10 \times 19$ mm. The da Vinci kinematic calibration and camera-to-tooltip error was 1.5 mm. The lowest single error was 0.6 mm. The correction factor matrix associated with the 0.6 mm error was used for the rest of the experiment. The overall system error was 5.1 mm.

3.2 Surgeon User Study

For the LUS only case, the planning and execution times were 2 min and 10 min 45 s, respectively. The excised tissue volume was 24 cm^3 and the volume of the tumour was 4 cm^3. Thus, the excised tissue volume to tumour volume ratio was 6:1. There was a gross margin and a separate microscopically (<1 mm) positive margin. The largest negative margin size was 24 mm.

For the LUS+ARUNS case, the planning and execution time were 1 min 57 s and 7 min 30 s respectively. The excised tissue volume was 16.5 cm^3, and the volume of the tumour was 5.5 cm^3. Thus, the excised tissue volume to tumour volume ratio was 3:1. There was a gross and a separate microscopically positive margin. The largest negative margin size was 12 mm. For both cases, the tumour was endophytic and the surgeon rated the R.E.N.A.L nephrometry score [22] as 12. In other words, a very difficult surgery was simulated.

After the user study, the surgeon reported that the ARUNS+LUS case provided more information for visualization of the tumour in the planning phase. The surgeon preferred the ARUNS+LUS case over the LUS case for visualizing the tumour in the execution phase. General comments about the ARUNS+LUS system include that the most useful guidance cue was that the screen flashed red once the instruments got to within a certain distance of the centre of the tumour. The warning aided the surgeon in avoiding the tumour and minimizing the healthy tissue excised. The surgeon found the top-down view easier to interpret than the side view. Video clips from the surgical resection performed for the ARUNS+LUS are included as supplementary material.

4 Discussion

The success of image-guided surgical systems is largely dependent on their accuracy, usability and the clinical need for the extra image guidance. Each of those aspects of the ARUNS will be addressed in turn in the discussion.

Both the ultrasound pinhead reconstruction precision error of 0.9 mm and the error of 1.5 mm for the da Vinci kinematics were consistent with error for similar experiments that have been reported in the literature of 1.2 mm [23] and 1.0 mm [20] respectively. The larger error in ARUNS may be because the gold standard used were optically tracked KeyDot® markers as opposed to an Optotrak® 3020 stylus (Northern Digital Instruments, Waterloo, ON, Canada), which has a reported tip error of 0.25 mm [20]. Given an ultrasound error of 0.9 mm and da Vinci kinematics error of 1.5 mm, the measured total system error of the ARUNS of 5.1 mm can be reduced through further refinement and testing. There is still error from optical tracking of both the LUS and the DART, manual pinhead segmentation, and an imprecise technique for touching the pinhead with the surgical instruments. Given that one of the end goals for ARUNS is to increase the amount of healthy kidney that is spared, it is important to reduce the total system error further. The standard of care recommendation for a kidney tumour resection is to leave a safety margin of 5 mm [3].

In terms of usability, the ARUNS orthogonal virtual camera viewpoint is different to other image guidance systems for abdominal surgery. The advantage of the orthogonal viewpoints is that it provides the surgeon a perspective they would not normally have without occluding the surgeon's view of the operative field. An additional advantage to the virtual viewpoints approach is that the lag, inevitably introduced by an image guidance system with graphical rendering, is much less of a distraction in the orthogonal view as opposed to the direct overlay view. However, further work is required in ARUNS for the positioning of the views, as the surgeon had difficulty orienting himself relative to given views. Additional simplistic cues such as rendering the camera, showing the centre line axis of the virtual viewpoints or letting the surgeon set the pose of the virtual viewpoints could help with minimize these issues. Using a colour gradient to represent the distance of the instrument to the tumour could improve the warning cue given to the surgeon as well.

The ARUNS differs from the work of Teber et al. [14] in the following ways: (1) only one surgical navigation marker, the DART, is inserted into the kidney, (2) the augmented reality image displayed is a 3D representation of the tumour generated by the intra-operative LUS scan, and (3) the surgical instruments and the display is presented to the surgeon via two orthogonal virtual camera viewpoints and a direct AR overlay (Fig. 4).

The ultimate goal is that the ARUNS will be used for human surgeries. To achieve that goal, the issues of ultrasound segmentation, possible tissue deformation relative to the DART, renal artery clamping, blood occlusion and seeding risk will have to be addressed. For simplicity, manual segmentation was performed. In practice, segmentation time can be minimised using (semi-)automatic algorithms that exist or using a bounding sphere approach for complex tumour geometry. However, *in vivo* automatic segmentation of tumours is more difficult than segmentation of phantoms. To account for tissue deformation, a FEM model of the tumour may be required [24] plus real-time surface geometry reconstruction. For renal artery clamping, the main issue is that, to minimize warm ischemia time, the ultrasound imaging should be performed prior to renal artery clamping. The shape of the kidney and tumour change when the perfusion pressure drops to zero. Insertion of the DART into the kidney yields a potential risk of seeding. According to preliminary tests, this may be prevented by using the stainless steel DART with electrocautery. It is also feasible that a range of DART geometries be available to the surgeon depending on tumour depth: long barbs for deep tumours, short barbs for shallow tumours and adhesive fixation for superficial tumours. Blood occlusion of the DART pattern can alleviated through an omniphobic coating to repel blood [25].

5   Future Work and Conclusion

Future studies are required with more users and more trials of the system. This will provide more robust results than the single surgeon/single phantom study performed, as well as provide a clearer understanding on usability and preference. For these studies, subsystem improvements and more rigorous validation can be performed.

The DART and ARUNS offer many interesting avenues for future research. One novel addition would be the incorporation of surface reconstruction. This can be facilitated by structured light using, for example, laser-based solutions [26] or projector-based solutions like the Pico Lantern [27]. A reconstructed surface mesh could be displayed in the orthogonal views to provide further depth cues. Furthermore, the surface could be used to provide the surgeon a true top-down view, as opposed to a view that is orthogonal to their camera viewpoint. Future work for ARUNS could also be the integration of the Pico Lantern for AR in MIS, such as the projection of the tumour outline onto the surface of the kidney. Using the generated surface mesh, an outline of the tumour from the perspective of the camera can be calculated and projected back onto the surface using the tracked projector.

There are also further extensions possible for the DART design and AR display. For example, customised tumour-based DARTs can be created from pre-operative imaging prior to surgery to handle tumours of varying geometries. For protruding tumours, instead of tracking the KeyDot® pattern on the DART optically, it could be used to brand a trackable pattern on the surface using electrocautery. Also, by using several unique DARTs, surgeons could insert them throughout surgery to provide persistent AR and overcome the line-of-sight issues. The virtual views are not limited to rendering one tumour mesh and the da Vinci tools. In practice, the AR display can be extended to include any model including blood vessels and other subsurface structures from pre-operative and intra-operative imaging sources. Leveraging the instrument tracking, a display of the path taken and the projected tool path can be shown as further guidance cues. The virtual views also let the surgeon see beyond their field of view, and localize tools or devices such as the LUS probe. These applications are all enabled by the relative tracking paradigm created by the DART. Finally, the DART and ARUNS concepts can be generalised to provide image guidance for standard non-robotic laparoscopy. In conclusion, the ARUNS is an innovative approach to surgical navigation for minimally invasive surgery and further investigation and user studies are warranted.

Acknowledgements. The authors gratefully thank Andrew Wiles of Northern Digital Inc. for support; Prof. Tim Salcudean for providing infrastructure and advice; Denise Kwok for graphics; and funding from the CIHR Vanier Scholarship, VCH-CIHR-UBC MD/PhD Studentship Award and the NSERC CGS-M Award.

References

1. Elhage, O., Murphy, D., Challacombe, B., Shortland, A., Dasgupta, P.: Ergonomics in minimally invasive surgery. Int. J. Clin. Pract. **61**(2), 186–188 (2007)
2. Sutherland, S.E., Resnick, M.I., Maclennan, G.T., Goldman, H.B.: Does the size of the surgical margin in partial nephrectomy for renal cell cancer really matter? J. Urol. **167**(1), 61–64 (2002)
3. Gill, I.S., Desai, M.M., Kaouk, J.H., Meraney, A.M., Murphy, D.P., Sung, G.T., Novick, A.C.: Laparoscopic partial nephrectomy for renal tumor: duplicating open surgical techniques. J. Urol. **167**(2), 469–476 (2002)
4. Hughes-Hallett, A., Mayer, E.K., Pratt, P., Mottrie, A., Darzi, A., Vale, J.: The current and future use of imaging in urological robotic surgery: a survey of the European Association of Robotic Urological Surgeons. Int. J. Med. Robot. Comput. Assist. Surg. **11**(1), 8–14 (2015)
5. Våpenstad, C., Rethy, A., Langø, T., Selbekk, T., Ystgaard, B., Hernes, T.A.N., Mårvik, R.: Laparoscopic ultrasound: a survey of its current and future use, requirements, and integration with navigation technology. Surg. Endosc. **24**(12), 2944–2953 (2010)
6. Su, L.M., Vagvolgyi, B.P., Agarwal, R., Reiley, C.E., Taylor, R.H., Hager, G.D.: Augmented reality during robot-assisted laparoscopic partial nephrectomy: toward real-time 3D-CT to stereoscopic video registration. Urology **73**(4), 896–900 (2009)
7. Schneider, C.M., Dachs II, G.W., Hasser, C.J., Choti, M.A., DiMaio, S.P., Taylor, R.H.: Robot-assisted laparoscopic ultrasound. In: Navab, N., Jannin, P. (eds.) IPCAI 2010. LNCS, vol. 6135, pp. 67–80. Springer, Heidelberg (2010)
8. Langø, T., Vijayan, S., Rethy, A., Våpenstad, C., Solberg, O.V., Mårvik, R., Johnsen, G., Hernes, T.N.: Navigated laparoscopic ultrasound in abdominal soft tissue surgery: technological overview and perspectives. Int. J. Comput. Assist. Radiol. Surg. **7**(4), 585–599 (2012)
9. Hughes-Hallett, A., Mayer, E.K., Marcus, H.J., Cundy, T.P., Pratt, P.J., Darzi, A.W.: Augmented reality partial nephrectomy: examining the current status and future perspectives. Urology **83**(2), 266–273 (2014)
10. Cheung, C.L., Wedlake, C., Moore, J., Pautler, S.E., Peters, T.M.: Fused video and ultrasound images for minimally invasive partial nephrectomy: a phantom study. In: Jiang, T., Navab, N., Pluim, J.P.W., Viergever, M.A. (eds.) MICCAI 2010. LNCS, vol. 6363, pp. 408–415. Springer, Heidelberg (2010)

11. Pratt, P., Di Marco, A., Payne, C., Darzi, A., Yang, G.Z.: Intraoperative ultrasound guidance for transanal endoscopic microsurgery. In: Ayache, N., Delingette, H., Golland, P., Mori, K. (eds.) MICCAI 2010. LNCS, vol. 7510, pp. 463–470. Springer, Heidelberg (2012)

12. Pratt, P., Jaeger, A., Hughes-Hallett, A., Mayer, E., Vale, J., Darzi, A., Peters, T., Yang, G.Z.: Robust ultrasound probe tracking: initial clinical experiences during robot-assisted partial nephrectomy. Int. J. Comput. Assist. Radiol. Surg. 10(12), 1905–1913 (2015)

13. Hughes-Hallett, A., Pratt, P., Dilley, J., Vale, J., Darzi, A., Mayer, E.: Augmented reality: 3D image-guided surgery. Cancer Imaging 15(Suppl. 1), O8 (2015)

14. Teber, D., Guven, S., Simpfendörfer, T., Baumhauer, M., Güven, E.O., Yencilek, F., Gözen, A.S., Rassweiler, J.: Augmented reality: a new tool to improve surgical accuracy during laparoscopic partial nephrectomy? Preliminary in vitro and in vivo results. Eur. Urol. 56(2), 332–338 (2009)

15. Schneider, C., Guerrero, J., Nguan, C., Rohling, R., Salcudean, S.: Intra-operative "Pick-Up" ultrasound for robot assisted surgery with vessel extraction and registration: a feasibility study. In: Taylor, R.H., Yang, G.-Z. (eds.) IPCAI 2011. LNCS, vol. 6689, pp. 122–132. Springer, Heidelberg (2011)

16. Yushkevich, P.A., Piven, J., Hazlett, H.C., Smith, R.G., Ho, S., Gee, J.C., Gerig, G.: User-guided 3D active contour segmentation of anatomical structures: significantly improved efficiency and reliability. Neuroimage 31(3), 1116–1128 (2006)

17. Geuzaine, C., Remacle, J.F.: Gmsh: a 3-D finite element mesh generator with built-in pre- and post-processing facilities. Int. J. Numer. Methods Eng. 79(11), 1309–1331 (2009)

18. Grenier, N., Gennisson, J.L., Cornelis, F., Le Bras, Y., Couzi, L.: Renal ultrasound elastography. Diagn. Interv. Imaging 94(5), 545–550 (2013)

19. Bouguet, J.Y.: Camera calibration toolbox for matlab (2004)

20. Kwartowitz, D.M., Herrell, S.D., Galloway, R.L.: Toward image-guided robotic surgery: determining intrinsic accuracy of the da Vinci robot. Int. J. Comput. Assist. Radiol. Surg. 1(3), 157–165 (2006)

21. Gooding, M.J., Kennedy, S., Noble, J.A.: Volume segmentation and reconstruction from freehand three-dimensional ultrasound data with application to ovarian follicle measurement. Ultrasound Med. Biol. 34(2), 183–195 (2008)

22. Kutikov, A., Uzzo, R.G.: The RENAL nephrometry score: a comprehensive standardized system for quantitating renal tumor size, location and depth. J. Urol. 182(3), 844–853 (2009)

23. Edgcumbe, P., Nguan, C., Rohling, R.: Calibration and stereo tracking of a laparoscopic ultrasound transducer for augmented reality in surgery. In: Liao, H., Linte, C.A., Masamune, K., Peters, T.M., Zheng, G. (eds.) MIAR 2013 and AE-CAI 2013. LNCS, vol. 8090, pp. 258–267. Springer, Heidelberg (2013)

24. Camara, M., Mayer, E., Darzi, A., Pratt, P.: Soft tissue deformation for surgical simulation: a position-based dynamics approach. Int. J. Comput. Assist. Radiol. Surg. 11(6), 919–928 (2016)

25. Leslie, D.C., Waterhouse, A., Berthet, J.B., Valentin, T.M., Watters, A.L., Jain, A., Kim, P., Hatton, B.D., Nedder, A., Donovan, K., Super, E.H.: A bioinspired omniphobic surface coating on medical devices prevents thrombosis and biofouling. Nat. Biotechnol. 32(11), 1134–1140 (2014)

26. Lin, J., Clancy, N.T., Stoyanov, D., Elson, D.S.: Tissue surface reconstruction aided by local normal information using a self-calibrated endoscopic structured light system. In: Navab, N., Hornegger, J., Wells, W.M., Frangi, A.F. (eds.) MICCAI 2015. LNCS, vol. 9349, pp. 405–412. Springer, Heidelberg (2015)

27. Edgcumbe, P., Pratt, P., Yang, G.Z., Nguan, C., Rohling, R.: Pico Lantern: surface reconstruction and augmented reality in laparoscopic surgery using a pick-up laser projector. Med. Image Anal. 25(1), 95–102 (2015)

Mobile Laserprojection in Computer Assisted Neurosurgery

Christoph Hennersperger[1]([⊠]), Johannes Manus[2], and Nassir Navab[1]

[1] Computer Aided Medical Procedures,
Technical University of Munich, Munich, Germany
christoph.hennersperger@tum.de
[2] Brainlab AG, Feldkirchen, Germany

Abstract. Neurosurgery is one of the key areas for computer-assisted navigation. By providing an intuitive visualization and feedback to the operator, augmented reality has the potential to provide improved clinical workflows and patient outcomes. In this work, a mobile augmented reality system for surgical neuronavigation is presented, allowing for a direct projection of anatomical information on both planar and non-planar surfaces. The system consists of a tracked mobile laser projector, integrated within a navigation system, providing registered patient surface and image data. Using this setup, image data can be corrected for distortions and displayed accurately on the body surface in relation to the patient. We present the overall system with an efficient distortion correction, and evaluate the accuracy with a series of experiments for point and surface projection errors, as well as the general clinical applicability. The system is demonstrated for the projection of craniotomy incision lines and general image data directly onto the surface of a human skull model, where an average error of 1.04 mm shows a sufficient accuracy with respect to the clinical application.

1 Introduction

Today, neurosurgery is commonly supported by computer-assisted navigation, providing visual feedback about the actual anatomy as well as guidance for instrument insertion (e.g. deep brain stimulation), or tissue removal (tumor resection) [10]. Thereby, a detailed surgical plan is constructed and executed, e.g. starting with an outline of the desired skull craniotomy along with potential targets for resection or stimulation. During the actual procedure, surgeons can rely on the plan and all available information on demand in order to request visual feedback or guidance whenever required. Although the technological developments significantly improved clinical workflows [10], emerging new technologies provide the potential to further ease these, especially by employing augmented and virtual reality [5, 15].

This work was partially supported by Brainlab AG, Feldkirchen. Experiments were performed using commercial and development equipment provided as such.

G. Zheng et al. (Eds.): MIAR 2016, LNCS 9805, pp. 151–162, 2016.
DOI: 10.1007/978-3-319-43775-0_14

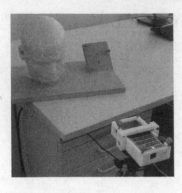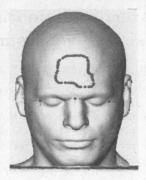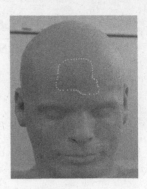

Fig. 1. Projection of a craniotomy line on a phantom head. The projector placed in a distance of approximately 60 cm (left) allows for an accurate projection of a planned trajectory (center) on the phantom model (right).

For brain surgery, skull incision lines are for example currently drawn manually on the patient's skin surface in reference to the actual surgical plan of a craniotomy displayed on a monitor on the side. Thereby, the respective shape and location of the incision is of high importance for the procedure, as deviations may negatively impact the working area of the surgeon in relation to structures deep to the brain surface. In this view, a direct and accurate projection of a previously planned craniotomy on the patient's skull in guaranteed accordance with the pre-operative plan could significantly increase the accuracy and further ease the actual skin marking. This work explores the potential of navigated projectors for the application in computer assisted neurosurgery, which is demonstrated for craniotomy incision planning. Beyond that, the system can also be used to project data on non-planar surfaces such as the human skull. While other surgical disciplines (e.g. abdominal surgery) would evenly benefit from such tools, neurosurgery provides a high level of technical integration by neuronavigation systems, which is the ideal basis for a facilitated clinical acceptance.

Despite advances in augmented reality for both head mounted displays as well as projection systems, to the best of our knowledge a *mobile* projection system for neurosurgery was not presented up to now. By extracting a mesh of the skin surface, geometrically undistorted images can be retrieved and projected directly on the target surface by means of a surface-based distortion correction. After positioning of the projector, the desired image is directly augmented on the patient's skin surface, before it can be removed again from the working space if required. Thus the system integrates well with the general workflow of navigated procedures and instruments. Our system uses a flexible optical tracking system as employed in most commercial neuronavigation systems together with a mobile pico-laser-projector, and provides for the first time an anatomically correct projection of planned data. Thereby, the projector is not fixed but can be dynamically moved, and the projected scene is updated with respect to the actual planned data in real-time.

2   Related Work in Medical Augmented Reality

Augmented reality techniques either utilize Head Mounted Displays (HMD) or a direct projection on target surfaces. The acceptance of HMDs in interventional settings is impaired due to a limited willingness of surgeons to wear these devices for multiple hours as well as further restrictions with respect to sterility. In contrast to an augmentation by HMDs, a direct projection of the information on the target area allows operators to interact with the system without the need to directly wear any of its components. Common systems relying on direct projection mostly achieve accuracies of about 1.5 mm target point deviation, which has not changed significantly within the last decade [6]. With respect to craniotomy planning, a distinct projection system developed for the visualization of a craniotomy directly onto the patient's head is presented in [3]. As the system does not include any patient registration or surface correction, an anatomically correct augmentation of information is not foreseen. First concepts towards surface-independent or distortion-corrected projections showed a promising direction [13], and more recently a pick-up projector for robotic surgery was introduced [2]. The device is tracked by a pattern attached to the projector to provide surgical overlay images for laparoscopic surgery.

With an application to neurosurgery, a direct projection of image data on skull surfaces is presented in [1,9], using segmented datasets for visualization. While this approach shows high accuracies of about 0.3 mm, the projector needs to be positioned and registered statically, which seems impractical in surgical environments because of line of sight issues. Another approach focuses on the projection using pico-projectors for surgical microscopes [14]. Finally, [8] shows a potential 3D surface reconstruction, combining a projector with an integrated camera system. With respect to the clinical application, however, the above mentioned works either suffer from a static registration or are targeted at applications (e.g. laparoscopic surgery) with different surgical requirements. The approach presented in this work introduces a tracked, mobile projector allowing for a distortion-corrected projection of image data in navigated procedures.

3   Mobile Projection System for CAS

A mobile projection system is developed, which can be introduced in the surgical space whenever required (on demand). Thereby, the introduction into and removal from the working area should not impose a significant overhead onto the clinical routine. In this work, the mobile projector is calibrated once with respect to an optical tracking mount. The calibrated projector and its pose are then used in order to provide augmented images directly on the surgical area. Figure 2 depicts a schematic overview of the involved components along with the data flow between these. In general, the overall system consists of (i) an optical tracking system (Northern Digital Inc, Waterloo, Ontario, Canada) to track instrument and tool poses in 3D space similar to most of the state-of-the-art neuronavigation systems, (ii) the projector (AAXA Technologies, Inc., Tustin,

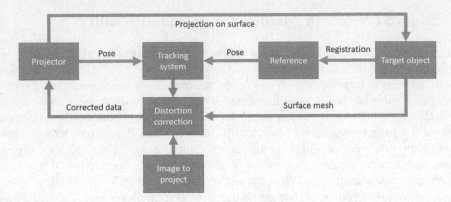

Fig. 2. Projection workflow. Both the projector as well as the reference frames registered to the target object are observed by the tracking system. Using this relation, the surface mesh is employed in order to correct the image data and project it on the surface in relation to the current projector position.

California, USA), which is mounted within a custom-designed tracking adapter and designed such that it can be utilized as a removable instrument, and (iii) a processing system utilizing all registered instruments to provide a distortion-corrected augmentation of image information onto the patient's skin surface. Similar to conventional neuronavigation systems, we introduce a reference frame (optical tracking marker), which is attached to the patient and allows for a registration of all other tools (e.g. pointer, projector) to the reference frame. The poses of the projector and the reference as tracked by the optical system are used as input for the distortion correction (Sect. 3.3) to be visualized by the projector.

3.1   Projector Integration

With respect to surgical applications, the projector technology is critical to ensure a sufficient accuracy especially with respect to the depth of field. Over the past years, laser projectors emerged as an attractive technology in this area. In contrast to other pico-projectors, laser-projectors stay in focus for arbitrary distances and thus enable an accurate projection not only on planar but also deformed surfaces such as the human skin. The projector employed in this work uses one LCoS element for each RGB-component in order to provide a 2D image projection. The small form-factor of pico-projectors allow for a direct utilization as mobile instruments, while the brightness (20 lumen for the AAXA L1) is still sufficient to visualize image data directly on the surgical area in proximity (<90 cm in our experiments) to the target. As a main advantage, such a mobile instrument allows to circumvent line-of-sight issues by changing its position, or removing it from the surgical area altogether if required.

In order to allow for a reliable tracking of the projector, a custom mount needs to be calibrated to the projected image geometry, such that points in

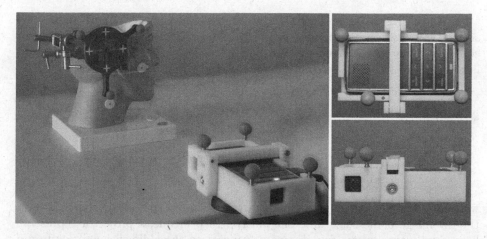

Fig. 3. Left: projection accuracy. For test purposes, four cross-hairs are projected on a calibrated tracking adapter used for intra-operative verification, demonstrating the projection accuracy. **Right: tracking mount.** The optical markers are placed asymmetrically to avoid ambiguous tracking estimates.

3D space can be used for a reliable projection on both planar and non-planar surfaces. The detection of individual optical markers is given directly by the optical system. The relation between the different marker spheres allows for an optimized design with respect to the tracking accuracy in relation to certain tool orientations. As shown in Fig. 3, our mount comprises of four spheres with a high pitch between the markers to minimize errors. The front spheres are elevated by 3.5 mm to account for the positioning of the optical camera above the scene.

3.2 System Geometry

Throughout this work, we define points in 3D space in homogeneous coordinates as $\bar{P} = [X, Y, Z, 1]^T$, with matrices and vectors indicated by bold capital and lower-case letters respectively. For points, vectors and matrices in reference to the different system components (projector, camera, reference), indices are introduced, where points in the 2D camera frame are defined as x_C, and reference and projector coordinates in 3D space as X_R and X_P accordingly. A transformation is always indicated from source to target, e.g. $P_R = \mathbf{T}_{CR} \cdot P_C$. Assuming a projective geometry for the projector, the camera-matrix defining the intrinsic parameters of the camera/projector is given by

$$\mathbf{C} = \begin{bmatrix} s_x & \theta & o_x \\ 0 & s_y & o_y \\ 0 & 0 & 1 \end{bmatrix} * \begin{bmatrix} f & 0 & 0 \\ 0 & f & 0 \\ 0 & 0 & 1 \end{bmatrix} = \begin{bmatrix} f*s_x & f*\theta & o_x \\ 0 & f*s_y & o_y \\ 0 & 0 & 1 \end{bmatrix}, \tag{1}$$

with f being the focal length of the camera, s_x, s_y the scaling from px to mm in x- and y-directions, o_x, o_y the offset from the image center to the top-left corner, and θ the skew-factor [4].

With respect to the observed scene, only the combination of both the intrinsic and extrinsic camera matrix defined by the transformation from the world coordinate system into camera coordinates can be observed. This combination is thereby defined as the projection matrix $\mathbf{P}$ of the scene

$$\lambda \cdot \bar{x}_C = \mathbf{P} \cdot \bar{X}_W \tag{2}$$

$$\lambda \cdot \bar{x}_C = \mathbf{C} \cdot [\mathbf{R}|\mathbf{t}] \cdot \bar{X}_W \tag{3}$$

$$\lambda \cdot \begin{bmatrix} x_C \\ y_C \\ 1 \end{bmatrix} = \begin{bmatrix} f*s_x & f*\theta & o_x \\ 0 & f*s_y & o_y \\ 0 & 0 & 1 \end{bmatrix} \cdot \begin{bmatrix} r_{11} & r_{12} & r_{13} & t_X \\ r_{21} & r_{22} & r_{23} & t_Y \\ r_{31} & r_{32} & r_{33} & t_Z \end{bmatrix} \cdot \begin{bmatrix} X_W \\ Y_W \\ Z_W \\ 1 \end{bmatrix} , \tag{4}$$

with $\mathbf{P} \in \mathbb{R}^{3 \times 4}$. Thus, it is possible to represent any spatial 3D coordinate on the 2D image plane using only one matrix. In principle, a projector represents here simply the inverse function of a camera; as three-dimensional points are illuminated from a two-dimensional ray, cast by the projected 2D pixel. Thus an accurate calibration of the projector ensures that points are correctly displayed in 3D space.

In order to estimate $\mathbf{C}$, $\mathbf{R}$, and $\mathbf{t}$ by a calibration, we follow a two-step approach. At first, the projection matrix $\mathbf{P}$ is determined using the Direct Linear transform, where we collect a series of correspondence pairs $\bar{X}_i \leftrightarrow \bar{x}_i$ between the 3D positions given by the optical tracking and the corresponding 2D projected image points

$$\bar{x}_i = \mathbf{P} \cdot \bar{X}_i = \begin{bmatrix} \mathbf{p}^{1T} \cdot \bar{X}_i \\ \mathbf{p}^{2T} \cdot \bar{X}_i \\ \mathbf{p}^{3T} \cdot \bar{X}_i \end{bmatrix} . \tag{5}$$

The actual projection matrix $\mathbf{P}$ can then be retrieved using the direct linear transformation with a least-squares approximation using the singular value decomposition [4]. Based on the retrieved projection matrix, the factorization of the intrinsic and extrinsic parameters can be performed in a second step by exploiting the orthogonality of the matrix $\mathbf{KR}$. Thereby, the factorization of $\mathbf{P}$ is especially beneficial for the direct integration of the visualization within OpenGL: Each matrix directly corresponds to a camera matrix defined in the OpenGL rendering pipeline, allowing for an efficient visualization of 3D scenes using the calibrated instrument. As $\mathbf{P} = \mathbf{C} \cdot [\mathbf{R}|\mathbf{t}]$, two submatrices $[\mathbf{CR}|\mathbf{Ct}] = [\mathbf{P}_1|\mathbf{P}_2]$ can be defined. Furthermore $\mathbf{C}$ is upper triangular and $\mathbf{R}$ is orthogonal. Thus the properties of the submatrix $\mathbf{CR}$ can be used to factorize $\mathbf{P}$

$$\mathbf{P}_1^{-1} = (\mathbf{CR})^{-1} = \mathbf{R}^{-1}\mathbf{C}^{-1} = \mathbf{R}^T\mathbf{C}^{-1} . \tag{6}$$

The QR-decomposition of $\mathbf{P}_1^{-1}$ provides $\mathbf{C}^{-1}$ and $\mathbf{R}^T$, allowing for a retrieval of $\mathbf{C}$ and $\mathbf{R}$ by inversion and transposition respectively, and $\mathbf{t} = \mathbf{C}^{-1}(\mathbf{Ct})$.

3.3 Distortion-Corrected Visualization

The aim of a surgical projection is to provide an accurate augmentation of anatomical or structural image information on surfaces in 3D space. For a correct spatial appearance, two factors impact the potential distortion of projected images. On the one hand, the orientation of the projector with respect to the target object surface and its surface normal may influence both the visibility and the quality of a projected image. On the other hand, objects on the projecting surface should be visualized in a geometrically correct fashion. To enable this, the actual geometry of the surface has to be considered and corrected for, such that the image appears spatially correct.

With respect to a view-dependent projection, the system in this work is based on similar work proposed in literature [13]. To allow for a low projection latency, however, modifications allowing for an efficient implementation of the projection scene directly in OpenGL are proposed. To correct for distortions based on the observer's viewpoint, a virtual plane is introduced, touching the projection surface at the center of the image to be projected. A simplified example of this concept is shown in Fig. 4a, where the red dots on the surface of the sphere correspond to the pixels of the virtual plane. By backprojecting a point on the sphere onto the virtual image plane, the latter can be used directly as image content to be displayed by the projector. The actual image information will be then visualized on the surface as a distortion-corrected image.

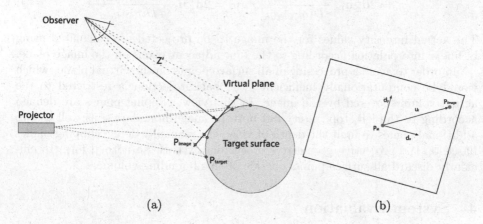

Fig. 4. (a) **Backprojection on virtual plane.** Objects to be displayed on the target surface are projected on a virtual image plane using central projection, where target points P_{target} are projected on an imaginary plane P_{image} to achieve distortion-correction. (b) **Retrieval of projection coordinates.** By using the direction vectors of the current image plane, image coordinates can be retrieved as offset vectors from the image center point.

To locate the corresponding points $\bar{P}_{target} \leftrightarrow \bar{P}_{image}$ for the distortion correction, every point on the surface needs to correspond to the respective image pixel. Thereby, the backprojection from the surface onto the virtual plane at a distance Z' prevents the creation of possible holes in the projected image content, as the backprojection on the virtual plane closer to the projection center ensures a dense sampling of the points. This relation can be directly expressed in homogeneous coordinates, allowing for an efficient online-visualization

$$\bar{X}' = \begin{bmatrix} X \cdot \frac{Z'}{Z} \\ Y \cdot \frac{Z'}{Z} \\ Z \cdot \frac{Z'}{Z} \\ 1 \end{bmatrix} = \begin{bmatrix} 1 & 0 & 0 & 0 \\ 0 & 1 & 0 & 0 \\ 0 & 0 & 1 & 0 \\ 0 & 0 & \frac{1}{Z'} & 0 \end{bmatrix} \cdot \bar{X} = \mathbf{S} \cdot \bar{X}\,, \tag{7}$$

where $\bar{X}$ and $\bar{X}'$ are the homogeneous coordinates of a 3D point and its projected counterpart, respectively. With respect to a geometrically correct projection of the image data, finally the coordinates $[x_i, y_i]^T$ of the actual point P_{Image} have to be determined, as shown in Fig. 4b. The point of contact $\bar{P}_M$ as well as the two directional vectors $\mathbf{d}_x$ and $\mathbf{d}_y$ are set based on the observer's viewpoint. $Dim_{X\,Image}$, $Dim_{Y\,Image}$ are defined by the original image size in px, and $Dim_{X\,Real}$, $Dim_{Y\,Real}$ defined by the object size in mm. Consequently, the coordinate vector of $P_{i\,Image}$ and the coordinates x_i, y_i are defined as

$$\mathbf{u}_i = \bar{P}_{i\,Image} - \bar{P}_M \tag{8}$$

$$x_i = 2\mathbf{d}_x^T \mathbf{u}_i \cdot \frac{Dim_{X\,Image}}{Dim_{X\,Real}}, \quad y_i = 2\mathbf{d}_y^T \mathbf{u}_i \cdot \frac{Dim_{Y\,Image}}{Dim_{Y\,Real}}\,. \tag{9}$$

The actual intensity values for the image to be projected are calculated using bi-linear interpolation according to the four adjacent pixels on the image plane.

In order to avoid a processing of all surface points on the virtual plane (which would be computationally inefficient), the backprojection is restricted to the actual volume covered by the image. In this view, clipping planes are defined according to the left, top, right, and bottom image boundaries, as well as two additional planes to limit the depth of view. We manually define clipping planes based on the projective geometry and evaluate the Hesse normal form to efficiently discard all surface points outside of this bounding volume.

4   System Evaluation

The accuracy of the overall system can be affected by various components, including the precision of the projector, the accuracy of the calibration as well as the geometrical layout of the actual marker spheres of the projector mount.

4.1   Projection Accuracy

The projection accuracy is evaluated by measuring the absolute point deviation of projected points from predefined ones, where the offset is measured manually. In order to do so, a reference tracking adapter is fixed on a planar surface with marked points in a known geometrical relation with respect to the reference frame (see Fig. 5 right). We perform the projector calibration using this plate by manually pointing to the respective calibration positions as numbered in Fig. 5

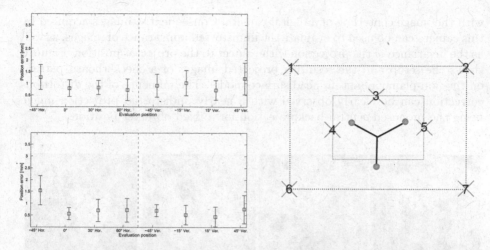

Fig. 5. Left: quantitative results. Accuracy of point measurements for different orientations of the evaluation plate in a distance of 35 cm (top) and 60 cm (bottom). **Right: evaluation pattern.** Overview of evaluation points on the reference plane, lying on two rectangles with the sizes 20 × 15 cm and 12 × 9 cm.

with an optically tracked pointer. Due to the focus on the projection accuracy, the intrinsic calibration and distortion of the projector is neglected here.

Thereby, six random plate positions including different translations and rotations are used to perform the calibration, resulting in a set of 42 correspondence pairs. The accuracy of projected points is then evaluated for varying distances (35 cm, 60 cm) and orientations (horizontal angles $-45°, 0°, 30°, 60°$, vertical angles $-45°, -15°, 15°, 45°$) between the planar surface and the projector. In order to achieve sufficient statistics, the experiment is repeated three times, resulting in a total of 168 evaluation points per distance (336 in total). The results for the point deviations for both 35 cm and 60 cm are shown in Fig. 5. The average error over all 336 measurements is 1.04 mm with a standard deviation of $\sigma = 0.54$ mm. A qualitative result of the projected point accuracy is further shown in Fig. 1 for the application of craniotomy planning. Based on an available surface model extracted from a phantom CT, a planned craniotomy line can be visualized accurately on the actual non-planar skull surface.

4.2 Surface Projection

In addition to the system point projection accuracy, the accuracy of distortion-corrected projection images is validated with respect to a predefined viewpoint in order to evaluate the general applicability of the developed system in a surgical setting. The patient calibration (surface mesh to patient head) is performed using a standard fiducial-based registration, where markers in the surface mesh are registered to positions as indicated by an optical pointer. The desired observer viewpoint is defined manually by the direction of an optical tracking pointer aligned with the image centerline of a digital camera. Consequently, images acquired by this camera can be used to evaluate the undistorted appearance of images, as well as the invariance of the projection with respect to the projector position. Figure 6 shows the setup and the resulting projected images of a checkerboard pattern on the non-planar phantom head surface model. The influence of the distortion-correction can be clearly observed with a nearly undistorted projection image using the proposed central-backprojection for a fixed observer position.

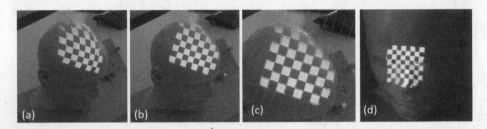

Fig. 6. Impact of distortion correction. The naive projection of images (a) shows significant distortions in comparison to the corrected projection (b). For qualitative evaluation, checkerboard edges are overlaid in (c), showing that distortion in the central area is minimal, with slightly noticeable distortions for regions with high angular orientation to the projection direction. Similar results can be obtained also for general high curvature surfaces, as for example in the facial area (d).

5 Discussion

In view of the quantitative and qualitative results of our evaluation, the proposed system allows for certain clinical applications in computer assisted surgery, and especially for the application of craniotomy planning. In comparison to other AR methods, the proposed system provides similar point accuracies, while being more flexible and adaptable to the actual clinical indication.

With respect to the projection of undistorted image data on non-planar surfaces, a summarizing statement seems to be slightly more complex. Our results show that the required accuracy for the projection of image data on surfaces can be achieved for both slightly curved as well as highly tortuous surfaces. However, based on the projection direction, the surface normal can result in a magnification-effect of potential inaccuracies: on surfaces which are nearly perpendicular to the projection direction, a slight offset can result in a significant distortion of the image data. This effect can be exacerbated for an imperfect registration of patients. Nonetheless, undistorted image data can be projected with a high precision for a realistic placement of the projector in relation to the target. Based on the surface mesh and its normals, potentially problematic settings with respect to projector and target position could further be automatically detected and considered in a clinical system. Thus the system is well-suited also for complex surface projections, e.g. for a projection of tumor data inside the brain.

Before a clinical integration of such systems can be targeted, however, also reliable systems for viewpoint-detection need to be integrated. In this work, the viewpoint of the operator was set manually by an optically tracked pointer. In view of an integration of such tools into clinical practice, however, manually setting the viewpoint is not feasible. We think that current developments such as new sensor-technology (integrated with microscopes, or surgical glasses) or external viewpoint trackings systems could potentially overcome the need for HMD or surgical glasses in the future and allow for a direct projection in a view-independent fashion.

Our evaluation of lighting conditions shows that projected patterns can be observed with moderate operation lighting, but get less visible on the skin surface especially for maximal operating light intensity. With respect to the presented application for craniotomy planning, this is not critical, as this is performed under normal room lighting during preparation. In view of future applications with direct operating light, however, improved projection technology will hopefully enable mobile laser projectors with higher brightness.

In terms of the overall system calibration, we recognized a certain variance of our calibration results based on the DLT algorithm and the correspondence matching in our experiments. In this view, future work will focus on an improved method to calibrate the projector and camera matrices directly, also including intrinsic calibration and rectification. Thereby, a recently proposed structured light approach [7] promises higher accuracies, using an integrated camera-projector combination. Such a combination could further allow for a direct 3D reconstruction of the anatomical surface during the surgery [11,12], which in turn could be also used to update the patient registration itself.

6   Conclusion

In this work, a mobile projection system for the application in computer assisted neurosurgery was presented. The system consists of a mobile tracked laser-projector, integrated with a navigation system using optical tracking. Surface data available in CAS-applications allows for a direct distortion correction based on extracted meshes online. The system not only allows for a projection of pre-interventionally planned points with high accuracy, but also for an undistorted projection of various image data directly onto non-planar and tortuous surfaces. With respect to the area of computer assisted neurosurgery, the system can be used to project craniotomy lines on the skull surface of the patient. In view of the presented system, we hope that this work facilitates a clinical acceptance of such systems, as well as the development of further applications for interventional augmented reality.

References

1. Besharati Tabrizi, L., Mahvash, M.: Augmented reality-guided neurosurgery: accuracy and intraoperative application of an image projection technique. J. Neurosurg. **123**(1), 206–211 (2015)
2. Edgcumbe, P., Pratt, P., Yang, G.-Z., Nguan, C., Rohling, R.: Pico lantern: a pick-up projector for augmented reality in laparoscopic surgery. In: Golland, P., Hata, N., Barillot, C., Hornegger, J., Howe, R. (eds.) MICCAI 2014, Part I. LNCS, vol. 8673, pp. 432–439. Springer, Heidelberg (2014)
3. Glossop, N., Wedlake, C., Moore, J., Peters, T., Wang, Z.: Laser projection augmented reality system for computer assisted surgery. In: Ellis, R.E., Peters, T.M. (eds.) MICCAI 2003. LNCS, vol. 2879, pp. 239–246. Springer, Heidelberg (2003)
4. Hartley, R., Zisserman, A.: Multiple View Geometry, 2nd edn. Cambridge University Press, New York (2010)
5. Helm, P.A., Teichman, R., Hartmann, S.L., Simon, D.: Spinal navigation and imaging: history, trends, and future. IEEE Trans. Med. Imaging **34**(8), 1738–1746 (2015)
6. Hoppe, H., Duber, S., Raczkowsky, J., Wrn, H.: Intraoperative visualization of surgical planning data using video projectors. In: Medicine Meets Virtual Reality 2001: Outer Space, Inner Space, Virtual Space, p. 206. IOS Press (2001)
7. Jiang, L., Zhang, S., Yang, J., Zhuang, X., Zhang, L., Gu, L.: A robust automated markerless registration framework for neurosurgery navigation. Int. J. Med. Robot. Comput. Assist. Surg. **11**(4), 436–447 (2015)
8. Leong-Hoï, A., Serio, B., Twardowski, P., Montgomery, P.: Three-dimensional surface reconstruction by combining a pico-digital projector for structured light illumination and an imaging system with high magnification and high depth of field. In: SPIE Photonics Europe, p. 913219. International Society for Optics and Photonics (2014)
9. Mahvash, M., Tabrizi, L.B.: A novel augmented reality system of image projection for image-guided neurosurgery. Acta Neurochir. **155**(5), 943–947 (2013)
10. Mezger, U., Jendrewski, C., Bartels, M.: Navigation in surgery. Langenbeck's Arch. Surg. **398**(4), 501–514 (2013)
11. Moreno, D., Taubin, G.: Simple, accurate, and robust projector-camera calibration. In: 2012 Second International Conference on 3D Imaging, Modeling, Processing, Visualization and Transmission (3DIMPVT), pp. 464–471. IEEE (2012)
12. Orghidan, R., Salvi, J., Gordan, M., Florea, C., Batlle, J.: Structured light self-calibration with vanishing points. Mach. Vis. Appl. **25**(2), 489–500 (2014)
13. Park, H., Lee, M.-H., Kim, S.-J., Park, J.-I.: Surface-independent direct-projected augmented reality. In: Narayanan, P.J., Nayar, S.K., Shum, H.-Y. (eds.) ACCV 2006. LNCS, vol. 3852, pp. 892–901. Springer, Heidelberg (2006)
14. Shi, C., Becker, B.C., Riviere, C.N.: Inexpensive monocular pico-projector-based augmented reality display for surgical microscope. In: 2012 25th International Symposium on Computer-Based Medical Systems (CBMS), pp. 1–6. IEEE (2012)
15. Wang, D., Ma, D., Wong, M.L., Wáng, Y.X.J.: Recent advances in surgical planning & navigation for tumor biopsy and resection. Quant. Imaging Med. Surg. **5**(5), 640 (2015)

Towards Augmented Reality Guided Craniotomy Planning in Tumour Resections

Marta Kersten-Oertel[3(✉)], Ian J. Gerard[1,3], Simon Drouin[1,3],
Kevin Petrecca[2,3], Jeffery A. Hall[2,3], and D. Louis Collins[1,2,3]

[1] Biomedical Engineering, McGill University, Montréal, Canada
[2] Neurology and Neurosurgery, McGill University, Montréal, Canada
[3] Montreal Neurological Institute and Hospital, Montréal, Canada
marta@bic.mni.mcgill.ca

Abstract. Augmented reality has been proposed as a solution to overcome some of the current shortcomings of image-guided neurosurgery. In particular, it has been used to merge patient images, surgical plans, and the surgical field of view into a comprehensive visualization. In this paper we explore the use of augmented reality for planning craniotomies in image-guided neurosurgery procedures for tumour resections. Our augmented reality image-guided neurosurgery system was brought into the operating room for 8 cases where the surgeon used augmented reality prior to tumour resection. We describe our initial results that suggest that augmented reality can play an important role in tailoring the size and shape of the craniotomy and for evaluating intra-operative surgical strategies. With continued development and validation, augmented reality guidance has the potential to improve the minimally invasiveness of image-guided neurosurgery through improved intraoperative surgical planning.

Keywords: Augmented reality · Tumour resection · Craniotomy · Image-guided neurosurgery

1 Introduction

An increasing amount of research has focused on using augmented reality (AR) in image-guided surgery (IGS) applications. In AR, real and virtual objects are combined into a comprehensive visualization. In image-guided surgery (IGS) the *virtual* objects correspond to patient-specific models, plans and preoperative images. The *real* world corresponds to the surgical field of view, which may be captured using an external camera, surgical microscope or endoscope. This real world is then merged with the virtual objects to create the augmented visualization. The motivation behind using augmented reality in IGS is twofold: (i) AR provides a visualization that maps the preoperative images from the IGS (or navigation) display onto the patient, and (ii) AR allows the surgeon to see pertinent anatomy below the visible surface of the patient. AR visualizations therefore, have the potential to improve the surgical workflow, allow for easier intraoperative planning, and improve surgical guidance to the anatomy of interest thus contributing to the minimization of the invasiveness of these procedures.

© Springer International Publishing Switzerland 2016
G. Zheng et al. (Eds.): MIAR 2016, LNCS 9805, pp. 163–174, 2016.
DOI: 10.1007/978-3-319-43775-0_15

Providing evidence that AR has these benefits in IGS, however, is a challenging task. Indeed, validation of AR IGS systems is one of the main elements lacking from this field of research; few groups have gone beyond testing in the laboratory to using their AR IGS systems in the operating room [1]. Given the constraints of the OR, accessibility to surgeons and clinical cases, and the challenge of determining suitable validation metrics for visualization techniques, this is not surprising. Over the last several years, we have been using our image-guided neurosurgery system, IBIS (Interactive Brain Imaging System) [2], in the operating room to evaluate how AR can impact image-guided neurosurgery (IGNS). In our previous work in image-guided neurovascular surgery, we gave preliminary evidence that the benefit of AR is very task specific [3]. We showed that for different neurovascular pathologies, AR is useful for vessel differentiation, localization of small and deep vessels, and craniotomy planning (i.e. the removal of the skull bone to expose the brain). In this paper, we explore the use of augmented for craniotomy planning in tumour resections. We provide examples from three of the eight surgical cases in which our system was used, and summarize the experiences the surgeons that have had using our AR IGS system in tumour resections.

The paper is organized as follows; first in Sect. 2 we describe related work in the area of augmented reality image-guided neurosurgery. In Sect. 3 we briefly describe our research neuronavigation software IBIS that allows for augmented reality visualization, how we create the augmented reality view, and the processing and visualization of preoperative patient images. In Sect. 4 we describe the use of augmented reality in real surgical cases for craniotomy planning, and we conclude and discuss avenues of future work in Sect. 5.

2 Related Work

One of the first clinical applications of AR and currently the most popular is neurosurgery [1]. In the 1990s, Gleason et al. [4] first proposed using AR in neurosurgery. In their system, live video images of the patient were augmented with 3D segmented virtual objects (e.g. tumours) from preoperative patient data. The MAGI (microscope-assisted guided intervention) neuronavigation system, developed by Edwards et al. [5, 6], allowed for stereo projection of virtual images into a neurosurgical microscope for ear, nose and throat (ENT) surgery and neurosurgery. Birkfellner et al. [7, 8] developed the Varioscope AR, a custom-built head-mounted operating microscope where virtual objects were combined with the surgical scene. Sauer et al. [9] developed a video see-through augmented reality display that provided a surgeon with stereo video view of patient anatomy, such as lesions, at the actual location inside the patient. Cabrilo et al. used the Zeiss OPMI Pentero's Multivision function that injects virtual images into one ocular of the neurosurgical microscope to carry in the context of neurovascular surgery [10, 11]. Mahvash and Tabrizi developed a projector-based AR system where images of the pertinent patient anatomy are project onto the skin, skull or brain surface in real-time [12]. Each of these systems has been tested on phantoms and some on patients, providing some evidence that AR can be useful for particular tasks in the OR. In our paper we examine how AR can be used in the specific task of craniotomy planning for tumour resections.

For more information as to the use of augmented reality in IGNS the reader is referred to a recent survey of the field [13].

3 Materials and Methods

3.1 IBIS System Overview

To create augmented reality visualizations in the OR, we used a custom-built research image-guide neurosurgery system, IBIS. For augmented reality three components are necessary: the IBIS neuronavigation workstation, an image-capture device (here a Sony HDR XR150 video camera was used), and a Polaris tracking system (Northern Digital, Waterloo, Canada), which is used to track the patient, surgical tools and the camera. The neuronavigation workstation runs Ubuntu 12.04 (64-bit), with an Intel Core i7-3820@3.6 GHz on a quad-core processor with 32 GB RAM. The graphics card is a GeForce GTX 670 and the video capture card is a Conexant cx23800. The custom-built software is written in C++ and uses the Visualization Toolkit (version 5.10), the Qt 4 user interface platform, and Insight Registration and Segmentation Toolkit (version 4.4). Previous publications using the IBIS software have focused on using intraoperative ultrasound (iUS) [14] for brain shift compensation, using AR in neurovascular surgery [2, 3, 15], and improving AR visualization accuracy with iUS [16].

3.2 Augmented Reality Visualization

To create AR visualizations in the operating room, live images of the surgical scene are augmented with pre-operative patient models (e.g. segmented tumours and vessels). The live images are captured by a calibrated Sony video camera and the virtual and real elements are merged and displayed on the neuronavigation system to inform and guide the surgeon.

There are three prerequisites for creating an AR view: (i) a camera must be calibrated, (ii) the calibrated camera must be spatially tracked, and (iii) a patient-to-image registration must be computed. These three elements give us the information needed to create a mapping between the virtual world and objects, and the real world. The *calibration* procedure involves computing the intrinsic (i.e. focus and image center) and extrinsic parameters of the camera, i.e. the transformation between the attached tracker and the optical center of the camera. Calibration is done using an implementation of Zhang's method [17], in which the edges of a planar calibration grid or checkerboard pattern of known size are detected using different poses of a camera. By calibrating the camera, the transform between the image and real world coordinates can be computed. Camera calibration is performed pre-operatively in the lab, and *tracking* the video camera ensures the position of the camera in the OR is known at all times. In the OR, the surgeon performs a *patient-to-image registration* by choosing, with a tracked surgical pointer, anatomical landmarks on the patient that correspond to those chosen preoperatively on the patients MR images [18]. This determines the mapping between the physical space of the patient and the virtual space of their preoperative images. The location of the camera, the camera calibration matrix and patient-to-image

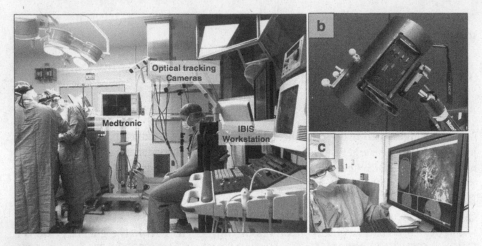

Fig. 1. The IBIS neuronavigation system in use in the OR: (a) The system is brought into the OR in parallel with the commercial Medtronic system. (b) A calibrated camera with an attached tracker is used to capture live images of the surgical scene. (c) The augmented reality visualization is displayed on the monitor of the IBIS workstation.

registration together provide us with the relationship between the pre-operative images and the live images of the surgical field of view, allowing for the creation of the AR visualization. In Fig. 1 we show the system being used in the operating room. For a more detailed description of the system, calibration and registration procedure, we refer the reader to [2].

3.3   MR Image Processing and Visualization

Data. In order to prepare for each case, the preoperative imaging data is processed to identify all structures and regions of interest. The data acquired for each of the patients was a gadolinium enhanced T1 weighted magnetic resonance image (MRI) obtained on a 1.5 T MRI scanner (Ingenia, Philips Medical Systems) at the Montreal Neurological Institute and Hospital (MNI/H). The MRI data was processed using a custom image-processing pipeline [4] that includes: de-noising [5], intensity non-uniformity correction [6] and normalization. As part of the pipeline, segmentation of cortical surface is done using the FACE method [7]. The automatic pre-processing is done using a local computing cluster at the McConnell Brain Imaging Centre (MNI) and takes 1–2 h.

The tumour is then manually segmented from the processed images using ITKSnap, and the visible vessels (typically the sinus and some large arteries and veins) are segmented using semi-automatic intensity thresholding also in ITKSnap. The processed images and patient-specific models are then imported into IBIS for visualization, planning and guidance (Fig. 2).

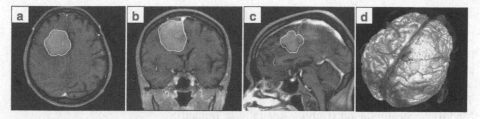

Fig. 2. Processed gadolinium T1 MRI from left to right: axial (a), coronal (b) and sagittal (c) slices showing the manually segmented tumour outline. (d) The 3D view shows the extracted cortical surface, vessels (purple) and segmented tumour (green). (Color figure online)

Visualization. Once the data has gone through the image-processing pipeline we create a 3D model with the cortical surface, extracted vessels and manually segmented brain tumour (i.e. Fig. 2(d)). During surgery, typically only the tumour and sometimes vessel virtual models are used in the AR view. Transparency is used to combine the virtual model with the real world such that the real world image is modulated to show the virtual objects below the surface in the region of interest (Fig. 3(c)). A typical problem with AR is that when transparency alone is used, i.e. the real and virtual objects are just alpha blended, then the virtual object appears to be floating above the real world. Therefore, to improve relative depth perception, we retain edges from the real world camera image (computed using a Sobel filter), so that the virtual object appears below the real world surface (Fig. 3(d)). For more information about our AR visualization the author is referred to [19].

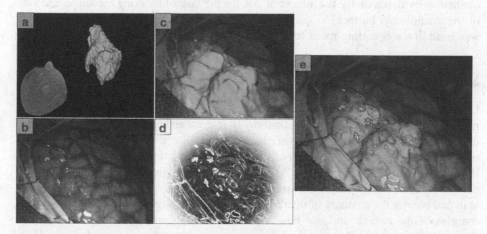

Fig. 3. (a) Segmented tumour and patient avatar. (b) Captured real world image of the cortical surface of a patient. (c) The transparency of the real world image is modulated to show the virtual segmented tumour object below the surface; however, the tumour appears to be coming out of the cortical surface, or possibly floating above it. (d) Edges of the image in (b) are computed using a Sobel filter and retained in the transparent part of the real world image, giving a correct perception of the relative depth between the real and virtual world (e).

3.4   OR Workflow

Camera calibration, image processing and the visualization of the patient-specific preoperative models are done prior to the surgical cases. As well, prior to surgery, patients consent to the use of our research neuronavgiation system, which has been approved by the Montreal Neurological Institute/Hospital Research and Ethics Board. The IBIS system is always brought into the OR in parallel with the commercial Medtronic StealthStation (Dublin, Republic of Ireland).

The system is set-up in the OR prior to the patient being brought in and therefore does not disrupt the OR workflow. The workflow is the same for each surgical case where augmented reality is used. Patient-to-image registration is performed after anaesthetization using the same anatomical landmarks at the same time on both systems (Medtronic and IBIS), in order to minimize disruption. Once the patient is registered the surgeon can use IBIS at any point in time during the surgery, AR visualization is always available and in our current protocol intraoperative ultrasound (iUS) is captured on the dura (to account for brainshift, i.e. the movement of the brain caused by the craniotomy and administrated drugs) both prior to and after resection.

Based on preliminary comments from the surgeons, we found that the task that may benefit most from AR visualization is craniotomy planning and therefore this is the focus of this paper. In this study, we asked the surgeon to use AR on the skin, bone, dura and cortex.

4   Results and Discussion

In the following section we describe the use AR in craniotomy planning, providing qualitative evidence on the usefulness of AR for the task of tailoring the shape and size of the craniotomy. Further, we present examples from three surgical cases where AR was used in the operating room for this task (Table 1).

4.1   Tailoring the Craniotomy

Determining the size and shape of a craniotomy is part of a planning process that takes into account both the location of the anatomy of interest and how the surgeon will access the anatomy through the opening of the skull. Ideally, the surgeon will design an opening that will allow access to all of the pertinent parts of the anatomy but minimize the amount of brain that is exposed. Augmented reality has the potential to facilitate this the task by allowing the surgeon to use "X-ray vision" to look through the surface of the skin and bone at the anatomy of interest. In doing so the surgeon can see the extent and margins of the tumour and use this to (1) plan the opening of the skin and (2) to determine the size and shape of the bone flap to be removed (e.g. Figs. 4, 5 and 6).

Planning the Skin Incision. By tailoring the skin incision to be smaller, there is less chance of infection and fewer stitches that are used, which can result in faster healing times. Of course, depending on the location and the size of the tumour the skin incision will vary in size however, smaller incisions are generally seen as optimal. Using

Table 1. Summary of the registration and calibration reprojection error and use of AR in each of three example cases. We focus on the technical details of the system, rather then the clinical details of the cases.

Case	Registration (RMS)[a]	Calibration error[b]	AR use
1 (Fig. 4)	3.7 mm	0.2 mm	The AR view was checked on the skin and bone after the surgeon traced the outline of the tumour. A good correspondence was found between the tracing and the AR view
2 (Fig. 5)	2.1 mm	0.18 mm	AR was used to trace the tumour on both the skin and cortex. A vessel was visible between the surface and tumour in the AR view that was taken into account during planning
3 (Fig. 6)	5.0 mm	0.2 mm	Due to a poor registration AR was used only after the surgeon traced the tumour using conventional neuronavigation and a discrepancy was seen between AR overlay and marked lines

[a]Patient-to-image fiducial registration error is calculated as root-mean square error on fiducial landmarks used to estimate the patient-to-image registration.
[b]Calibration error is computed as the average reprojection error between 3D points and their 2D projections in the AR display.

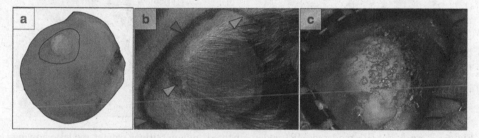

Fig. 4. (a) Case 1: 3D rendered MRI skin surface (from the back, with the patient's neck directed towards the top of the image) and segmented tumour virtual patient model, showing position of patient head and approximate location of the planned craniotomy. (b) In this case the tumour outline indicated by the orange arrow was done using the Medtronic system and checked using AR. There was a good correspondence between the AR view and the outlined tumour. The blue arrow indicates the boundary of the tumour and overlaps with the contour of the planned skin incision. The pink arrow indicates the superior boundary of the planned skin incision. (Color figure online)

augmented reality, the surgeon can trace the extent of the tumour on the skin using a sterile marker and plan as minimal a skin incision as possible.

When a good calibration and initial registration, are achieved, the AR view is deemed accurate and can be used by the surgeon for intraoperative planning. Currently, we access the accuracy of the AR view using the commercial system. In Fig. 4(b) we

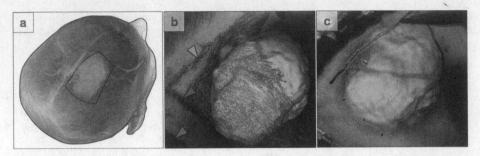

Fig. 5. Case 2: (a) 3D rendered MRI and segmented tumour virtual patient model, showing position of patient head and location of the planned craniotomy. (b) The surgeon uses AR to determine the location and extent of the tumour. The blue arrow indicates the posterior boundary of a bounding box around the tumour and the pink arrow indicates the planned posterior boundary of the craniotomy that will allow resection of the tumour. The orange arrow shows the medial extent of the bounding box around the tumour, which is also the planned craniotomy margin. (c) The surgeon uses the AR view to trace around the tumour (see the felt marker in the top right of the image) in order to determine the size of the bone flap. Note the vessel (in purple) that was visualized in the AR view and was taken into account for the craniotomy. (Color figure online)

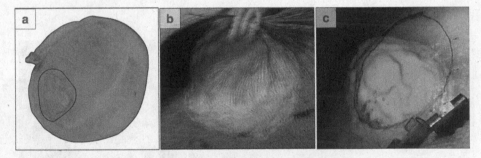

Fig. 6. Case 3: (a) 3D rendered MRI and segmented tumour virtual patient model, showing position of patient head and location of the craniotomy planned. (b) Tumour projected onto the scalp, due to a poor registration results in IBIS the surgeon used traditional the Medtronic system to trace the tumour. (c) A discrepancy can be seen (1–2 cm) between the outlined tumour, which was drawn using the Medtronic system, and the AR overlay given in IBIS.

show a good correspondence between real and virtual elements of the AR view. In Fig. 5(b) we show a case where the surgeon used IBIS AR to define the boundaries of the tumour and then based on this and his plan on how the tumour will be resected, determined the extent of the skin incision. Unfortunately, due to the compounding of errors from tracking, registration and camera calibration, the mapping between real and virtual models is not always accurate. In Fig. 6(b) we given an example of a case where, due to a poor registration result on our research system, the AR overlay is misaligned with the drawn tumour boundary, which was planned using the commercial navigation system.

Planning the Bone Flap to Be Removed. The size and shape of the bone flap to be removed is smaller than the skin incision and is planned to facilitate access to the pertinent anatomy. A surgeon can make use of AR visualization to trace around the points of the virtual tumour in order to determine the location, as well, as the shape and size of the bone flap to be removed. In Fig. 5(c) we see how the surgeon had used dots to outline the tumour and then connects these to create the contour of the tumour on the bone, in order to plan the surgical approach[1]. In this case, the accuracy of the AR overlay was deemed high based on a comparison with the commercial navigation system, which we use as a silver standard. In our third case in which there was a poor initial registration, the misalignment between the overlay and the planned craniotomy using the Medtronic system can be seen on the bone (Fig. 6(c)).

4.2   Other Uses of AR in Tumour Resections

Although in this paper we have focused on using AR for craniotomy planning, we've also explored the use of AR on the dura to plan the dural incision and on the cortex to plan the resection corridor and surgical approach (Fig. 7). By combining iUS that is taken on the dura, and updating the MRI images to account for brain shift and mis-registration errors we can use AR to visualize the preoperative patient images and segmented tumour which have been correctly re-aligned to the reality of the patient [16].

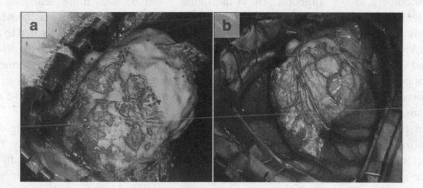

Fig. 7. Augmented reality visualization can be used on the dura (a) to plan the dural incision and on the cortex (b) to plan the resection corridor and surgical approach. This is the same case as in Fig. 5.

4.3   Qualitative Results

Comments from the surgeons suggest that an accurate AR overlay, can be beneficial and facilitate craniotomy planning particularly for smaller lesions. Furthermore, AR overlays can be useful in showing anatomy, such as vessels, in the surgical field of

---

[1] A video of the surgeon using AR in this surgical case can be viewed at: https://www.youtube.com/watch?v=tru4uwQIvyI.

view that may impact the surgical plan (as in Fig. 5(c)) and help facilitate describing the surgical plans and patient anatomy to colleagues, residents and the OR staff. For example, in a case not presented here, a dural vessel inhibited the safe and complete removal of the dura. The AR view allowed for visualization of this vessel on the surface of the dura that in turn allowed for appropriate intraoperative planning and avoidance of a minor bleed during surgery.

We have found that although there is a learning curve to understanding augmented reality visualizations, as a surgeon becomes accustomed to these visualizations they find it can aid in intraoperative surgical planning. Whereas in the first cases we asked the surgeons to use augmented reality at particular points in surgery, in later cases, the surgeon (who had used AR the most) asked to see the AR visualizations at different points in surgery and suggested when and how it could be most useful.

5 Conclusions and Future Work

In this preliminary study we have looked at the possible benefit of using augmented reality in craniotomy planning for tumour resections. Our initial results suggest that with a good initial alignment between patient models and the real world, AR visualization of the tumour and vessels below the surface is useful in planning a craniotomy that may minimize the exposure of the brain.

According to the surgeons, AR visualization could be even more beneficial for smaller lesions where it may not be as evident how small the craniotomy may be while still allowing access for resection. The usefulness of this system is intimately tied to the accuracy of the AR visualization, which can vary widely by case. In order for widespread use of this technique more stable initial accuracy will be pivotal. Furthermore, the impact of the perception of the depth of the tumour in the AR view needs to be explored. In order to ensure an accurate overlay, in the future, we will explore the use of transcranial US to account for initial patient-to-image misregistration errors.

In future work, we propose to quantitatively determine the effect of using AR visualization on the size and shape of a planned craniotomy in a prospective study. In a recent study by Mahvash et al. [20], which compared craniotomy planning with no image-guidance to planning with guidance, the authors showed that all ten neurosurgeons in the study changed the craniotomy localization and skin incision initially planned with no guidance when image-guided tumour visualization was shown. Furthermore, the size of the craniotomy was significantly larger ($p < 0.035$) when no image-guidance was used. We would expect even more significant results with the use of reliable and accurate AR. One can imagine doing a similar study in which a surgeon first plans the craniotomy using traditional image-guidance and is then shown the AR view. We posit that the craniotomy plan would change to be smaller with this type of visualization.

In order to improve the surgical workflow, we plan to expand IBIS to allow for AR on a tablet device for in-situ visualization. This will obviate the need for the surgeon to look away from the operating field to the neuronavigation system and the visualization to be in front of the surgeon and above the patient, facilitating the marking of lesion boundaries and surgical plans on the surface of the patient.

Augmented reality visualization offers a promising avenue of research that has the potential to improve surgical workflows and further minimize the invasiveness of neurosurgery.

References

1. Kersten-Oertel, M., Jannin, P., Collins, D.L.: The state of the art of visualization in mixed reality image guided surgery. Comput. Med. Imaging Graph. **37**, 98–112 (2013)
2. Kersten-Oertel, M., Gerard, I., Drouin, S., Mok, K., Sirhan, D., Sinclair, D.S., Collins, D.L.: Augmented reality in neurovascular surgery: feasibility and first uses in the operating room. Int. J. Comput. Assist. Radiol. Surg. **10**(11), 1823–1836 (2015)
3. Kersten-Oertel, M., Gerard, I.J., Drouin, S., Mok, K., Sirhan, D., Sinclair, D.S., Collins, D.L.: Augmented reality for specific neurovascular surgical tasks. In: Linte, C.A., Yaniv, Z., Fallavollita, P. (eds.) AE-CAI 2011. LNCS, vol. 9365, pp. 92–103. Springer, Heidelberg (2015)
4. Gleason, P.L., Kikinis, R., Altobelli, D., Wells, W., Alexander III, E., Black, P.M., Jolesz, F.: Video registration virtual reality for nonlinkage stereotactic surgery. Stereotact. Funct. Neurosurg. **63**, 139–143 (1994)
5. Edwards, P., Hawkes, D., Hill, D., Jewell, D., Spink, R., Strong, A., Gleeson, M.: Augmentation of reality using an operating microscope for otolaryngology and neurosurgical guidance. J. Image Guid. Surg. **1**, 172–178 (1995)
6. Edwards, P.J., King, A.P., Hawkes, D.J., Fleig, O., Maurer Jr., C.R., Hill, D.L., Fenlon, M.R., de Cunha, D.A., Gaston, R.P., Chandra, S., Mannss, J., Strong, A.J., Gleeson, M.J., Cox, T.C.: Stereo augmented reality in the surgical microscope. Stud. Health Technol. Inform. **62**, 102–108 (1999)
7. Birkfellner, W., Figl, M., Matula, C., Hummel, J., Hanel, R., Imhof, H., Wanschitz, F., Wagner, A., Watzinger, F., Bergmann, H.: Computer-enhanced stereoscopic vision in a head-mounted operating binocular. Phys. Med. Biol. **48**, N49–N57 (2003)
8. Birkfellner, W., Figl, M., Huber, K., Watzinger, F., Wanschitz, F., Hummel, J., Hanel, R., Greimel, W., Homolka, P., Ewers, R., Bergmann, H.: A head-mounted operating binocular for augmented reality visualization in medicine - design and initial evaluation. IEEE Trans. Med. Imaging **21**, 991–997 (2002)
9. Sauer, F., Khamene, A., Bascle, B., Rubino, G.J.: A head-mounted display system for augmented reality image guidance: towards clinical evaluation for iMRI-guided neurosurgery. In: Niessen, W.J., Viergever, M.A. (eds.) MICCAI 2001. LNCS, vol. 2208, pp. 707–716. Springer, Heidelberg (2001)
10. Cabrilo, I., Bijlenga, P., Schaller, K.: Augmented reality in the surgery of cerebral arteriovenous malformations: technique assessment and considerations. Acta Neurochir. (Wien) **156**, 1769–1774 (2014)
11. Cabrilo, I., Bijlenga, P., Schaller, K.: Augmented reality in the surgery of cerebral aneurysms: a technical report. Neurosurgery **10**(Suppl. 2), 252–260 (2014). Discussion 260-1
12. Mahvash, M., Besharati Tabrizi, L.: A novel augmented reality system of image projection for image-guided neurosurgery. Acta Neurochir. (Wien) **155**, 943–947 (2013)
13. Meola, A., Cutolo, F., Carbone, M., Cagnazzo, F., Ferrari, M., Ferrari, V.: Augmented reality in neurosurgery: a systematic review. Neurosurg. Rev. 1–12 (2016). [epub ahead of print]

14. Mercier, L., Del Maestro, R.F., Petrecca, K., Kochanowska, A., Drouin, S., Yan, C.X., Janke, A.L., Chen, S.J., Collins, D.L.: New prototype neuronavigation system based on preoperative imaging and intraoperative freehand ultrasound: system description and validation. Int. J. Comput. Assist. Radiol. Surg. **6**, 507–522 (2011)
15. Kersten-Oertel, M., Gerard, I., Drouin, S., Mok, K., Sirhan, D., Sinclair, D., Collins, D.: Augmented reality in neurovascular surgery: first experiences. In: Linte, C.A., Yaniv, Z., Fallavollita, P., Abolmaesumi, P., Holmes III, D.R. (eds.) AE-CAI 2014. LNCS, vol. 8678, pp. 80–89. Springer, Heidelberg (2014)
16. Gerard, I.J., Kersten-Oertel, M., Drouin, S., Hall, J.A., Petrecca, K., De Nigris, D., Arbel, T., Louis Collins, D.: Improving patient specific neurosurgical models with intraoperative ultrasound and augmented reality visualizations in a neuronavigation environment. In: Oyarzun Laura, C., et al. (eds.) CLIP 2015. LNCS, vol. 9401, pp. 28–35. Springer, Heidelberg (2016). doi:10.1007/978-3-319-31808-0_4
17. Zhang, Z.: A flexible new technique for camera calibration. IEEE Trans. Pattern Anal. Mach. Intell. **22**, 1330–1334 (2000)
18. Gerard, I.J., Collins, D.L.: An analysis of tracking error in image-guided neurosurgery. Int. J. Comput. Assist. Radiol. Surg. **10**, 1579–1588 (2015)
19. Kersten-Oertel, M., Gerard, I., Drouin, S., Mok, K., Sirhan, D., Sinclair, D., Collins, D.L.: Augmented reality in neurovascular surgery: feasibility and first uses in the operating room. Int. J. Comput. Assist. Radiol. Surg. **10**, 1–14 (2015)
20. Mahvash, M., Boettcher, I., Petridis, A.K., Besharati Tabrizi, L.: Image guided versus conventional brain tumor and craniotomy localization. J Neurosurg Sci. (2015). http://europepmc.org/abstract/med/25600554, PMID:25600554

Augmenting Scintigraphy Images with Pinhole Aligned Endoscopic Cameras: A Feasibility Study

Peter A. von Niederhäusern[1]([✉]), Ole C. Maas[2], Michael Rissi[3],
Matthias Schneebeli[3], Stephan Haerle[1], and Philippe C. Cattin[1]

[1] Department of Biomedical Engineering, University of Basel,
Basel, Switzerland
{peter.vonniederhaeusern,stephan.haerle,philippe.cattin}@unibas.ch
[2] Radiology and Nuclear Medicine Clinic, University Hospital of Basel,
Basel, Switzerland
[3] DECTRIS Ltd., 5405 Baden, Switzerland

Abstract. Morbidity of cancer is still high and this is especially true for squamous cell carcinoma in the oral cavity and oropharynx which is one of the most widespread cancers worldwide. To avoid spreading of the tumor, often the lymphatic tissue of the neck is removed together with the tumor. Such neck dissections are inherently dangerous for the patient and only required in roughly 30 % of the patients as has been shown by studies. To prevent overtreatments, sentinel lymph node biopsy is used where the first lymph node after the tumor is probed for cancerous cells. The lymphatic tissue is then only completely removed when tumor cells are found. This sentinel node is localized by means of detecting a radioactive tracer that is injected near the tumor. Its uptake is then measured and observed. State-of-the-art support for the specialist is a 1-dimensional audio-based gamma detection unit which makes it challenging to detect and excise the true sentinel lymph node for an effective histologic examination and therefore correct staging.

This feasibility study presents the working principles and preliminary results of a scintigraphy device that is supported by augmented reality to aid the surgeon performing sentinel lymph node biopsy. Advances in detector- and sensor technology enable this leap forward for this type of intervention. We developed and tested a small-form multi-pinhole collimator with axis-aligned endoscopic cameras. As these cameras and the pinholes provide the same projective geometry, the augmentation of the gamma images of tracer enriched lymph nodes with optical images of the intervention site can be easily done, all without the need for a 3D depth map or synthetic model of the surgical scene.

Keywords: Scintigraphy · Sentinel lymph node biopsy · Radioguided surgery · Augmented reality · Field of view · Projective geometry

1 Introduction

Cancer is one of the main causes of death worldwide. In the case of head and neck squamous cell carcinoma (HNSCC) the correct staging includes the careful

© Springer International Publishing Switzerland 2016
G. Zheng et al. (Eds.): MIAR 2016, LNCS 9805, pp. 175–185, 2016.
DOI: 10.1007/978-3-319-43775-0_16

examination of the nearby lymphatic system. As the current clinical and radiological assessment procedures are limited in their accuracy [1], many specialized centers still focus solely on the complete removal of all lymph nodes in the head-and neck area [2]. This procedure is called elective neck dissection (END) and is often not necessary and harbors the risk to damage the complex intricate nervous and lymphatic systems near the intervention site [3]. An alternative is sentinel lymph node biopsy (SLNB), often used in breast cancer surgery and melanoma, which is a minimal invasive standard staging procedure based on radioactive tracers (*i.e.* 99m technetium; 99Tc). It has also been successfully applied for selected head and neck tumors and is the most accurate histologic staging procedure with the highest success rate [4–6]. The goal of SLNB is to examine the first draining lymph node after a tumor site. This sentinel lymph node (SLN) is most likely the first to receive metastases [7]. If the SLN is tumor free, no END needs to be carried out and the specialist speaks of a "clinically negative neck" (cN0-neck). It is therefore of utmost importance that SLNB be as accurate as possible in order to correctly stage the malignancy in the subsequent histopathologic work-up of the excised lymph nodes.

Current preoperative HNSCC assessment is performed using either lymphoscintigraphy (LS) or more recently single photon emission tomography (SPECT) combined with computed tomography (CT). Thanks to the integration of SPECT/CT into the procedure a higher spatial resolution and therefore a better anatomical orientation is achieved compared to the classical LS alone. SPECT/CT is nowadays considered the standard method for preoperative imaging before any SLNB [2]. During an SLNB procedure the specialist is guided by a handheld 1-dimensional audio-based gamma detection probe (HGDP) indicating activity of the radioactive tracer in the lymphatic system. For the intervention to be effective, the surgeon relies on the SPECT/CT images from the preoperative assessment. As not only the target node (5 mm–10 mm in diameter) is infiltrated and made visible by the tracer, the identification proves to be especially challenging. This is accentuated where there are no prominent visible anatomic landmarks. The general consensus is that the lymph node with the highest noise-to-background ratio in gamma radiation is the true SLN. Therefore, the need for more sophisticated imaging devices and better data visualization arises given these intricacies of SLNB.

The company SurgicEye[1] sells a commercially available system based on freehand SPECT (fhSPECT) that solves some of the aforementioned problems of SLNB. Freehand SPECT depends on a preparation step needed to register the gamma probe with the patient followed by gamma activity acquisition in order to build a correct synthetic 3D model of the tumor and its location. This model is then used to produce the augmentation of the surgical scene, displayed on an external screen. After each tissue removal, the model needs to be updated by a consecutive gamma activity acquisition in order to correct the augmentation [8].

---

[1] http://www.surgiceye.com/en/declipseSPECT/openSurgery.html.

The research group of Prof. Dr. Nassir Navab from the TU in Munich has a strong background in augmented reality (AR) for radioguided surgery in general and sentinel lymph node biopsy in particular.

The approach of fhSPECT was developed by these researchers [9]. One of their recently published review articles compares clinical applications of 3D scintigraphic imaging (fhSPECT) and navigation in radioguided surgery [10].

An overview of the current technologies, different modalities, devices, tools and staging procedures to treat each type of malignancy is also provided by the IAEA's Guided Intraoperative Scintigraphic Tumour Targeting (GOSTT) [2] report.

The *aim* of this research project is to develop an advanced mobile hand-held scintigraphy unit with AR capabilities (Fig. 1). This unit fuses or augments directly gamma activity images with optical images of the incision for better localization and identification of tracer enriched lymph nodes during SLNB. These augmented images are then displayed on a tablet computer or similar device attached to the unit. To the best of our knowledge, such an intraoperative AR representation of the surgical scene of an SLNB intervention is unique. The presented preliminary results show the potential of our concept.

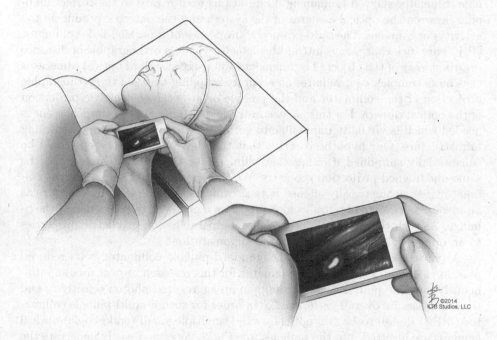

Fig. 1. Artistic rendering of an intraoperative setup of the mobile hand-held scintigraphy unit (*e.g.* tablet computer). The collimator and its endoscopic cameras on the back of the unit are pointing towards the patient. A live view of the patient's tracer enriched SLN, overlaid on top of the incision, is presented to the surgeon on the display.

---

[2] http://www-pub.iaea.org/books/IAEABooks/10661/Guided-Intraoperative-Scintig-raphic-Tumour-Targeting-GOSTT

2   Materials and Methods

In this study, we used endoscopic cameras NanEye[3] that measure only 1 mm × 1 mm × 1.7 mm in width, depth and height, respectively. Their pixel resolution is 250 × 250 pixels with a pixel size of 3 μm × 3 μm and thus an aspect ratio of 1:1. The effective focal length is 660 μm. The built-in optics are fisheye-based lenses with an f-number of 2.7, an aperture of 244 μm and a depth of focus between 8 mm–75 mm.

Our industrial collaborator DECTRIS[4] provided us with a gamma detector prototype with a native resolution of 487 × 195 pixels and a pixel size of 172 μm × 172 μm. DECTRIS' detector technology is based on Hybrid Photon Counting (HPC) and cadmium telluride (CdTe) sensor material. Furthermore, a Linux PC based data processing unit as well as the necessary software packages to operate the detector were part of their contribution.

To effectively detect high energy photon (γ-ray) sources and to be able to correctly map the tracer enriched target tissue, a γ-detector also depends on a particular collimator design. In a preliminary study [11], the used parallel-hole collimator showed fundamental limitations with regard to the correct mapping between the optical cameras of the system and the detector producing the activity- or γ-image. The opto-geometric properties of a parallel-hole collimator (PHC) are such that γ-rays hitting the detector yield an orthographic or distance invariant view of the object. The augmentation using standard optical cameras is thus more complex as it requires an accurate mapping between the orthographic projection of the collimator and the pinhole or projective geometric projection of the optical camera. For this, an accurate 3D depth map of the surgical scene is needed which is virtually impossible to get in the OR, without using a tracking infrastructure. Our hypothesis states that the above mentioned steps could be substantially simplified if either the collimator or the optical camera had the same and aligned projection geometry. We thus propose on using a pinhole collimator with geometrically aligned optical cameras. A pinhole collimator acts as an idealized "camera obscura" which produces a perspective projection of the γ-image. As such the pinhole approach has comparable opto-geometric properties to an optical camera simplifying image augmentation.

A particular disadvantage of the standard pinhole collimator is its reduced photon yield. Our custom built collimator for this research project uses simultaneously multiple pinholes which results in an aggregated photon sensitivity and thus increases its overall performance. In order for such a multi-pinhole collimator (MPC) design to be still optically valid, multiple small (endoscopic) optical cameras are inserted into the pinholes, see Fig. 2. As γ-rays easily penetrate the relatively small cameras, no significant attenuation is to be expected. The overlap of the field of view of the endoscopic cameras will in the future be exploited by stitching algorithms to present a unified image. The optical parameters of the endoscopic cameras are such that their diagonal field of view (FOV) is 90°,

---

[3] http://www.cmosis.com/products/product_detail/naneye_module.
[4] DECTRIS Ltd., 5405 Baden, Switzerland.

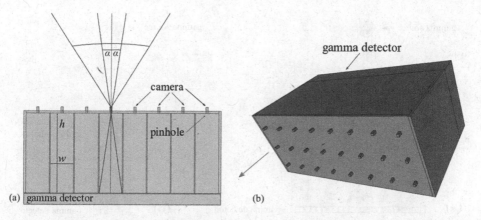

Fig. 2. (a) Pinhole compartment of a multi-pinhole collimator with its field of view (FOV, $2 \times \alpha$), given the specific geometric properties. The FOV of a miniature camera is drawn in comparison. (b) Rendering of the used camera placement layout with respect to the pinholes of the collimator. The endoscopic optical cameras are 1 mm × 1 mm in length, width and 1.7 mm in height. The collimator has dimensions 85.9 mm × 36 mm × 36 mm, pointing towards the surgical scene (arrow).

which corresponds to a vertical and horizontal FOV of approx. 71°, given an aspect ration of 1:1. The half-angle α of the FOV of an idealized pinhole camera thus given by

$$\tan(\alpha) = \frac{w}{2} \times \frac{1}{h}$$

where w denotes the width and h the height of the pinhole compartment. This model is adequate for the envisioned solution to combine the two modalities (*i.e.* γ- and optical images), see Fig. 2a.

The septae (vertical compartment separations along h) and the front- and side plates need to be thick enough in order to absorb γ-rays which do not pass through the pinholes. This avoids the generation of an unwanted background signal on the actual detector. Our calculations suggest a thickness of 1 mm for the front- and side plates and a thickness of 0.25 mm for the septae. As such only 5 % of the emitted photons are able to penetrate the shielding. Lead and Tungsten are standard materials in nuclear medicine to build collimators [12]. Tungsten has very good mechanical properties and a high specific density of 19.25 g/cm³ and is thus used for our collimator. The assembled multi-pinhole collimator and the cameras are shown in Fig. 2b.

The basic workflow and the specific challenges to combine a PHC produced γ-image with an optical camera image shall be presented qualitatively in Fig. 3. The two gamma sources shown in the image (originating from *i.e.* two neighboring lymph nodes) are mapped on-top of each other in the orthographic projection of the PHC. As they do not share the same depth in the tissue, the detected gamma activity should be split in two in the optical cameras looking from one side. This, however, can only be resolved with accurate depth information of the tracer activity which is not available (Fig. 3a).

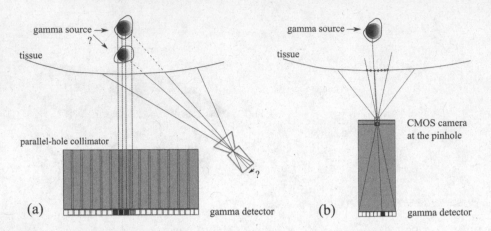

Fig. 3. (a) Optical camera with its view cone, perspective projection. Parallel-hole collimator, orthographic (parallel) projection. The two γ-sources are at an unknown depth which cannot be measured. (b) Our approach: both view cones of the camera and the pinhole overlap symmetrically. An incident γ-ray is seen by the detector under the same viewing angle as the corresponding object point seen by the camera. No depth information is needed for the augmentation.

Our approach is based on the hypothesis that similar opto-geometric properties of pinhole modeled cameras yield similar or identical projections. Any detection of an incident γ-ray on the MPC detector belongs to the same homogeneous trace as the corresponding pixel on the optical image (Fig. 3b). As long as both viewing axes are properly aligned, and hence there is a symmetric overlap of the FOV of the pinhole and the optical camera, the activity and the pixels are correlated and provide a correct registration. *A priori* depth information is therefore not needed.

To test and verify our assumption on fusing the two modalities, we set up an experiment consisting of a vial filled with 0.1 ml of metastable technetium (99Tc). The liquid in the tip of the inner tube served as an idealized point source with a radioactivity of 15 MBq. This technetium isotope is a standard tracer for SPECT/CT and LS and is therefore routinely used in the domain of nuclear medicine. The vial was then placed at specific distances (*i.e.* 3 cm, 5 cm, 7 cm) from the combined γ-detector/camera unit and observed using different exposure times (Fig. 4). The distances where chosen such that they correspond to the expected distance from the device to the surgical site (neck of patient).

In this experiment *one* endoscopic camera/pinhole pair was used to present the working principle. The camera was calibrated in a separate step using Zhang's algorithms [13] and a chessboard pattern to obtain its intrinsic and extrinsic parameters. The intrinsic parameters of an optical camera need to be known in order to compensate for lens distortions and to obtain the principal point. The principal point is at the center of the projection of the image and often offset with respect to the optical axis due to imperfections in the alignment between the camera chip and the optics.

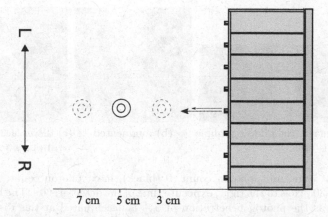

Fig. 4. Setup of the experiment on.the workbench, as seen from above. The vial is placed at a distance of 5 cm and roughly aligned with an endoscopic camera, which is slightly offset to the axis of the pinhole (smaller arrow), due to manual placement. Other measured distances are also indicated (dashed circles). The photon acquisition time for each position is 30 s and 60 s, respectively.

The pinhole image patch, as it is acquired through the ideal camera model of the pinhole, does not suffer from distortion or shifts and can serve as ground truth orientation for the scintigraphy device. Therefore, the center of the pinhole image patch can be further used to fine tune the alignment of both images. As the point sources (vials, Fig. 4) and the optical camera were manually placed and inserted, offsets between both images are inevitable and need to be corrected by the algorithm. Currently, each off-line augmentation or fusion uses a specific offset correction factor.

Implementation. A basic off-line image overlay algorithm is used to translate an image patch $\mathbf{P_n}$ of $pinhole_n$ from the γ-detector to the principal point of the optical image $\mathbf{I_n}$ of the corresponding $camera_n$. $\mathbf{P_n}$ has size 60×64 pixels, $\mathbf{I_n}$ has size 250×250 pixels. As the pinhole characteristics are such that the pinhole image $\mathbf{P_n}$ is mirrored, a rotation of $180°$ around its center needs to be applied. Let $\mathbf{t}$ be the translation vector $:= principalPoint(\mathbf{I_n}) - \mathbf{P_n}/2$ and $\mathbf{R}$ the rotation matrix, we obtain for every pixel $\mathbf{p}$ of $\mathbf{P_n}$

$$\mathbf{p'} = \mathbf{t} + \mathbf{R} * \mathbf{p}$$

where $\mathbf{p'}$ indicates an activity in the coordinate system of $\mathbf{I_n}$. Correction factors $s * e_x, s * e_y$ can be added to $\mathbf{t}$ to visually align the activity image in case of slight offsets. For every $\mathbf{p'}$ its activity value is evaluated by a hard-coded color look-up table. The augmentation is thus $\mathbf{I_n}(\mathbf{p'}) = color(\mathbf{p'})$.

3   Results

The following image series (Figs. 5, 6, 7, 8) show the augmentation or fusion of an optical image with the corresponding γ-image. The distances from the detector

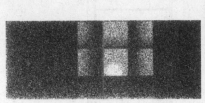
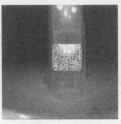

(a) activity image, the middle pinhole image patch is used   (b) augmented   (c) thresholded, median filtered with a 3 × 3 kernel

Fig. 5. Vial at 3 cm, min. photon count: 0 (black), max. photon count: 21 (white), pinhole offset: 30 pixels to the right, exposure time of the detector: 60 s. The background signal is high as the photon penetration of 5 % is accentuated at this distance. The pinhole cannot fully capture the source as it is partially out of its view cone.

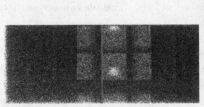
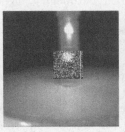
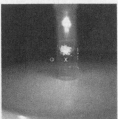

(a) activity image, the middle pinhole image patch is used   (b) augmented   (c) thresholded, median filtered with a 3 × 3 kernel

Fig. 6. Vial at 5 cm, min. photon count: 0 (black), max. photon count: 19 (white), pinhole offset: 30 pixels to the right, exposure time of the detector: 60 s. With increasing distance, less unwanted photons hit the shielding and thus their absorption probability is higher. The source is now completely in the view cone.

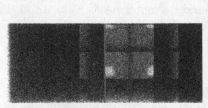
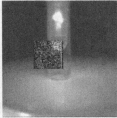
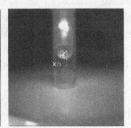

(a) activity image, the middle pinhole image patch is used   (b) augmented   (c) thresholded, median filtered with a 3 × 3 kernel

Fig. 7. Vial at 5 cm, min. photon count: 0 (black), max. photon count: 16 (white), pinhole offset: -10 pixels to the left, exposure time of the detector: 30 s. The pinhole cannot fully capture the source as it is partially out of its view cone.

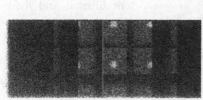
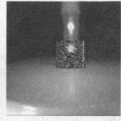

(a) activity image, the middle pinhole image patch is used   (b) augmented   (c) thresholded, median filtered with a 3 × 3 kernel

Fig. 8. Vial at 7 cm, min. photon count: 0 (black), max. photon count: 14 (white), pinhole offset: 30 pixels to the right, exposure time of the detector: 60 s. At larger distances the other pinholes also begin to capture the source, given the opening angles of their view cone.

to the vial are given, following the experimental setup according to Fig. 4. The same middle pinhole/camera pair was used throughout the experiments.

Each experiment was done with the same radioactive source of approx. 15 MBq, measured at the start of the first experiment. The fusion algorithm presented in the Implementation Section was applied. The images to the right (c) show the principal point (white circle) as well as the pinhole center (white x). The difference is the offset applied to match the activity pixels $\mathbf{p}'$ with the vial inner tube where the tracer (99m technetium; 99Tc) liquid is stored. No scaling of either image is applied. The γ-detector has some defective cells (middle gray column, a). Specific observations are given for each augmentation run.

4   Discussion and Conclusion

First tests with our device show promising results. Our hypothesis of using a multi-pinhole based collimator with axis-aligned endoscopic cameras can explain the good spatial matching of the γ-activity images with the corresponding optical images. This can be seen in the Results section. However, the background signal at short distances is considerably high and challenges image segmentation to properly display SLNs. Further, the augmentation depends on a proper axis alignment between pinhole and camera. Compared to the state-of-the-art, the image quality of the endoscopic cameras for the envisioned operating distances is at least as good as with normal cameras for capturing the patient's neck, given sufficient illumination is provided. The sensitivity of the gamma detector is superior in terms of photon conversion rate as what is currently available on the market. This particular combination makes it possible to provide a system that meets the criteria to advance SLNB in a truly AR fashion.

Current limiting factors of sentinel lymph node biopsy are its strong dependence on accurate preoperative imaging modalities and the crude orientation provided by 1-dimensional audio-based gamma detectors for the localization of sentinel lymph nodes. The augmentation of the gamma activity of the tracer enriched lymph nodes with the optical images of the surgical scene, as presented in this feasibility study, helps the surgeon to better orient himself and focus the biopsy towards the relevant regions of the intervention site. A more targeted biopsy enables a more reliable post-operative histopathologic staging and therefore a more effective analysis of potential cancerous tissue. Breast cancer and melanoma staging based on SLNB face similar challenges. Our approach is therefore also applicable in these domains and could provide a step forward for sentinel lymph node biopsy in general.

Next development steps of the project focus on building an improved collimator shielding to better constrain unwanted photons to reduce the background signal. Furthermore, clustering and stitching algorithms need to be developed in order to take advantage of the multiple pinhole configuration and the endoscopic camera array to improve the capturing process of the gamma activity as well as the incision. To correct for any axis misalignments between the harboring pinholes and their cameras, we envision a calibration scheme to further improve the augmentation process. A chessboard patterned object combined with a weak radioactive source and radioactive transparent corner points could be used to establish a correct point-to-point correspondence between the optical cameras and the γ-detector. The vision to provide a truly mobile hand-held device, as shown in Fig. 1, lastly needs integration of the crucial hardware parts into a relatively small form factor.

References

1. Abdul-Rasool, S., Kidson, S.H., Panieri, E., Dent, D., Pillay, K., Hanekom, G.S.: An evaluation of molecular markers for improved detection of breast cancer metastases in sentinel nodes. J. Clin. Pathol. **59**(3), 289–297 (2006)
2. Haerle, S.K., Stoeckli, S.J.: SPECT/CT for lymphatic mapping of sentinel nodes in early squamous cell carcinoma of the oral cavity and oropharynx. Int. J. Mol. Imaging **2011**, 106068 (2011)
3. Kowalski, L.P., Sanabria, A.: Elective neck dissection in oral carcinoma: a critical review of the evidence. Acta otorhinolaryngologica Italica : organo ufficiale della Società italiana di otorinolaringologia e chirurgia cervico-facciale **27**(3), 113–117 (2007)
4. Husarik, D.B., Steinert, H.C.: Single-photon emission computed tomography/ computed tomographyfor sentinel node mapping in breast cancer. Semin. Nucl. Med. **37**(1), 29–33 (2007)
5. Keski-Säntti, H., Mätzke, S., Kauppinen, T., Törnwall, J., Atula, T.: Sentinel lymph node mapping using SPECT-CT fusion imaging in patients with oral cavity squamous cell carcinoma. Eur. Arch. Oto-Rhino-laryngol.: Official J. Eur. Fed. Oto-Rhino-Laryngol. Soc. (EUFOS): Affiliated Ger. Soc. Oto-Rhino-Laryngol. - Head Neck Surg. **263**(11), 1008–1012 (2006)
6. Haerle, S.K., Hany, T.F., Strobel, K., Sidler, D., Stoeckli, S.J.: Is there an additional value of SPECT/CT over planar lymphoscintigraphy for sentinel node mapping in oral/oropharyngeal squamous cell carcinoma? Ann. Surg. Oncol. **16**(11), 3118–3124 (2009)
7. Sobin, L., Wittekind, C.: International Union Against Cancer: TNM Classification of Malignant Tumours, 6th edn. Wiley, Hoboken (2002)

8. Okur, A., Ahmadi, S.A., Bigdelou, A., Wendler, T., Navab, N.: MR in OR: first analysis of AR/VR visualization in 100 intra-operative Freehand SPECT acquisitions. In: 10th IEEE International Symposium on Mixed and Augmented Reality, ISMAR 2011, pp. 211–218 (2011)
9. Wendler, T., Herrmann, K., Schnelzer, A., Lasser, T., Traub, J., Kutter, O., Ehlerding, A., Scheidhauer, K., Schuster, T., Kiechle, M., Schwaiger, M., Navab, N., Ziegler, S.I., Buck, A.K.: First demonstration of 3-D lymphatic mapping in breast cancer using freehand SPECT. Eur. J. Nucl. Med. Mol. Imaging 37(8), 1452–1461 (2010)
10. Bluemel, C., Matthies, P., Herrmann, K., Povoski, S.P.: 3D scintigraphic imaging and navigation in radioguided surgery: freehand SPECT technology and its clinical applications. Expert Rev. Med. Devices 13(4), 339–351 (2016)
11. Kistler, B.: Master Thesis: Augmented Reality for Radio-guided Surgery (2015)
12. Azazrm, A., Gharapapagh, E., Islamian, J., Mahmoudian, B.: Advances in pinhole and multi-pinhole collimators for single photon emission computed tomography imaging. World J. Nucl. Med. 14(1), 3 (2015)
13. Zhang, Z.: A flexible new technique for camera calibration. IEEE Trans. Pattern Anal. Mach. Intell. 22(11), 1330–1334 (2000)

Tactile Augmented Reality for Arteries Palpation in Open Surgery Training

Sara Condino[1], Rosanna Maria Viglialoro[1(✉)], Simone Fani[2],
Matteo Bianchi[2,3], Luca Morelli[1], Mauro Ferrari[1,5], Antonio Bicchi[2,3],
and Vincenzo Ferrari[1,4,5]

[1] EndoCAS Center, Department of Translational Research and New
Technologies in Medicine and Surgery, University of Pisa, Pisa, Italy
{sara.condino,rosanna.viglialoro,vincenzo.
ferrari}@endocas.org,
{luca.morelli,mauro.ferrari}@med.unipi.it
[2] Research Center "E.Piaggio" Faculty of Engineering,
University of Pisa, Pisa, Italy
simonefani89@gmail.com, {matteo.bianchi,
antonio.bicchi}@centropiaggio.unipi.it
[3] Department of Advanced Robotics, Istituto Italiano di Tecnologia, Genoa, Italy
[4] Department of Engineering Information, University of Pisa, Pisa, Italy
[5] Vascular Surgery Unit, Cisanello University Hospital AOUP, Pisa, Italy

Abstract. Palpation is an essential step of several open surgical procedures for locating arteries by arterial pulse detection. In this context, surgical simulation would ideally provide realistic haptic sensations to the operator. This paper presents a proof of concept implementation of tactile augmented reality for open-surgery training. The system is based on the integration of a wearable tactile device into an augmented physical simulator which allows the real time tracking of artery reproductions and the user finger and provides pulse feedback during palpation. Preliminary qualitative test showed a general consensus among surgeons regarding the realism of the arterial pulse feedback and the usefulness of tactile augmented reality in open-surgery simulators.

1 Introduction

In open surgery, surgeons rely heavily on haptics, including kinesthetic (force) and cutaneous (tactile) feedback, e.g. when palpating tissue to distinguish healthy from diseased and to localize hidden anatomical structures [1]. The haptic feedback can enable the identification of anatomical landmarks such as muscle, bones and blood vessels [2]. For all this reasons, the haptic sense plays a paramount role in many surgical procedures allowing the surgeon to avoid damages to healthy tissues and/or unintentional perforations/ruptures of blood vessels and life-threatening exsanguination. In particular, palpation is an essential step of several surgical procedures for locating arteries, hidden beneath tissues, by arterial pulse detection. Surgical simulation would ideally provide realistic haptic sensations to the operator. At the current time, arterial palpation is mostly neglected in medical training simulators, with the exception of very specialized simulators [3]. These latter can be grouped into three main classes: physical

G. Zheng et al. (Eds.): MIAR 2016, LNCS 9805, pp. 186–197, 2016.
DOI: 10.1007/978-3-319-43775-0_17

simulators such as life-sized anatomical human models (i.e. SimMan® by Laerdal, HPS by CAE) with simulated feel able arterial pulse (i.e. carotid, femoral and brachial pulse), virtual simulators with haptic interfaces for simulation of pulse palpation in a virtual environment [3, 4], hybrid simulators with a physical replica of a pulsating arterial vessel and augmented reality functionalities (i.e. to improve the simulation realism by adding a "virtual jet" of blood in case of a possible needle insertion after pulse palpation) [5, 6]. Examples of implementing a pulse simulator include: using an hydraulic interface (with an hydraulic pump to inflate a tube) to provide a physical replica of a pulsating vessel [5, 6]; using the acoustic Radiation Pressure (ARP) phenomena generated by focusing multiple ultrasonic transducers to create perceivable vibrations trough an haptic interface [7, 8]; integrating different tactile devices, based on a piezoelectric pads, a micro speakers, or a pin array, into a commercial force feedback device (Falcon by Novint Technologies, Inc.) [4]. In this work we propose a tactile augmented reality system for open-surgery simulation. The main idea is to merge benefits of haptic feedback in surgical training with those offered by an augmented physical simulator comprising high-fidelity physical models of the human anatomy and augmented reality functionalities. This paper presents a proof-of-concept implementation of the afore-mentioned approach for the simulation of artery pulse palpation. The system is based on the integration of a wearable haptic device into an augmented physical simulation platform allowing the real time tracking and augmented reality visualization of deformable tubular structures [9, 10]. In particular, we propose a method to accurately track the arterial replicas and the user finger [11] and to provide pulse feedback during palpation through a wearable haptic device. As detailed in the following paragraphs, we have chosen cholecystectomy simulation for the preliminary demonstration of the proposed concept. During this surgical procedure, pulse palpation is an essential step for the recognition of the cystic and right hepatic artery.

2 Materials and Methods

The following paragraphs briefly describes the augmented physical simulation platform and the haptic interface used for the proof of concept demonstration of the tactile augmented reality concept.

2.1 Augmented Reality Simulator (AR-Sim) for Laparoscopic Cholecystectomy

The AR-Sim, is an augmented physical simulator to train some important steps of the cholecystectomy procedure: the exposition of gallbladder, and the exposition/dissection of Calot's triangle (Fig. 1).

This latter, which is the most challenging step of the entire procedure, requires a meticulous dissection of the Calot's triangle contents [12] for a proper ligation and division of the cystic artery and cystic duct. The simulation platform comprises: realistic physical replicas of the involved anatomical structures, an electromagnetic (EM) tracking system, an optical calibration-acquisition system, and a laptop.

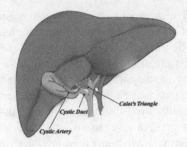

Fig. 1. Anatomy of Calot's triangle.

In particularly the AR-Sim includes patient-specific physical replicas of: liver, gall-bladder, pancreas, abdominal aorta, stomach, duodenum (fabricated as described in [9, 10]) and realistic physical replicas of biliary ducts, arterial tree and connective tissue (fabricated as described in [9, 10]). All the anatomical replicas match the shape, geometry and consistency of real human organs to enable a realistic interaction between the surgical tools/surgeon hand and the simulated anatomy (Fig. 2). The biliary ducts and arterial tree are sensorized with EM sensors and tracked in real time for the implementation of augmented reality functionalities: tactile augmented reality and visual augmented reality. Indeed, the current version of the simulator, which was originally design for laparoscopic procedures, includes visual augmented reality information (Fig. 2), displayed on a laptop screen, to aid the trainee in the recognition of the Calot's triangle, covered by connective tissue. In this work, this visual cue is integrated with the tactile augmentation: the surgeon can not only visualize the position of the cystic artery through the AR scene but can also feel its pulse by means of the haptic device.

The optical calibration-acquisition system has a twofold function indeed it allows the user to perform a calibration routine, and it acquires the real scene and displays it on the laptop screen.

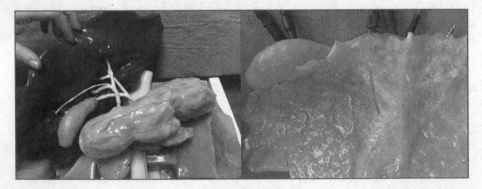

Fig. 2. The AR-Sim simulator: (a) patient-specific physical replicas; (b) augmented reality scene allowing the trainee to visualize the current position of the cystic artery and biliary tree (respectively represented by the red and green virtual structures) which are covered by the synthetic connective tissue. (Color figure online)

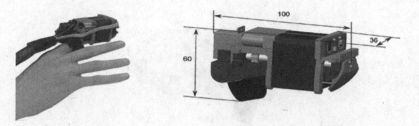

Fig. 3. W-FYD on a user's finger (on the left): W-FYD CAD design and dimensions (in mm) – weight 100 g.

2.2 Wearable Fabric Yielding Device W-FYD

W-FYD (Wearable Fabric Yielding Device) (Fig. 3) is a tactile display for softness rendering and multi-cue delivery that can be worn on user's finger [13]. The mechanical structure, inspired by the grounded version of the device [14–17], is also similar to the one reported in [18], where two DC motors can vary the stiffness of the fabric stretching it, if independently controlled, provide tangential force (Fig. 4). The fabric is wrapped around two pins connected to the frame through suitable supports.

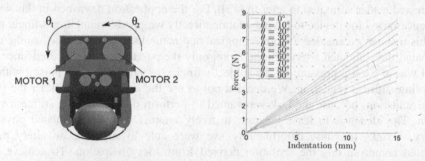

Fig. 4. Representation of a finger interacting with the W-FYD (on the left); characterization curves for different motor positions ($\theta 1$ and $\theta 2$) (on the right).

When the user's finger is inserted inside the device, two different interaction modes can be used: active one, where the finger actively explores the fabric surface for softness, and passive mode, where the finger pad interacts with the fabric passively, thanks to the lifting mechanism that put the fabric, whose stiffness is regulated using the two DC motors, in contact with user's finger, which is still. In the active mode, the device is attached to the back of the finger, hence the only movement the user can perform is the flexion of the distal phalanx, which provokes the indentation of the fabric.

To enable also passive mode, a lifting system is implemented trough a servomotor and a camshaft-based lifting mechanism, which puts the fabric in contact with the user's finger pad, making the platform where the fabric is wrapped around moving vertically of distance h_p (Fig. 5).

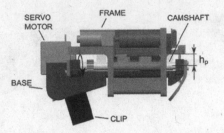

Fig. 5. Passive mode: the fabric frame is put in contact by the camshaft lifting mechanism and servo-motor, inducing a variation of the height hp of the frame.

The fabric stretching system is actuated separately from the indentation mechanism, hence it is possible to change the fabric stiffness independently from the force exerted on the finger of the user. Different levels of stiffness can be generated changing the stretching state of the fabric, obtained changing the relative angle between the two DC motors. The control of the stretching state of the fabric, and hence of the stiffness stimulus to be delivered, relies on the characterization of the system (Fig. 4 right side). Finally, thanks to the presence of the two independently controlled DC motors, W-FYD is endowed with an additional translational degree of freedom, which can induce a sensation of sliding/slipping on the user's fingertip (for further details the interested reader is invited to refer to [13]). For the application described in this work, we customized the device to have the fabric directly wrapped around user's finger pad. In this manner we enabled a more ecological and naturalistic interaction when the user palpated the simulated artery. Furthermore, only the passive mode was used since the goal was to exert a pressure on the subject's finger (to simulate artery pulse), without enabling stiffness rendering. We decided not to use the active mode, neither the stiffness rendering, because the task we wanted to perform did not require stiffness variation. The idea was to leave the user to freely interact with the simulated physical artery. Thanks to fabric deformability, we were able to superimpose artery pulse without compromising the sensation derived from artery palpation. To achieve this goal, we commanded a saw-tooth height variation to the lifting mechanism, in order to induce a deformation of the finger pad that simulates the pulsing artery. We sew a load cell (FSR model 400 round, thickness 0.1–0.3 mm) on the part of the fabric that was not in contact with the finger pad: the goal was to detect the pressing force exerted by the user. Future works will aim at investigating multi-digit implementation of the device and other haptic effects.

2.3 Wearable Haptic Device Sensorization and Calibration

The Wearable Haptic Interface was sensorized with a 6DOF EM Aurora Sensor positioned as illustrated in Fig. 6.

A calibration procedure is required to precisely derive the position of the user finger from the EM sensor data so that to activate the pulse simulation when the user fingertip touches the artery models. At this aim a simple method based on static digitization was employed. In particular, at each time t the position of the user fingertip, $^{GRF}\vec{p}(t)$, can be calculated as:

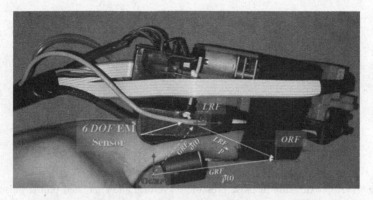

Fig. 6. W-FYD sensorized with a 6DOF EM Aurora sensor.

$$^{GRF}\vec{p}(t) = {}^{GRF}\vec{o}(t) + {}^{GRF}R_{LRF}(t)^{LRF}\vec{p} \tag{1}$$

Where:

GRF indicates the Aurora Reference Frame (Global Reference Frame);

LRF indicates a Local Reference Frame at the EM coil center;

$^{GRF}\vec{o}(t)$ is a 3D vector expressing the position at time t of the Local Reference Frame origin in the Aurora Reference Frame (GRF);

$^{GRF}R_{LRF}(t)$ is a 3-by-3 rotation matrix which indicates the orientation of the Local Reference Frame with respect to the Aurora Reference Frame (GRF) at time t;

$^{LRF}\vec{p}$ is a 3D vector expressing the position of the user fingertip in the Local Reference Frame.

$^{GRF}\vec{o}(t)$ and $^{GRF}R_{LRF}(t)$ are directly derived from the 6DOF EM sensor which is tracked in real time. $^{LRF}\vec{p}$ can be considered constant over a simulation session (since the EM sensor is rigidly attached to the Wearable Haptic Interface) and it can be evaluated at the beginning of each session by positioning the tip of a digitizer at the user fingertip. $^{LRF}\vec{p}$ indeed can be calculated as follow:

$$^{LRF}\vec{p} = {}^{GRF}R_{LRF}^{-1}(k)\left({}^{GRF}\vec{p}(k) - {}^{GRF}\vec{o}(k)\right) \tag{2}$$

where k denotes the calibration time instant, $^{GRF}\vec{p}(k)$ is the digitized position (it is a 3D vector expressing the position at time k of the Digitizer Tip in the Aurora Reference Frame).

2.4 Arterial Pulse Simulation

The human pulse wave has different shapes depending on the patient constitution and medical conditions, and also on the pulse region [6, 19]. In this paper, as a first approximation of the pulse pressure waveform, we have used a saw-tooth waveform model. Figure 7 shows a typical arterial pressure waveform and the simulated pulse

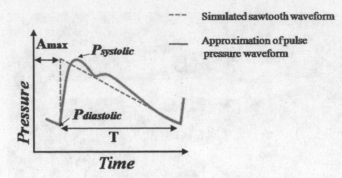

Fig. 7. Approximation of pulse pressure waveform and simulated profile pulse.

profile used in this study. The simulated wave form is characterized by the pulse period T and by the maximum amplitude A_{max}.

The length of the pulse period T can be varied to simulate different heart rate. The normal resting heart rate for adults ranges from 60 to 100 beats per min (BPM), although this can vary depending on different circumstances. During a cholecystectomy procedure the heart rate changes depending on the patient decubitus, drug effects and carbon dioxide insufflation (in case of laparoscopic interventions), and it ranges from 70 to 90 beats per min [20].

A_{max} is calculated as:

$$A_{max} = [(F_{measured} - F_{min})/(F_{max} - F_{min})] \times \mu \tag{3}$$

Where:
$F_{measured}$ is the pressing force exerted by the user (measured by the force sensor)
μ is the coefficient corresponding to the maximum deformation induced on the finger pad by the device
F_{max} and F_{min} are the force bounds (see below).

In our simulation a pulsating force feedback is rendered when two criteria, based on a proximity condition between the user fingertip and artery and on the force exerted by the user on the artery, are contemporaneously satisfied. As for the proximity condition, we employed a "bang-bang" control model making use of a threshold to take into account the Aurora sensor accuracy and precision. In particular, the pulse simulation is activated when the distance between the user fingertip and the sensorized artery satisfies:

$$d \leq R_{artery} + h_{tissue} + \delta_{Aurora} \tag{4}$$

Where:
d is distance between the user fingertip and the sensorized artery
R_{artery} is the sensorized artery radius
h_{tissue} is the sensorized thickness of the connective tissue which cover the artery
δ_{Aurora} is the Aurora dynamic accuracy which is 0.5 mm [21].

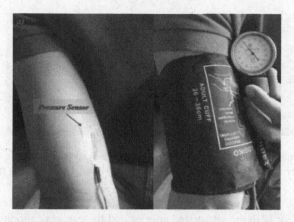

Fig. 8. Calibration procedure: (a) positioning of the pressure sensor, (b) manual sphygmo-manometer used for the sensor calibration.

The pulse is deactivated when:

$$d \geq R_{artery} + h_{tissue} + \delta_{Aurora} + \varepsilon_{Aurora} \tag{5}$$

where ε_{Aurora} is the Aurora dynamic precision which is 0.57 mm [21].

As regards to the force exerted by the user on the artery the following criteria should be satisfied:

$$F_{min} \leq F \leq F_{max} \tag{6}$$

where F_{max} and F_{min} are the forces measured by the pressure sensor corresponding respectively to a standard systolic (120 mmHg) and diastolic (60 mmHg) pressure. These values were defined by using the following simple calibration procedure. The pressure sensor was attached to the skin of a volunteer in correspondence to the brachial artery (Fig. 8). The cuff of the sphygmomanometer was then positioned over the sensor; the cuff was inflated to a pressure of 60 mmHg and to a pressure 120 mmHg and the forces measured by the pressure sensor were recorded.

3 Experimental Design

Qualitative tests were performed to preliminary assess the proposed simulation concept.

3.1 Experimental Set-up

The experimental set-up included the W-FYD and a simplified version of the AR-Sim simulator comprising only a sensorized arterial tree replica covered with synthetic connective tissue (Fig. 9). To preliminary test the system the arterial tree and the connective tissue were positioned over a box (made of expanded polystyrene) as

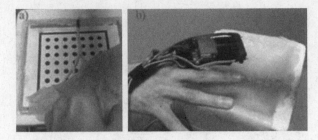

Fig. 9. Experimental set-up: (a) sensorized arterial tree covered with synthetic connective tissue and positioned over a box (with the calibration grid). (b) A surgeon wearing the W-FYD.

showed in Fig. 9. The box was used as a spacer over the EM field emitter and as a physical support for both the sensorized arteries and the camera calibration grid [9, 10].

3.2 Qualitative Evaluation

A total of ten surgeons (eight general surgeons and two vascular surgeons) participated in this study. All participants were asked to try the simulator and to complete a questionnaire. The surgeons were asked to wear the tactile display and to palpate the mockup for the recognition of the cystic or right hepatic artery. During palpation, the W-FYD conveyed a pulse feed-back on user's finger. The questionnaire comprises 6 items (listed in Table 1) assessed using a five point Likert scale (1 = strongly disagree to 5 strongly agree). Participants were also asked to comment on any other aspect of the simulator which they felt was important but had not been directly included in the questionnaire, and to list any suggestion to improve the simulation realism. Statistical analysis of data was performed using the SPSS® Statistics Base 19 software. The central tendencies of responses to a single Likert item were summarized by using median, with dispersion measured by interquartile range. The Wilcoxon signed-ranks test was used to determine the significance of the responses to each item evaluating if the operators were significantly more likely to agree or disagree with each of the statements. A p-value < 0.05 was considered statistically significant.

Table 1. Surgical simulator questionnaire: preliminary results. The central tendency of responses is summarized by using median with dispersion measured by IQR ($25° \sim 75°$)

QUESTIONNAIRE ITEM	Median (IQR)	P
1. The pulse feedback is realistic	3.50 (3.00;4.00)	0.025
2. The location of the arterial pulse in the real environment is correct and realistic	4.00 (3.00;4.25)	0.034
3. The arterial pulse is felt on the user fingertip	4.00 (2.00;4.25)	0.317
4. The pulse magnitude is realistic	4.00 (3.50;4.00)	0.058
5. The integration of W-FYD in the surgical simulator is useful	4.00 (4.00;5.00)	0.003
6. The integration of W-FYD in the laparotomic cholecystectomy simulator is useful for the recognition of the arterial tree	4.00 (4.00;4.00)	0.003

4 Results and Conclusions

Table 1 summarizes results of preliminary qualitative evaluation indicating that there is overall significant agreement with the following statements: "The pulse feedback is realistic", "The location of the arterial pulse in the real environment is correct and realistic", "The integration of the W-FYD in the surgical simulator is useful", "The integration of W-FYD in the laparotomic cholecystectomy simulator is useful for the recognition of the arterial tree". Moreover participants agreed with items 3 and 4 even if a larger study is required for statistical evidence. Pulse palpation, as well as pulse diagnosis, is a subjective process depending on a practitioner's palpatory skill and ability to discriminate changes in pulse variables. For this reason, the variability among the surgeons responses may reflect differences in user's ability and sensitivity. Obtained results, however are very positive and encourage further studies to develop the proposed simulation platform. Responses to item 2, validate the accuracy of the user fingertip localization (which depends on the accuracy of the EM tracking system and of the haptic device calibration), since the pulse is correctly perceived when the user touches the physical arterial replica.

The most prevalent theme within participants comments was the need for: reducing the dimension of the haptic interface to improve the human factor, and enabling a multi-digit implementation allowing the trainee to palpate the pulse with two fingers. Moreover participants suggested to add the possibility of differentiating the amplitude of the simulated arterial pulse according to the palpated artery. Indeed, whereas the mean arterial pressure is known to be identical in all parts of the arterial tree, the pulse pressure has a greater amplitude in peripheral than in central arteries due to the buffering function of the arteries [22, 23]. More particularly, one surgeon suggested to reduce the minimum force to be exerted by the user on the artery to feel the pulse. No concerns were raised on the realism of the synthetic tissue whose constructive materials were selected to feel natural to the touch according to the surgeon feedback [10]. To conclude, the benefit of haptic feedback in surgical training has been already recognized by several research groups and companies working in this field (e.g. Immersion Medical, Surgical Science and Mentice). Most of the work is focused on haptic rendering for simulation of tool–tissue interactions in virtual reality simulators for training of minimally invasive surgical procedures. In this work we firstly present a proof-of-concept implementation of tactile augmented reality for open-surgery training. Preliminary qualitative test showed a general consensus among surgeons regarding the realism of the arterial pulse feedback and the usefulness of integrating this kind of haptic interface in open-surgery simulators. In the future the W-FYD will be optimized according to the surgeon feedback, enabling a multi-digit implementation while reducing the haptic device size. Moreover future studies will address ergonomics and human factors issues in the design of the augmented reality functionalities, considering the possibility to integrate an head-mounted display in the surgical training platform.

Acknowledgements. Work supported by the SThARS project (funded by the Italian Ministry of Health and Regione Toscana through the call "Ricerca Finalizzata 2011–2012"); the European Research Council under the Advanced Grant Soft Hands "A Theory of Soft Synergies for a New Generation of Artificial Hands" (No. ERC-291166), the EU H2020 projects "SoftPro:

Synergy-based Open-source Foundations and Technologies for Prosthetics and Rehabilitation" (No. 688857), and the EU FP7 project (No. 601165) "WEARable HAPtics for Humans and Robots (WEARHAP)".

References

1. Poorten, V.E., Demeester, E., Lammertse, P.: Haptic feedback for medical applications, a survey. In: Proceedings of the Actuator, pp. 18–20 (2012)
2. Hu, J., Chang, C.Y., Tardella, N., Pratt, J., English, J.: Effectiveness of haptic feedback in open surgery simulation and training systems. Stud. Health Technol. **119**, 213–218 (2006)
3. Ullrich, S., Kuhlen, T.: Haptic palpation for medical simulation in virtual environments. IEEE Trans. Vis. Comput. Graph. **18**, 617–625 (2012)
4. Coles, T., John, N.W., Gould, D.A., Caldwell, D.G.: Haptic palpation for the femoral pulse in virtual interventional radiology. In: Second International Conferences on Advances in Computer-Human Interactions, ACHI 2009, pp. 193–198 (2009)
5. Luboz, V., Zhang, Y., Johnson, S., Song, Y., Kilkenny, C., Hunt, C., Woolnough, H., Guediri, S., Zhai, J., Odetoyinbo, T., Littler, P., Fisher, A., Hughes, C., Chalmers, N., Kessel, D., Clough, P.J., Ward, J., Phillips, R., How, T., Bulpitt, A., John, N.W., Bello, F., Gould, D.: ImaGiNe Seldinger: first simulator for Seldinger technique and angiography training. Comput. Methods Programs Biomed. **111**, 419–434 (2013)
6. Coles, T.R., John, N.W., Gould, D.A., Caldwell, D.G.: Integrating haptics with augmented reality in a femoral palpation and needle insertion training simulation. IEEE Trans. Haptics **4**, 199–209 (2011)
7. Iwamoto, T., Tatezono, M., Shinoda, H.: Non-contact method for producing tactile sensation using airborne ultrasound. In: Ferre, M. (ed.) EuroHaptics 2008. LNCS, vol. 5024, pp. 504–513. Springer, Heidelberg (2008)
8. Hung, G.M., John, N.W., Hancock, C., Hoshi, T.: Using and validating airborne ultrasound as a tactile interface within medical training simulators. In: Bello, F., Cotin, S. (eds.) ISBMS 2014. LNCS, vol. 8789, pp. 30–39. Springer, Heidelberg (2014)
9. Ferrari, V., Viglialoro, R.M., Nicoli, P., Cutolo, F., Condino, S., Carbone, M., Siesto, M., Ferrari, M.: Augmented reality visualization of deformable tubular structures for surgical simulation. Int. J. Med. Robot. Comput. Assist. Surg. **12**, 231–240 (2016)
10. Maria Viglialoro, R., Condino, S., Gesi, M., Ferrari, M., Ferrari, V.: Augmented reality simulator for laparoscopic cholecystectomy training. In: De Paolis, L.T., Mongelli, A. (eds.) AVR 2014. LNCS, vol. 8853, pp. 428–433. Springer, Heidelberg (2014)
11. Viglialoro, R., Condino, S., Gesi, M., Ferrari, M., Ferrari, V., Freschi, C., Cutolo, F.: AR visualization of "synthetic Calot's triangle" for training in cholecystectomy. In: 12th IASTED International Conference on Biomedical Engineering, BioMed 2016 (2016)
12. Abdalla, S., Pierre, S., Ellis, H.: Calot's triangle. Clin. Anat. **26**, 493–501 (2013)
13. Bianchi, M., Battaglia, E., Poggiani, M., Ciotti, S., Bicchi, A.: A wearable fabric-based display for haptic multi-cue delivery. In: 2016 IEEE Haptics Symposium (HAPTICS), pp. 277–283 (2016)
14. Bianchi, M., Scilingo, E.P., Serio, A., Bicchi, A.: A new softness display based on bi-elastic fabric. In: EuroHaptics Conference, 2009 and Symposium on Haptic Interfaces for Virtual Environment and Teleoperator Systems, World Haptics 2009, Third Joint, pp. 382–383 (2009)
15. Bianchi, M., Serio, A., Scilingo, E.P., Bicchi, A.: A new fabric-based softness display. In: 2010 IEEE Haptics Symposium, pp. 105–112 (2010)

16. Serio, A., Bianchi, M., Biechi, A.: A device for mimicking the contact force/contact area relationship of different materials with applications to softness rendering. In: 2013 IEEE/RSJ International Conference on Intelligent Robots and Systems, pp. 4484–4490 (2013)
17. Bianchi, M., Serio, A.: Design and characterization of a fabric-based softness display. IEEE Trans. Haptics **8**, 152–163 (2015)
18. Minamizawa, K., Fukamachi, S., Kajimoto, H., Kawakami, N., Tachi, S.: Gravity grabber: wearable haptic display to present virtual mass sensation. In: ACM SIGGRAPH 2007 Emerging Technologies, San Diego, California, p. 8. ACM (2007)
19. Ullrich, S., Mendoza, J., Ntouba, A., Rossaint, R., Kuhlen, T.: Haptic pulse simulation for virtual palpation. In: Tolxdorff, T., Braun, J., Deserno, T.M., Horsch, A., Handels, H., Meinzer, H.-P. (eds.) Bildverarbeitung für die Medizin 2008: Algorithmen — Systeme — Anwendungen Proceedings des Workshops vom 6. bis 8. April 2008 in Berlin, pp. 187–191. Springer, Heidelberg (2008)
20. O'Leary, E., Hubbard, K., Tormey, W., Cunningham, A.J.: Laparoscopic cholecystectomy: haemodynamic and neuroendocrine responses after pneumoperitoneum and changes in position. Br. J. Anaesth. **76**, 640–644 (1996)
21. Nafis, C., Jensen, V., Beauregard, L., Anderson, P.: Method for estimating dynamic EM tracking accuracy of surgical navigation tools - art. no. 61410K. In: Medical Imaging 2006: Visualization, Image-Guided Procedures, and Display, vol. 6141, pp. 152–167 (2006)
22. Bia, D., Aguirre, I., Zocalo, Y., Devera, L., Cabrera Fischer, E., Armentano, R.: Regional differences in viscosity, elasticity and wall buffering function in systemic arteries: pulse wave analysis of the arterial pressure-diameter relationship. Rev. Esp. Cardiol. **58**, 167–174 (2005)
23. Benetos, A., Laurent, S., Hoeks, A.P., Boutouyrie, P.H., Safar, M.E.: Arterial alterations with aging and high blood pressure. A noninvasive study of carotid and femoral arteries. Arterioscler. Thromb. J. Vasc. Biol./Am. Heart Assoc. **13**, 90–97 (1993)

Augmented Reality Guidance with Electromagnetic Tracking for Transpyloric Tube Insertion

Jordan Bano[1(✉)], Tomohiko Akahoshi[2], Ryu Nakadate[1], Byunghyun Cho[2], and Makoto Hashizume[1]

[1] Center for Advanced Medical Innovation, Kyushu University, Fukuoka, Japan
jordan.bano@gmail.com
[2] Department of Advanced Medical Initiatives, Faculty of Medical Sciences, Kyushu University, Fukuoka, Japan

Abstract. Transpyloric tube insertion is a commonly intervention which consists in inserting a tube through the nose, the oesophagus and the stomach until the pylorus. This procedure can be done blindly if no licensed physician operator is available. Thus, the caregivers have to insert the tube without any visual feedbacks. The position of the tube has also to be conformed to avoid any issues.

We proposed a guidance system for the insertion of this tube through an augmented reality application using an electromagnetic tracker. The trajectory and the orientation of the tube were visualized on a screen to monitor the tube insertion but also to conform the position of the tube tip inside the pylorus. This monitoring was improved by adding preoperative landmarks coming from a CT image or intraoperative landmarks obtained with ultrasound. Finally, the display was overlaid on a camera view to match the tube trajectory on the patient during the insertion so the clinicians directly visualized anatomical landmarks to guide themselves during the tube insertion.

Preliminary results on one phantom showed the usefulness of our guidance system for blindly tube insertion. Further evaluations have to be realized on animals and on patients to validate these results.

Keywords: Augmented reality · Transpyloric tube insertion · Guidance system · Electromagnetic tracking

1 Introduction

Transpyloric tube insertion is a commonly procedure done to provide nutritional support for injured patient in the intensive care unit [ICU]. In this procedure, a tube has to be inserted through the nose, oesophagus, stomach and pylorus. The main difficulty is to enter through the pylorus which can be thin (diameter: 2 to 5 mm). Afterwards, a verification is done to conform the tube tip position.

The methods used for this insertion can greatly differ: in the best case, an endoscope can be used to monitor the insertion inside the pylorus. But otherwise, the insertion is done blindly without any guidance and visual feedbacks.

© Springer International Publishing Switzerland 2016
G. Zheng et al. (Eds.): MIAR 2016, LNCS 9805, pp. 198–207, 2016.
DOI: 10.1007/978-3-319-43775-0_18

In the case of an insertion using an endoscope, an expert must be available to manipulate it which limits the number of interventions.

Nurses can also insert the tube without the use of endoscope and so without any visual feedbacks. The main indication used by caregivers in this case is the length of tube to insert. Before insertion, clinicians have to estimate this length with two measurements: the first one corresponds to the distance between the nose, the ear and the xiphoid process (gastric mark) and the second one is the distance between the gastric mark and the left or right costal margin (pyloric mark).

During the insertion, the tube is inserted and the collision with stomach makes it possible to attain the pylorus. But in some cases, the tube is looping inside the stomach and the main indication (i.e. the length of the inserted tube) is not any more reliable (see Fig. 1).

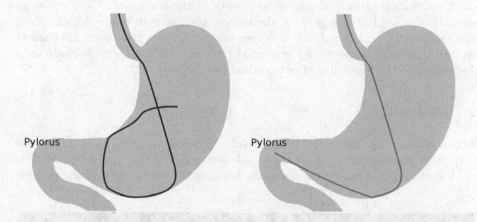

Pylorus   Pylorus

Fig. 1. One can see on the left an example of a tube inserted that makes a loop inside the stomach. On the right, the tube was successfully inserted inside the pylorus. On both cases, the tube was pushed on the stomach wall and was deviated on different directions.

The confirmation of the tip tube position is also crucial to avoid any mistakes such as inserting the tube in the lungs which can cause the patient's death [15, 16]. The gold standard is fluoroscopy which means to be at proximity of one scanner that can be unavailable in some clinics. Moreover, this technique exposes the patients to radiation and can be expensive.

In resume, in this clinical context, two mains issues can be tackled: the guidance during the tube insertion and the verification of the position of the tube. Three main systems are currently available to guide the tube insertion.

Electromagnetic guidance has been widely evaluated and already showed his relevancy compared to blindly procedure [12,20]. A commercial system (Cortrak Enteral access system) is mainly used which consists in a dedicated tube with an electromagnetic sensor at its tip. This system can provide a monitoring of the tube trajectory and have been well evaluated [3,5,6,11,13,14,19,22]. It has been shown that the trajectory is useful to guide the insertion of the tube. Moreover, the display of the trajectory can be enough to conform the position of the tube tip which means that the confirmation with an X-ray could be unnecessary. One limitation of this system is that no landmark can be displayed during the tube insertion.

Magnetic system consists in the use of a magnetic probe to attract a magnet included in the tube [1,2,7,18]. This probe needs to be pushed in the patient which can be no reliable for obese patients. Moreover, the exact position of the tube cannot be known with this kind of device.

Finally, ultrasound have been used to detect the tip tube and to monitor its position [8–10]. The tracking is done manually which means that the clinicians have to move the US probe and find the tip tube on the US images by himself.

In this paper, we propose to guide the tube insertion using electromagnetic tracking: its use already shown good results in the literature. We propose to improve this kind of system with the use of landmarks to guide the clinicians and the overlay on the patient' skin (see Sect. 2). Afterwards, our experiments on two different phantoms are presented (see Sect. 3). We then conclude on a discussion on the feasibility of our method (see Sect. 4).

2   Method

In this section, the augmented reality display is described (see Fig. 2): firstly, the trajectory monitoring, secondly the supplementary data that could be added on the monitoring and finally, the matching between the trajectory and the patient.

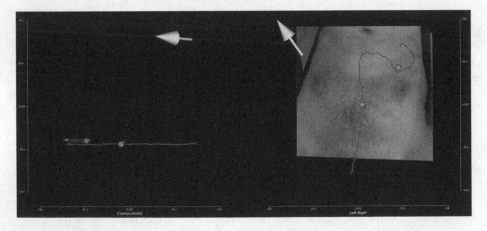

Fig. 2. Example of the full guidance system with: a sagittal view (left) and a coronal view (right), the tube tip trajectory (red), the orientation of the tip (yellow), the landmarks (green) and the patient's picture. We outline that this picture was not taken during a real tube insertion. (Color figure online)

2.1   Trajectory Tracking

The trajectory view was divided in a sagittal and a coronal views. The orientation of the tube tip was also displayed so the caregiver can know how to rotate the tube. Indeed, this information is crucial to know if the tube is in a wrong direction which happened when a loop occurred.

The guidance system was based on Visualization Toolkit (VTK) and Qt and could be used on a laptop or a tablet device at the convenience of the clinicians. The electromagnetic tracking was done using an Aurora system (Northern Digital Inc., Waterloo, Ontario, Canada) with a 6-DOF sensor.

2.2   Supplementary Data

The guidance of the tube insertion could be improved with a target point to let know where the pylorus was. Two kinds of data were added to extract this target: preoperative and intraoperative ones.

Preoperative Data. ICU patients generally underwent a medical image for the diagnosis. This image contains useful information that can be displayed in the software. Before or during procedure, clinicians could select landmarks on the medical image to guide the tube insertion. We outline three important landmarks:

- the gastroesophageal junction that is required to know quickly if the tube was inserted or not in the lungs,
- the pylorus that is the target during the insertion (see Fig. 3),
- the sternum that is required for the registration between the CT world and the virtual world.

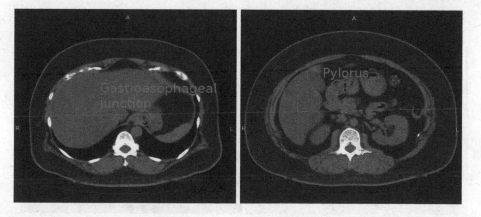

Fig. 3. Example of the position of the gastroesophageal junction and the pylorus on CT axial slices.

Indeed, this registration was realized when the electromagnetic sensor was put on the patient' sternum and that a manual selection of the sternum was done on the CT image. A transformation matrix between the CT world and the virtual world was then computed to translate the other landmarks in the virtual world.

Intraoperative Data. In the case that no preoperative data is available for one patient, intraoperative data can be acquired.

Ultrasound can be used to detect landmarks such as the pylorus. This device is well-known for its cost-effectiveness but can be difficult to manipulate. Thus, we focused on easily identifiable landmarks such as the gallbladder. Indeed, this organ is located near the pylorus which can be a close landmark to the pylorus to guide during the tube insertion.

2.3   AR on the Patient' Skin

An overlay of the guidance system on the patient' skin was proposed to provide anatomical landmarks such as the xiphoid process or the costal margin that could be directly seen to support the guidance. We remind that these landmarks are usually used to estimate the length of tube to insert inside the patient.

Augmented reality on the patient' skin have already been tackled in other clinical contexts. It have shown great advantage for laparoscopic surgery where trocars have to been inserted through the patient' skin [17, 21].

In our case, the goal is to provide a view of the patient during insertion. A picture of the patient was taken with the tablet camera and was used as a background for the coronal trajectory view. Recording during the procedure could also be done but the camera had to be fixed close to the patient which can be cumbersome.

The camera has to be calibrated to fit the same coordinate world than the guidance system. A calibration using a chessboard was realized to take the intrinsic parameters of the camera into account. A perspective transformation was also

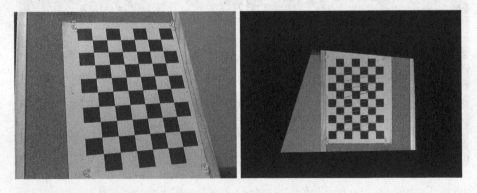

Fig. 4. One can see on the left a picture of a checkerboard. On the right, this picture was transformed to keep a point of view orthogonal to the surface.

applied to the video frame in order to always keep a point of view orthogonal to the surface (i.e. the patient's bust). These two steps were done using OpenCV library (Fig. 4). This transformation was based on the positions of the corners of the chessboard. Finally, the position of the electromagnetic sensor was manually localized on the image to register the tube tip position on the video world.

3 Experiments and Results

First trials have been done on commercial phantoms (EsophagoGastroDuodenocsopy simulator and ESD Training Model ©Koken). In both cases, the landmarks (green spheres) were acquired manually with the EM sensor before the insertion. The first phantom consisted in a set of organs (nose, oesophagus, stomach, pylorus) and the second one (a stomach model only) made possible to conform visually where the tube was through small holes. One can see on Fig. 5 that the trajectory of the tube fits the shape of the phantom.

An evaluation was done using the second phantom in three different protocols (see Fig. 6): (1) without the guidance system, (2) with the simple guidance system (i.e. without our proposed improvements) and (3) with the full guidance system (i.e. with the landmarks, the patient's picture and a clear view of the tip orientation). The second phantom only was used to be able to see if a loop has happened or not which was not possible with the first phantom.

Participants had to insert the tube and stopped the insertion when they believed that the tube was close enough to the pylorus. Then, the distance between the tube tip and the pylorus positions was measured according to the electromagnetic tracking. We outline that the position of the pylorus was chosen and fixed before the experiments.

The average distance for the five participants were: 79.7 mm for protocol (1), 47.8 mm for protocol (2) and 41.2 mm for protocol (3). The tube tip was positioned closest to the pylorus (45 %) with the visual feedback (conditions (2) and (3)) which confirms the usefulness of the guidance system. A less significant improvement can be observed between conditions (1) and (2) (15 %). The remaining distance between the tip and the pylorus was due to some parts of the phantom that were sticky. Moreover, it was difficult to manipulate the tube in particular to change the orientation of the tip.

Loops occurred only without the guidance system (40 %) because the participant could not see when the tip was stuck. Indeed, when the tube was inserted whereas the tip was stuck, the tube looped inside the phantom.

Overall, the participants were more confident using protocol (3) that provided a target to reach. The trajectory only was helpful but it was difficult to find a way without this target and to know if the target was reached or not.

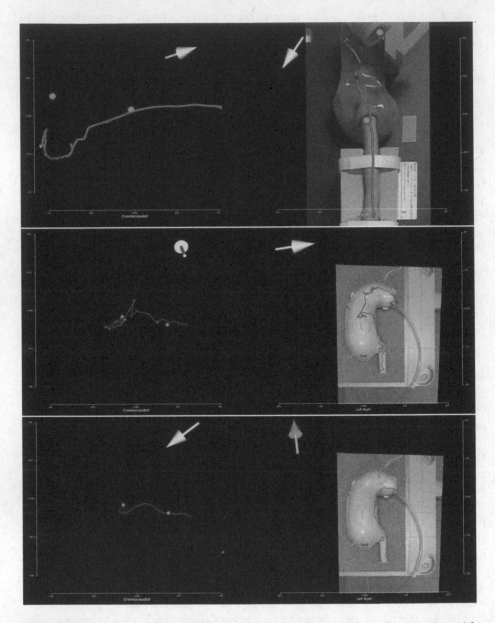

Fig. 5. Three examples of the augmented reality guidance of the tube insertion with: the trajectory (red), the orientation of the tip (yellow) and the landmarks (green sphere). On the top, an example when the tube stayed blocked by a part of the stomach on the first phantom. This can be seen by looking at the orientation of the tube. On the middle, a successful insertion is illustrated and on the bottom, one can see the trajectory of the sensor when we removed it from the tube: this trajectory can be enough to confirm the good position of the tube. (Color figure online)

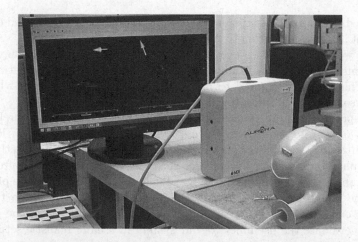

Fig. 6. One can see the setup of our system: the participant was aside of the phantom, a screen was put in front of him to display the guidance system and finally, the electromagnetic tracking device was put aside the phantom.

4   Discussion

Our method was based on an electromagnetic device and a tablet only. Both of these devices can be easily installed in a patient's room. However, the price of the electromagnetic device can reduce the availability of our method. We outline that the electromagnetic sensor can be reused several times and can avoid costs due to X-ray.

In the case where intraoperative data have to acquire, an US probe is also required which is commonly available in ICU department. Another possible limitation is the fact that the probe can be difficult to manipulate for novices. But in this work, we focused on organ that one can easily identify such as the gallbladder.

We tackled in this paper the blindly insertion of the transpyloric tube but this guidance system can also be useful when an endoscope is used. In this case, after the tube insertion, the electromagnetic sensor can be inserted through the tube and its trajectory can conform the good placement of the tube.

The pylorus entry position was localized according to a preoperative medical image. However, it is difficult to know if its position is the same than during intervention. A study on 3D+t medical images of the same patient have to be realized to oversee if this landmark is reliable to guide during transpyloric tube insertion. At our knowledge, the only study related to these landmarks is the one of Cohen et al. [4]. This study was done on 200 children (classified into 4 age groups) and aims to study if the gastro-esophageal junction can be find according to other landmarks. For that, they compared different distances such as the one between the gastroesophageal junction and the spine or the one between the pylorus and the spine. This paper outlined that the pylorus can generally be find between the 11th and 12th thoracic vertebra. This point can be interesting because a fast identification of these vertebra can be done on the patient just before the insertion. This identification can provide a margin area where the pylorus can be localized and be displayed in our guidance system. These results have to be validated on adult cases but it is a first indication to find robust landmarks.

In our work, we chose to overlay the tube trajectory on a picture of the patient's bust. Another solution is to project the trajectory on the patient' skin directly. This solution required to fix a projector above the patient which can be cumbersome but will be tested in the future.

Our experiments were done on a phantom which provided a preliminary evaluation only. The conditions are not the same than a real insertion on a patient. Firstly, organs of interest (stomach and oesophagus) were directly visible using the phantom which is unrealistic. Secondly, the tube tip was often stuck because of the rigidity of the phantom and the lack of liquids inside the phantom. Finally, the phantom did not deform like a human's stomach when the tube touched it or because of the breathing. The next experiments will be done on animals to evaluate the usefulness of our system in a more realistic setup.

5   Conclusion

In this paper, we have presented a full guidance system for transpyloric tube insertion. This guidance system was based on an electromagnetic tracking to monitor the tube trajectory and its tip orientation. Preoperative or intraoperative landmarks could then be added to guide the insertion. Finally, this system was overlaid on a picture of the patient's bust to clearly see where the tube tip was according to the patient's anatomy. This method was tested on one phantom and promising results were outlined. Further experiments on animals and after on patients will be done to assert this method usefulness.

Acknowledgments. This work was supported (in part) by JSPS Grant-in-Aid for Scientific Research on Innovative Areas (Multidisciplinary Computational Anatomy) JSPS KAKENHI Grant Number 26108010.

References

1. Akers, A.S., Pinsky, M.: Placement of a magnetic small bowel feeding tube at the bedside the syncro-bluetube. J. Parenter. Enteral Nutr. 0148607115594235 (2015)
2. Boivin, M., Levy, H., Hayes, J., Magnet-Guided Enteral Feeding Tube Study Group, et al.: A multicenter, prospective study of the placement of transpyloric feeding tubes with assistance of a magnetic device. J. Parenter. Enteral Nutr. 24(5) 304–307 (2000)
3. Boyer, N., McCarthy, M.S., Mount, C.A.: Analysis of an electromagnetic tube placement device versus a self-advancing nasal jejunal device for postpyloric feeding tube placement. J. Hosp. Med. 9(1), 23–28 (2014)
4. Cohen, M.D., Ellett, M.L.C., Perkins, S.M., Lane, K.A.: Accurate localization of the position of the tip of a naso/orogastric tube in children; where is the location of the gastro-esophageal junction? Pediatr. Radiol. 41(10), 1266–1271 (2011)
5. Deane, A.M., Fraser, R.J., Young, R.J., Foreman, B., O'Conner, S.N., Chapman, M.J., et al.: Evaluation of a bedside technique for post-pyloric placement of feeding catheters. Crit. Care Resusc. 11(3), 180 (2009)

6. Dolan, A.M., O'Hanlon, C., O'Rourke, J.: An evaluation of the cortrak enteral access system in our intensive care. Ir. Med. J. (2012)
7. Gabriel, S.A., Ackermann, R.J.: Placement of nasoenteral feeding tubes using external magnetic guidance. J. Parenter. Enteral Nutr. 28(2), 119–122 (2004)
8. Gubler, C., Bauerfeind, P., Vavricka, S.R., Mullhaupt, B., Fried, M., Wildi, S.M.: Bedside sonographic control for positioning enteral feeding tubes: a controlled study in intensive care unit patients. Endoscopy 38(12), 1256–1260 (2006)
9. Hernandez-Socorro, C.R., Marin, J., Ruiz-Santana, S., Santana, L., Manzano, J.L.: Bedside sonographic-guided versus blind nasoenteric feeding tube placement in critically ill patients. Crit. Care Med. 24(10), 1690–1694 (1996)
10. Kim, H.M., So, B.H., Park, K.N., Choi, S.M., Jeong, W.J.: The effectiveness of ultrasonography in verifying the placement of a nasogastric tube in patients with low consciousness at an emergency center. J. Emerg. Med. 43(5), 918 (2012)
11. Kline, A.M., Sorce, L., Sullivan, C., Weishaar, J., Steinhorn, D.M.: Use of a non-invasive electromagnetic device to place transpyloric feeding tubes in critically ill children. Am. J. Crit. Care 20(6), 453–460 (2011)
12. Koopmann, M.C., Kudsk, K.A., Szotkowski, M.J., Rees, S.M.: A team-based protocol and electromagnetic technology eliminate feeding tube placement complications. Ann. Surg. 253(2), 297–302 (2011)
13. Mathus-Vliegen, E.M.H., Duflou, A., Spanier, M.B.W., Fockens, P.: Nasoenteral feeding tube placement by nurses using an electromagnetic guidance system (with video). Gastrointest. Endosc. 71(4), 728–736 (2010)
14. Metheny, N.A., Meert, K.L.: Effectiveness of an electromagnetic feeding tube placement device in detecting inadvertent respiratory placement. Am. J. Crit. Care 23(3), 240–248 (2014)
15. Metheny, N.A., Meert, K.L.: A review of published case reports of inadvertent pulmonary placement of nasogastric tubes in children. J. Pediatr. Nurs. 29(1), e7–e12 (2014)
16. Milsom, S.A., Sweeting, J.A., Sheahan, H., Haemmerle, E., Windsor, J.A.: Naso-enteric tube placement: a review of methods to confirm tip location, global applicability and requirements. World J. Surg. 39(9), 2243–2252 (2015)
17. Nicolau, S., Soler, L., Mutter, D., Marescaux, J.: Augmented reality in laparoscopic surgical oncology. Surg. Oncol. 20(3), 189–201 (2011)
18. Ozdemir, B., Frost, M., Hayes, J., Sullivan, D.H.: Placement of nasoenteral feeding tubes using magnetic guidance: retesting a new technique. J. Am. Coll. Nutr. 19(4), 446–451 (2000)
19. Powers, J., Luebbehusen, M., Spitzer, T., Coddington, A., Beeson, T., Brown, J., Jones, D.: Verification of an electromagnetic placement device compared with abdominal radiograph to predict accuracy of feeding tube placement. J. Parenter. Enteral Nutr. 35(4), 535–539 (2011)
20. Smithard, D., Barrett, N.A., Hargroves, D., Elliot, S.: Electromagnetic sensor-guided enteral access systems: a literature review. Dysphagia 30(3), 275–285 (2015)
21. Volonté, F., Pugin, F., Bucher, P., Sugimoto, M., Ratib, O., Morel, P.: Augmented reality and image overlay navigation with Osirix in laparoscopic and robotic surgery: not only a matter of fashion. J. Hepato-Biliary-Pancreat. Sci. 18(4), 506–509 (2011)
22. Windle, E.M., Beddow, D., Hall, E., Wright, J., Sundar, N.: Implementation of an electromagnetic imaging system to facilitate nasogastric and post-pyloric feeding tube placement in patients with and without critical illness. J. Hum. Nutr. Diet. 23(1), 61–68 (2010)

Exploring Visuo-Haptic Augmented Reality User Interfaces for Stereo-Tactic Neurosurgery Planning

Ulrich Eck[1(✉)], Philipp Stefan[1], Hamid Laga[2], Christian Sandor[3],
Pascal Fallavollita[1], and Nassir Navab[1]

[1] Chair of Computer Aided Medical Procedures,
Technische Universität München, Munich, Germany
`ulrich.eck@tum.de`
[2] School of Engineering and Information Technology,
Murdoch University, Perth, Australia
[3] Nara Institute of Science and Technology,
Interactive Media Design Lab, Ikoma, Japan

Abstract. Stereo-tactic neurosurgery planning is a time-consuming and complex task that requires detailed understanding of the patient anatomy and the affected regions in the brain to precisely deliver the treatment and to avoid proximity to any known risk structures. Traditional user interfaces for neurosurgery planning use keyboard and mouse for interaction and visualize the medical data on a screen. Previous research, however, has shown that 3D user interfaces are more intuitive for navigating volumetric data and enable users to understand spatial relations more quickly. Furthermore, new imaging modalities and automated segmentation of relevant structures provide important information to medical experts. However, displaying such information requires frequent context switches or occludes otherwise important information.

In collaboration with medical experts, we analyzed the planning workflow for stereo-tactic neurosurgery interventions and identified two tasks in the process that can be improved: volume exploration and trajectory refinement. In this paper, we present a novel 3D user interface for neurosurgery planning that is implemented using a head-mounted display and a haptic device. The proposed system improves volume exploration with bi-manual interaction to control oblique slicing of volumetric data and reduces visual clutter with the help of haptic guides that enable users to precisely target regions of interest and to avoid proximity to known risk structures.

Keywords: Augmented reality · Haptics · Neurosurgery · Planning

1 Introduction

Stereo-tactic neurosurgery is a form of minimally invasive surgery that uses a stereo-tactic frame to locate targets inside the brain. This method enables

G. Zheng et al. (Eds.): MIAR 2016, LNCS 9805, pp. 208–220, 2016.
DOI: 10.1007/978-3-319-43775-0_19

interventions that require highly precise targeting, like biopsy, ablation, lesion, injection, stimulation, implantation, and radio-surgery. The two most important criteria when planning such interventions are: to precisely deliver the treatment at the desired target, and to avoid proximity to any risk structures along the trajectory, such as blood vessels or critical brain regions.

The planning of trajectories for a stereo-tactic neurosurgery procedure is a highly complex task, which requires good understanding of the location and structure of the targeted brain regions, as well as all regions affected by any planned trajectory. Neurologists and neurosurgeons explore the original image datasets and segmented volumetric structures to gain understanding about the patient's anatomy. They perform trajectory planning before a surgery to identify target regions and possible paths, and during surgery, where the pre-planned trajectories are refined and verified to avoid any proximity to risk structures. The intra-operative planning procedure is performed while the patient is under full anesthesia, after the stereo-tactic frame was mounted, and after the pre-operative images are registered with an intra-operative CT scan so that the planned trajectories can be computed in frame coordinates. The intra-operative planning can take up to two hours while the patient is in the operating theatre. In this paper we propose a novel Visuo-Haptic Augmented Reality (VHAR) user interface for neurosurgery planning, which reduces the required time for planning and therefore reduces the negative impact on the patient and makes the procedure more cost-effective.

Volumetric image data exploration and trajectory planning in medical practice is typically done using desktop-based workstations with mouse and keyboard. Specialized planning software provides 2D/3D views onto the available patient image data. Operators define trajectories in slice views onto the medical volumes. During planning, they iterate between volume exploration using mouse and keyboard, relocating trajectory points with the mouse to avoid proximity with identified risk structures, and verifying that the recently changed path does not interfere with previously identified risk areas. They also switch often between different image modalities, since not all structures are visible in all images. The type and amount of information available to neurosurgeons and neurologists has vastly increased. This includes new imaging modalities [6], improved computer assisted segmentation of volumetric data [4], computer assisted risk assessment [15], and automated trajectory planning [3–5]. Selecting the appropriate data and visualizing it still remains a challenge especially since additional visual overlays often interfere with the requirement to see the original image dataset with all the details.

The VHAR user interface of our neurosurgery planning application integrates a force feedback haptic device into an Augmented Reality (AR) system. Operators see patient data visualization using a Head-Mounted Display (HMD) and can intuitively explore it using bi-manual 3D interaction (see Fig. 1). The haptic device provides force feedback that enables precise 3D targeting and informs operators about nearby risk structures. By providing haptic guides, we can reduce visual clutter while still providing sufficient information to efficiently plan the required trajectories.

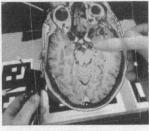 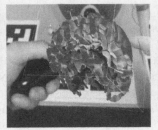 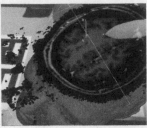

(a) Oblique volume slicing.   (b) Segmented structures.   (c) Trajectory verification.

Fig. 1. The Visuo-Haptic Augmented Reality (VHAR) user interface of the neurosurgery application enables users to naturally interact with medical volume datasets: (a) Users explore volumetric data using oblique slicing and bi-manual interaction. (b) Segmented structures and planned trajectories (yellow lines) are displayed. (c) Users inspect and refine trajectories to avoid proximity to risk structures using an oblique slice plane that is perpendicular to the trajectory. (Color figure online)

2   Related Work

Neurosurgical intervention planning requires precise understanding of spatial relations between target areas, access paths, and critical regions. Current planning systems often use slice visualization for volumetric data and user interfaces with keyboard and mouse for navigation and planning, but previous research has shown that 3D user interfaces can greatly enhance the spatial understanding for such tasks. Goble et al. [9] presented a novel user interface for neurosurgical visualization. Their system tracks passive interface props like a solid sphere, cutting plane, and pointer for user interaction. They found that medical experts prefer the intuitive bi-manual 3D interaction over traditional slice viewers. Our planning system improves on their work so that the medical visualization appears co-located with the interface props using an AR display. Eagleson et al. [7] presented an interactive neurosurgery planning system where multiple users can explore and annotate patient datasets using a tabletop display with a touch surface. They use a haptic device that is placed onto the display to provide 3D input for volume exploration, but their system does not provide any haptic feedback.

Researchers have also studied the benefits of AR for surgery planning. Abhari et al. [1] evaluated user performance during the planning of a brain tumor resection. Such tasks require a good understanding of the spatial relationships between relevant anatomy like tumors and risk-structures. They compared task performance of medical experts when using different visualization techniques. In a preliminary study they showed that users performed as good or better in AR than in all other modes. The benefits of AR are however larger for novices than for experts. Shamir et al. [14] presented an augmented reality user interface for improved risk assessment in image guided keyhole surgery. They augment the risk of all possible trajectories onto the surface of a head phantom. Based on an expert review they conclude that the proposed AR user interface is beneficial for planning of difficult operations and for education. Our system builds upon and enhances their interaction techniques, and adds haptic feedback as another modality to display important information.

Recent advances in image registration and segmentation algorithms enable researchers to build complete image processing pipelines. D'Albis et al. [4] presented a fully integrated and automated planning solution for deep-brain stimulation (PyDBS). Their workflow automates pre-operative, intra-operative, and post-operative imaging tasks, such as registration and segmentation. Our neurosurgery planning system integrates the data generated by PyDBS.

Researchers are also working on automated trajectory planning systems for neurosurgery interventions [2,5,15], which autonomously suggest candidate trajectories to operators. These systems can reduce planning times and help users to better estimate the risk of the planned trajectory. However, such automated planning methods require a broad body of medical knowledge in digital form and accurately segmented and labeled patient data in order to produce acceptable results.

Information generated by automated trajectory planning systems can be either used to suggest trajectories, or to improve guidance of users during the planning procedure. During interviews with medical experts we realized that they often prefer access to additional information over automated processes, which they are not fully in control of. Operators can for example be guided during trajectory planning using visual and haptic guides that use data extracted from automated pipelines. Such guides inform operators about accessibility and the risk of certain configurations in real-time.

The contributions of our work are improved interaction techniques for neurosurgery planning using VHAR, which combine bi-manual volume exploration with haptic visualization and guides. The intuitive positioning and slicing of medical volumes and segmented structures helps operators to better understand the spatial relations, which reduces the time required to identify target regions and risk structures. The application provides haptic guides that display context-dependent constraints as forces in addition to the visual rendering of medical image data and segmented structures in AR. Replacing some of the visual information with haptic feedback reduces visual clutter while still providing the required information. The presented trajectory planning method further reduces the required time for planning of trajectories by reducing the number of iterations needed for refining and verifying trajectories.

3   System Design

This section presents the system design of the proposed user interface for neurosurgery planning that simplifies the exploration of medical datasets and the trajectory planning procedure. When using the planning system, users wear a HMD and hold a haptic stylus with their dominant hand. In the other hand, they hold a tracked handle with buttons used as secondary input to the application. As shown in Fig. 1, a patient dataset consisting of volumetric images and segmented structures is displayed in the haptic workspace. The proposed application allows users to pick up, transform, and place the patient dataset with the tracked handle in order to adjust the viewing angle. They use the haptic stylus to control slicing operation during exploration and verification, and to define trajectories.

3.1 Volume Exploration

The volume exploration component visualizes volumetric and geometric information interactively. During volume exploration, users mainly need control over the displayed content, effective ways to locate regions of interest inside the volume, and views that allow them to understand spatial relations between risk structures and planned trajectories.

In the proposed planning tool, users can directly manipulate the pose of the volume using the tracked handle, which gives them an intuitive way to place and orient the medical dataset as needed, similar to [9]. At the same time, they operate the haptic stylus with their dominant hand to interactively explore the volume using slice views on the volumetric data.

The visual augmentations are rendered using a multi-volume raycaster for volumetric image datasets (see Fig. 1a) and a geometry renderer for segmented structures (see Fig. 1b). Users inspect data using the oblique slicing method [13], which is a generic version of the typically used axis-aligned slice planes. In contrast to axis-aligned slice planes, users can additionally control the orientation of the slice. The combination of oblique slicing with the two-handed interaction allows operators to quickly change volume pose and slice properties. Preliminary reviews with medical experts showed that the proposed method reduces the required time to find regions of interest and help to understand spatial relations within the volume.

The concept of the oblique slicing technique is shown in Fig. 2a. Users place a volume V at a convenient pose O_V and control the slice plane SP using a haptic stylus S. The plane $SP(p, n)$ is defined by a point p, which is controlled by the position of the haptic stylus S, and a normal vector n. The normal vector is selected depending on the current task and the user's preference. Currently, the oblique slicing component supports three viewing modes, which differ only by the data source for the plane normal n:

- **View-Aligned:** The slice plane is always parallel to the view plane of the current camera and therefore provides the most detailed view onto the current slice. Users can additionaly use head movement to control the slicing. The plane normal n is the normal of the camera view-plane.
- **Stylus-Aligned:** The slice plane is controlled by the haptic stylus, which gives the operator maximum control over the slicing operation. The plane normal n is the unit-vector along the longitudinal axis of the haptic stylus S.
- **Trajectory-Aligned:** The slice plane is always perpendicular to the current trajectory. This mode was suggested by medical experts for trajectory verification. The plane normal n is the unit-vector along the current trajectory T.

The oblique slice view is automatically activated once the stylus tip S is inside the volume bounding box (V). The slice plane is computed every frame relative

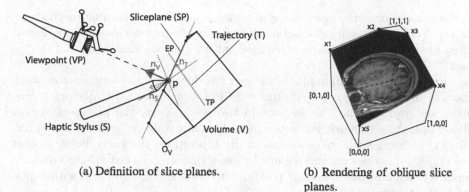

(a) Definition of slice planes.

(b) Rendering of oblique slice planes.

Fig. 2. Oblique slicing of medical datasets in AR: (a) Slice plane SP is defined using point p and normal vector n. The plane normal can be controlled by the view plane of the current camera n_V, the haptic stylus n_S, or the trajectory n_T. (b) Volumetric medical dataset with oblique slice plane. Vertices x_i of the slice plane and their corresponding texture coordinates are computed for real-time rendering using OpenGL shaders.

to the volume origin O_V using the current pose of the haptic stylus and the selected plane normal. The slice plane SP controls a clipping plane, which hides unwanted geometry and volumetric image data. Additionally, the locations of three to six vertices, x_i, are computed that define a polygon, which represents the intersection of the slice plane with the volume bounding box. In addition to the vertex locations, we determine their texture coordinates in relation to the volume bounding box (see Fig. 2b). The polygon is textured using a OpenGL shader by interpolating over data from a three-dimensional texture that represents the medical volume.

Once users have found the desired view on the data, they can lock the slice plane. A locked slice plane enables a haptic plane effect, which attracts the stylus tip to the slice plane if close enough. The haptic feedback guides users to stay on the selected plane, for example when placing points for trajectory planning.

3.2 Trajectory Planning

A trajectory is defined by two 3D positions in a pre-defined reference frame: the target point (TP) and the entry point (EP). The target point is located near or inside the region of interest and the entry point is placed on the upper surface of the skin of the head. While defining these two points initially is straightforward once a promising trajectory was identified, the refinement of the trajectory is not. When modifying entry or target position to adjust the trajectory, previous checks about risk structures in proximity are invalidated in every iteration. Therefore, the verification of the trajectory requires users to revisit again all previously identified areas.

The planning procedure can be optimized if previously known information about risk is used to guide operators. Risk structures can be manually identified in the dataset or determined using automated trajectory planning methods [2, 12,15]. Such additional information is typically displayed visually, but then it often obstructs the view onto other relevant information that is needed for the task.

Our proposed system improves the user interface for trajectory planning with the aim to reduce the required number of iterations between trajectory refinement and verification. This is done in two ways. First, the proposed system allows operators to mark safe zones in problematic areas near the planned trajectory. Defining such zones automatically repositions the entry point so that the trajectory passes critical regions in zones that are marked safe. Second, we replace visual information about proximity to marked risk structures with haptic guides to reduce visual clutter.

Mark Safe Zones: Users specify one or more safe zones near risk structures in proximity while verifying the trajectory using the trajectory-aligned oblique slice view. Safe zones have the shape of a circular disc and are defined with a center (RP_i) and a radius (r_i) in the currently displayed slice (see Fig. 5e). A trajectory intersects all planes that contain safe zones at an intersection point (IP_i). Valid trajectories must intersect with each safe zone at a distance d_i from IP_i to RP that is less or equal to r_i. To achieve this, the entry point EP is moved to a new location EP' to change the trajectory accordingly (see Fig. 3). Users also define an initial confidence radius (r_t) when specifying EP to limit the area in which the entry point can be repositioned.

Reposition the Entry Point: The goal when repositioning the entry point is that a refined trajectory should pass only through areas that are marked as safe. This is achieved using springs that pull the trajectory towards the safe zone centers. The proposed algorithm simulates the trajectory as pendulum with the springs attached at equilibrium to calculate the new entry point EP' using the constraints specified as safe zones. The application invokes the algorithm whenever a trajectory point was modified. Prior to invocation, the target point,

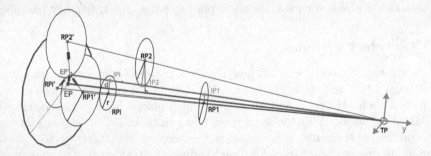

Fig. 3. The initial (blue) trajectory TP—EP is optimized with three refinement points $RP1$, $RP2$, RPi. Safe zones are defined as conic volumes around the refinement points with an additional radius. A new (red) trajectory TP—EP' is calculated where the mass-spring system defined by the projected points $RP1'$, $RP2'$, RPi' is at equilibrium. (Color figure online)

the entry point, and all centers of safe zones are transformed into a reference frame (I) with TP as its origin and the negative y-axis pointing towards the entry point. From this definition follows that $TP = [0, 0, 0]$ and $EP = [0, -l_t, 0]$, where l_t is the length of the trajectory. The position of the new entry point EP' is defined in generalized coordinates α_0 and β_0.

$$EP' = \begin{bmatrix} l_t \sin(\alpha_0) \\ -l_t \cos(\alpha_0) \cos(\beta_0) \\ -l_t \sin(\beta_0) \cos(\alpha_0) \end{bmatrix} \tag{1}$$

To complete the definition of the pendulum, a rigid sphere with mass m_1 is attached at the location of EP' and a link between TP and EP' is defined with mass m_2. Without considering any safe zones and assuming normal gravity $g = [0, -1, 0] \times 9.81 \frac{m}{s^2}$, the pendulum is in a stable state at $\alpha = 0$ and $\beta = 0$.

Safe zones affect the trajectory as follows. First, all centers of safe zones $RP_i = [x_i, y_i, z_i]$ and their radii (r_i) are projected onto a plane defined by the point EP and the vector $[0, -1, 0]$ as its normal.

$$RP'_i = RP_i \frac{-l_t}{y_i} \tag{2}$$

$$r'_i = r_i \frac{-l_t}{y_i} \tag{3}$$

Springs between the projected centers RP'_i and EP' pull the trajectory away from nearby risk structures by applying forces (F_i) to the pendulum as shown in Fig. 3. The springs are parameterized using a stiffness factor (k) and the ratio between the initial confidence radius (r_t) and r'_i.

$$F_i = k\frac{r_t}{r'_i}(EP' - RP'_i) \tag{4}$$

The motion of the pendulum is limited using a damping force (F_d) with the factor (c) that is calculated using the current velocity (V) of EP'.

$$F_d = -cV \tag{5}$$

The effects of all forces that are applied to the pendulum are simulated using Kane's method [11] to calculate the new location of EP' where all forces are at equilibrium. The static parameters used in the current system are: $m_1 = 0.1$ kg, $m_2 = 0.01$ kg, $c = 5$, and $k = 25$. With these parameters, the duration of the simulation can be limited to 0.3 s to reach the equilibrium. The new location EP', however, can be computed faster than real-time so that the position updates are supplied without noticeable delay in the current implementation. The final entry point for the surgical procedure is located at the intersection of the refined trajectory and the patient's head surface.

Haptic Guides for Safe Zones: Safe zones are also used to visualize the boundaries of safe corridors using force feedback. Such haptic guides help operators to

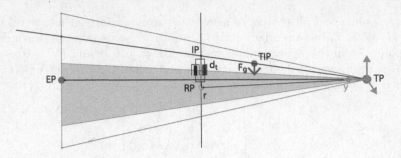

Fig. 4. Haptic guides are computed based on the specified trajectory and the marked safe zones. This example shows a trajectory with one safe zone that is defined by its center RP and its radius r. A conical volume defined by RP, TP, r marks a safe corridor. If the haptic stylus TIP is outside the safe corridor, a spring-damper system is activated that pulls the stylus back into the area marked grey. The conic volumes are intersected if multiple refinement points are active.

stay within previously defined safe zones while editing the trajectory or to identify impossible configurations earlier in the planning procedure. Impossible configurations exist when no trajectory passes safe zones within the defined distance to the center and therefore no safe path with the current configuration is possible.

Figure 4 shows an example how haptic guides are calculated using a single refinement point. The haptic stylus TIP is placed near the trajectory. A safe zone is defined by its center RP and a radius r. In this example the TIP is outside of the conical volume (grey) described by TP, RP, and r. In this case, a haptic guide is activated that pulls the stylus back into the safe zone by displaying a force. The force is generated using a spring-damper system that pulls the TIP towards the safe volume (blue arrow). Multiple safe zones generate multiple overlapping conical volumes. The intersection of these volumes is visualized using force feedback.

Feedback forces to display haptic guides are computed as follows. First, for each safe zone, we transform the TIP position (T), the target point (TP), the entry point (EP), and the center (RP) into a reference frame with TP as its origin and the positive y-axis pointing towards the entry point. The trajectory is therefore defined by $TP = [0, 0, 0]$ and $EP = [0, l_t, 0]$, where l_t is the length of the trajectory. Then, we define a ray from the origin TP through $T = [x_t, y_t, z_t]$ and compute the intersection point (IP) of the ray with the plane that is defined by the center RP and the normal $[0, 1, 0]$.

$$IP = T\frac{l_t}{y_t} \tag{6}$$

Then, we compute the distance d_t from IP to RP. If d_t is larger than the radius (r) of the current safe zone, the system activates the haptic guide. Finally, we calculate the guide force F_g using the unit vector $v_g = \frac{RP-IP}{\|RP-IP\|}$, the magnitude $m_g = d_t - r$, and a stiffness factor k.

$$F_g = k(m_g v_g) \tag{7}$$

To ensure stability of the system, a damping force is displayed if any haptic guide is active. The damping force (F_d) is computed using the velocity (V) of the *TIP* and a damping factor (c) (see Eq. 5). The stiffness factor k and the damping factor c need to be adapted to the properties of the haptic device and the end-to-end latency of the haptic rendering component.

Finally, all forces that are generated by active haptic guides are added and divided by the number of active guides. Then, we add the damping force, transform the resulting force vector back into world coordinates, and display the haptic feedback to the user. The feedback forces are disabled if the distance of the *TIP* to the closest safe corridor is above an activation distance to avoid unwanted forces when moving the haptic stylus. Furthermore, the haptic effect is disabled if the *TIP* is too close to *TP* since the safe corridor becomes too narrow to render stable forces.

4 Implementation

We implemented our system for exploring and evaluating novel interaction techniques in neurosurgery trajectory planning. The system was developed with H3DAPI for visual and haptic rendering. We integrated the tracking and sensor-fusion library Ubitrack [10] and calibrated the complete system using the calibration method presented by Eck et al. [8]. The remaining registration errors between haptic and visual stimuli are typically between $1 - 2$ mm after calibration. The target environment for running the application is a VHAR workspace that consists of a custom HMD, an AR-Tracking DTrack system, a PHANToM Premium haptic device, and a tracked Kensington Wireless Presenter.

As previously discussed in Sect. 3, the user interface consists of two main components: volume exploration and trajectory planning. Both components access a shared model consisting of all volumetric images and segmented structures including their attributes and spatial relations. The implemented planning workflow guides operators through the planning process and provides sensible defaults for the visibility of information in the visual and haptic channels. Patient data is loaded from PyDBS [4] datasets.

Figure 5 presents screen shots from the different trajectory planning stages: (a) The planning process starts with volume exploration. Users can attach the dataset to the sub-dominant hand controller to alter its position and orientation. With the haptic stylus tip they control the oblique slicing with viewpoint alignment to explore the volume and to identify the region of interest. (b) A target point is specified on a locked slice plane near or inside the region of interest. (c) The display switches to rendering risk structures for identifying possible entry point regions. Once found, the entry point and its confidence region are defined. Users receive haptic feedback when they hit the head surface. (d) Verification is required after each modification of the trajectory. Operators load different image modalities and inspect the regions near the planned trajectory using the trajectory-aligned slice view. (e) if they find any risk structures nearby they mark a safe corridor near the identified risk, which alters the planned trajectory.

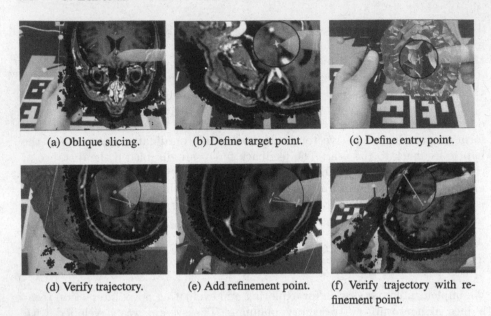

(a) Oblique slicing.   (b) Define target point.   (c) Define entry point.

(d) Verify trajectory.   (e) Add refinement point.   (f) Verify trajectory with re-
                                                                 finement point.

Fig. 5. Screenshots from the application. (b–f) area of interest is magnified for better visibility (not part of the visualization).

(f) Operator is inspecting a refined trajectory. Note how the trajectory does not directly pass the defined trajectory points anymore, but shows the result of the physics-based optimization.

Haptic feedback is generated with context-dependent force effects. These effects receive the haptic pose in real-time and display guide forces. The following effects generate haptic feedback:

- **Plane Constraints** are active when oblique slice planes are locked or during interaction with other planar user interface elements like menus. They are defined by a plane, force calculation parameters (stiffness and damping), and an activation distance that disables the force effect if the distance of the haptic stylus exceeds the limit. Once the haptic stylus is close enough, the force effect pulls the haptic stylus towards the plane.
- **Rigid Surfaces** are rendered for selected segmented structures like the head surface during entry point definition. Such guides help during 3D point placement, because operators do not need to verify the placement from different perspectives.
- **Safe Corridors** are defined by safe zones. Section 3.2 provides details about haptic guides for safe corridors.

During interviews with medical experts, we gathered feedback in various stages during the development. The volume exploration component received positive feedback during reviews with junior and senior medical experts. The experts did not require any training to use the system and stated that navigating the medical dataset is very intuitive and efficient. They suggested to extend the current implementation with capabilities for scaling the dataset and to provide magnification lenses so that operators can interact more precisely and get a more detailed view on the patient data. The final review with a junior medical expert showed that the current application provides a useful interface for trajectory planning that should be further evaluated with a group of more experienced neurosurgeons and neurologists to validate the utility of the proposed planning tool. During the review, the junior expert tested the trajectory planning workflow by performing several planning tasks. He found that the haptic guide that displays the head surface is very useful to correctly position the initial entry point. The proposed method to improve the trajectory refinement looks promising, however, the definition of safe zones using a disc-like shape could be improved by enabling operators to mark them with a more flexible approach like free-hand segmentation.

5   Conclusions and Future Work

The neurosurgery planning application provides a novel user interface for trajectory planning in stereo-tactic interventions. The intuitive user interface simplifies volume exploration. The additional haptic guides reduce visual clutter and help operators to efficiently plan trajectories. The interactive refinement approach reduces the number of iterations that are required for editing and refining trajectories by optimizing the entry point using manually defined safe corridors.

In future work, we plan to evaluate the VHAR user interface for trajectory planning with a group of medical experts. Such evaluation would include the comparison of user performance and accuracy for systems with and without haptic risk guides, comparing the proposed oblique slicing method with traditional cross-section slices, studying the benefits of the proposed viewing modes for the interactive volume exploration component, and comparing the proposed system to current state-of-the-art desktop based planning systems.

Furthermore, we plan to extend the algorithms that refine the trajectory and provide haptic guides to support more flexible shapes for marking safe zones during the planning process. A possible approach is to allow operators to draw safe zones in the slice images instead of specifying a center and a radius. With more detailed information about risk structures in patient datasets such as blood vessels and critical brain regions, the haptic guides could also be automatically generated once a target point has been defined, similar to Shamir et al. [15].

Finally, the work presented in this paper enables the evaluation of 3D user interfaces for trajectory planning. The presented interaction techniques can potentially improve the outcome of stereo-tactic interventions for patients by reducing the required time for planning and by increasing the safety of the planned trajectories.

References

1. Abhari, K., Baxter, J.S.H., Chen, E.S., Khan, A.R., Wedlake, C., Peters, T., Eagleson, R., de Ribaupierre, S.: The role of augmented reality in training the planning of brain tumor resection. In: Liao, H., Linte, C.A., Masamune, K., Peters, T.M., Zheng, G. (eds.) MIAR 2013 and AE-CAI 2013. LNCS, vol. 8090, pp. 241–248. Springer, Heidelberg (2013)
2. Bériault, S., Al Subaie, F., Collins, D.L., Sadikot, A.F., Pike, G.B.: A multi-modal approach to computer-assisted deep brain stimulation trajectory planning. Int. J. Comput. Assist. Radiol. Surg. **7**(5), 687–704 (2012)
3. Bériault, S., Subaie, F.A., Mok, K., Sadikot, A.F., Pike, G.B.: Automatic trajectory planning of DBS neurosurgery from multi-modal MRI datasets. In: Fichtinger, G., Martel, A., Peters, T. (eds.) MICCAI 2011, Part I. LNCS, vol. 6891, pp. 259–266. Springer, Heidelberg (2011)
4. Albis, T.D., Haegelen, C., Essert, C., Fernandez-Vidal, S., Lalys, F., Jannin, P.: PyDBS: an automated image processing workflow for deep brain stimulation surgery. Int. J. Comput. Assist. Radiol. Surg. **10**(2), 117–128 (2015)
5. De Momi, E., Caborni, C., Cardinale, F., Castana, L., Casaceli, G., Cossu, M., Antiga, L., Ferrigno, G.: Automatic trajectory planner for stereo-electro-encephalography procedures: a retrospective study. IEEE Trans. Biomed. Eng. **60**(4), 986–993 (2013)
6. Dormont, D., Seidenwurm, D., Galanaud, D., Cornu, P., Yelnik, J., Bardinet, E.: Neuroimaging and deep brain stimulation. Am. J. Neuroradiol. **31**(1), 15–23 (2010)
7. Eagleson, R., Wucherer, P., Stefan, P., Duschko, Y., de Ribaupierre, S., Vollmar, C., Fallavollita, P., Navab, N.: Collaborative table-top VR display for neurosurgical planning. In: Proceedings of the IEEE Virtual Reality Conference, pp. 169–170 (2015)
8. Eck, U., Pankratz, F., Sandor, C., Klinker, G., Laga, H.: Precise haptic device co-location for visuo-haptic augmented reality. IEEE Trans. Comput. Graph. Vis. **21**(12), 1427–1441 (2015)
9. Goble, J.C., Hinckley, K., Pausch, R., Snell, J.W., Kassell, N.F.: Two-handed spatial interface tools for neurosurgical planning. IEEE Comput. **1**(7), 20–26 (1995)
10. Huber, M., Pustka, D., Keitler, P., Echtler, F., Klinker, G.: A system architecture for ubiquitous tracking environments. In: Proceedings of the 6th IEEE and ACM International Symposium on Mixed and Augmented Reality, pp. 211–214. IEEE Computer Society, Nara (2007)
11. Kane, T.R., Levinson, D.A.: Dynamics, Theory and Applications. McGraw-Hill Book Company, New York (1985)
12. Khlebnikov, R., Kainz, B., Muehl, J., Schmalstieg, D.: Crepuscular rays for tumor accessibility planning. IEEE Trans. Vis. Comput. Graph. **17**(12), 2163–2172 (2011)
13. Preim, B., Bartz, D.: Visualization in Medicine. Morgan Kaufmann, Burlington (2007)
14. Shamir, R.R., Horn, M., Blum, T., Mehrkens, J.H., Shoshan, Y., Joskowicz, L., Navab, N.: Trajectory planning with augmented reality for improved risk assessment in image-guided keyhole neurosurgery. In: Proceedings of the 8th IEEE International Symposium on Biomedical Imaging, pp. 1873–1876 (2011)
15. Shamir, R.R., Joskowicz, L., Tamir, I., Dabool, E., Pertman, L., Ben-Ami, A., Shoshan, Y.: Reduced risk trajectory planning in image-guided keyhole neurosurgery. Med. Phys. **39**(5), 2885–2895 (2012)

Interactive Depth of Focus for Improved Depth Perception

Megha Kalia$^{(\boxtimes)}$, Christian Schulte zu Berge, Hessam Roodaki,
Chandan Chakraborty, and Nassir Navab

Technische Universität München, Arcisstraße 21, 80333 Munich, Germany
kalia.megha84@gmail.com

Abstract. The need to look into human body for better diagnosis,
improved surgical planning and minimally invasive surgery led to breakthroughs in medical imaging. But, intra-operatively a surgeon needs to
look at multi-modal imaging data on multiple displays and to fuse the
multi-modal data in the context of the patient. This adds extra mental effort for the surgeon in an already high cognitive load surgery. The
obvious solution to augment medical object in the context of patient suffers from inaccurate depth perception. In the past, some visualizations
have addressed the issue of wrong depth perception, but not without
interfering with the natural intuitive view of the surgeon. Therefore, in
the current work an interactive depth of focus (DoF) blur method for
AR is proposed. It mimics the naturally present DoF blur effect in a
microscope. DoF blur forces the cue of accommodation and convergence
to come into effect and holds potential to give near metric accuracy; its
quality decreases with distance. This makes it suitable for microscopic
neurosurgical applications with smaller working depth ranges.

Keywords: Interactive DoF · Medical AR · Perception

1 Introduction

Augmented reality (AR) is a technology where 3D computer generated images
are superimposed on real-world images [16], ideally giving the perception of co-
existence of real and virtual components in the same space [15]. The idea of
application of AR in medical applications is not new [1,2,15,17,20]. Numerous
image-guided surgery systems have appeared in order to reduce surgical time
and to increase the understanding of the patient's anatomy intra-operatively
[18,19]. Despite remarkable improvements in calibration accuracy, these systems
still suffer from incorrect depth perception of the augmented object [6]. This
has made it difficult to integrate medical AR technology into natural surgical
workflow.

The problem of wrong depth perception in medical augmented reality is well
documented where the augmented object, despite being rendered at the correct
depth, seems to be pasted over the real scenario instead of being perceived as a

© Springer International Publishing Switzerland 2016
G. Zheng et al. (Eds.): MIAR 2016, LNCS 9805, pp. 221–232, 2016.
DOI: 10.1007/978-3-319-43775-0_20

part of the anatomical context [2]. Taking lessons from psychology, researchers have tried to use monocular depth cues to address the problem of wrong depth perception. For example, occlusion is used by Bajura et al. to improve depth perception by deploying a pit-like synthetic hole on the patient's body [2], while Bichlmeier et al. used parallax cue for the same problem by using a virtual window [17]. Although these groups addressed the problem of depth perception, the natural and intuitive anatomical view of the surgeon was hindered. Some other groups attempted to solve the spatial depth perception issue by using other depth cues like fog, partial occlusion and task-based visualization in neurosurgery [15]. Although these techniques have the potential to give a good spatial understanding of surgical field, the problem of relative depths between different layers of anatomy is still unaddressed. Augmenting too much information at various levels can also cause the problem of cluttering.

In the current work, the interactive depth of focus (DoF) blur, as a function of distance, is proposed and evaluated as a possible source of information about relative depths between various anatomical structures in intra-operative settings. The DoF blur effect forces the accommodation cue to come into play. The cue has potential to give depth information with metric accuracy, but is effective only within a limited distance range [8]. This makes the DoF technique suitable in microscopic surgical tasks, which naturally has DoF blur effect and works within a limited distance range. Another limitation of DoF blur is that it fails many times at giving ordinal depth information [8]. Therefore, the idea to combine this cue with the cue of occlusion, which inherently suffers from lack of quantitative depth information, is proposed.

2   Background and Related Work

To overcome the problem of wrong depth perception several research groups used and evaluated different depth cues. But the use of various depth cues is very much task dependent in medical AR. Therefore, in the current section we intend to briefly explain and mention the related state of the art, about the depth cues which are relevant to microsurgical tasks.

2.1   Depth of Focus

In optics, the amount of blur introduced in an image, depends on how far the image is formed from the imaging plane, as shown in Fig. 1 (left). This blur is quantified in the form of circle of confusion (CoC) which in turn depends on other factors. This effect is quite commonly encountered in normal photography and microscopy while trying to focus objects at different depths.

It is actually the cue of accommodation and convergence which is being simulated in optics of human visual system through DoF. Convergence, however comes into picture under stereoscopic vision. Accommodation is the change in the shape of eye lens to keep retinal image sharp. Ciliary muscles control the accommodation [24, 25]. Therefore, the information about the amount of move-ment of ciliary muscles to adjust eye lens thickness, while trying to focus on objects at different depths, goes to brain and is interpretted as depth informa-tion. Thus, even in monocular vision the cue of accommodation can give near metric depth accuracy. But the cue fails to give ordinal depth information, since objects both in front and at back, are out of focus. Also, this cue is effective only up to a limited threshold distance. In medical AR, Ropinski et al. [4] used DoF in CT vessel angiography data. The effect was applied to add depth percep-tion to angiography data which is usually devoid of any spatial depth cues. The accuracy was improved but an increase in response time was recorded. They heuristically defined a depth threshold to apply different amounts of blur at different depths. There was an inherent assumption that viewer is looking at the vessels nearby. Therefore, blur was applied at the far away vessels. This assumption and static blur might cause discomfort for viewer which could be of consideration, especially in surgical cases.

2.2 Occlusion

Occlusion is said to be the strongest among all the depth cues [5]. Though, the use of term *occlusion* as a depth cue is ambiguous, since occlusion does not provide depth information per se. Occlusion is the source of ordinal depth information [7]. The cue is equally effective at varied distances [8]. Therefore, the cue rather asserts the depth order information in case of ambiguous depth cues.

The cue of occlusion is stronger than other depth cues and turns out to be the perpetrator for wrong depth perception in most of the cases. Even when the object is rendered at the correct depth, the mind perceives the object to be pasted or floating over background context because of occlusion. Therefore, numerous groups have tried partial occlusion to overcome this issue. Some groups tried to use curvature values to manipulate transparency for partial occlusion [3] while others tried to extract edge data from background. For visualization of vessel data in neurosurgery, Kersten-Oertel et al. [15] extracted sobel edges on GPU from background and manipulated the alpha values according to that. All the mentioned techniques although gave good visualization results they were very much task dependent.

2.3 Color

For hundreds of years, color has been used in pictures, art and paintings to add depth information. It is reported that color act as a depth cue because differ-ent colors have different wavelengths [9]. Colors having higher wavelengths are diffracted less than the colors having lower wavelengths and therefore, different colors are focused at different depths due to chromatic aberration. Thus, while looking at equidistantly different colored objects, it is not possible to perceive both the objects at same depth [9]. In medical AR community colors of rendered objects are chosen without much pre-thought. This not only can cause wrong depth perception but also inattention blindness [10]. Railey et al. [11] showed the effect of color on perceived depth of object by paired comparison test. The results complied by the known effect of warm and cool colors on depth perception, i.e. warm colors are perceived as nearer whereas cool color objects recede in perception [11,21].

3   Methods

3.1   Depth of Focus Blur Rendering

DoF focus rendering was performed using OpenGL framework using GLSL and C++. MRI and CT brain data was used for the purpose of visualization. From segmented tumor data, surface meshes were generated. The z-coordinates of these surface meshes were scaled to render different meshes at different depths in world coordinate space.

For DoF rendering according to depth, blurring was implemented according to CoC calculation. CoC was calculated according to thin lens model [14], [Fig. 1 (right)]. Here, a is the height of object, d is the distance of object from lens. f is the focal length of the lens and s is the screen position at which the image of object will be formed, whereas, x and x' are the de-focused images of the object. The difference of $|x - x'|$ is responsible for the diameter of CoC and hence, the amount of blur.

As can be seen in Fig. 1 (right), from the similarity of triangles we have

$$x/a = s/d \tag{1}$$

and

$$x'/a = (s - f)/f \tag{2}$$

which gives $x' = a(s/f - 1)$. Therefore, CoC diameter can be computed as,

$$CoC = |(x - x')|$$
$$= \left| a \left[s \left(\frac{1}{f} - \frac{1}{d} \right) - 1 \right] \right| \tag{3}$$

For the current implementation, focal length of human eye at infinity was taken as $f = 16.7$ mm and approximate normal aperture size of human eye was taken as $a = 7$ mm. After, CoC calculation at each depth point, it was converted to pixel coordinates. Gaussian kernel is applied for blurring whose kernel size was taken as half of the CoC in pixel coordinates.

Using render-to-texture approach each object was rendered as different layer in the form of a separate texture. This would allow to use each texture independent of others. Thus, each object's properties could be manipulated multiple times, without affecting other objects for the purpose of validation. Each object was also rendered in a depth texture. Depth values were sampled in a shader using GPU. In fragment shader, depth values were converted to object space by taking Z-near and Z-far planes. This step was important for CoC rendering in OpenGL since all depth values from various layers should be in the same depth range. The object space depth values were also scaled in the range of 0 to 150. The idea was to simulate interactive DoF and see its effect in the distance usually encountered in surgical scenario. CoC calculation was automatically performed according to depth where depth values were inputted from keyboard interactively.

The amount of blur was applied according to the function shown in Fig. 1 (right), where variation of CoC diameter was plotted with distance. It can be noticed that the relationship of amount of blur with distance is not linear and achieves plateau as the distance increases.

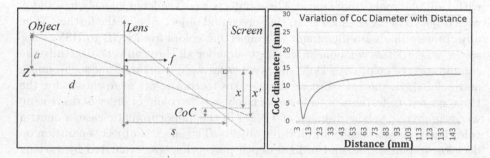

Fig. 1. (*left*) Thin lens model [14]. (*right*) Variation of CoC with depth

3.2 Eliminating the Effect of Other Depth Cues

For the purpose of evaluation of DoF blur, the influence of other depth cues was negated. For example, x and y-coordinates of two object meshes were scaled in the same range even when rendered at different depths to eliminate the effect of relative size cue. Similarly, to eliminate the influence of illumination-contrast, in HSV color-space *saturation* and *value* components were kept same changing only *hue* component for all rendered objects.

3.3 Experiments

In intra-surgical settings, the relative depth information between various anatomical layers is important for surgical planning and decision making. In a surgical microscope, the relative depth information is naturally present in the form of defocus blur. Therefore, experiments were designed to evaluate the effect of DoF blur with color and occlusion cue.

Objects were not rendered in real surgical image to evaluate DoF blur independent of other factors and depth cues, which otherwise were difficult to control, e.g. specular light, illumination contrast, color contrast and relative size cue. Though, if found relevant, the technique can easily be integrated in medical AR pipeline within human brain context.

Experiment 1: The purpose of the first experiment was the evaluation of effect of DoF blur with color cue on ordinal depth judgements. DoF blur mimics optical effects of accommodation, thus holds potential to give quantitative depth information. But as stated by Cutting et al. [8], the accommodation cue fails to give accurate ordinal depth judgments since farther as well as nearer objects are out of focus. This makes it difficult for the brain to make a decision.

The decision to supplement DoF blur with color cue information was taken since, in the field of medical AR, augmented objects are always presented in some color on surgical background. The ambiguous color selection can not only create conflict of cues but may also lead to inattention blindness [10], risking the complete defeat of the purpose of AR. Thus, studying the effect of color combined with DoF blur makes more sense. Three objects were rendered, namely a, b and c, with object a being the nearest to the screen and object c being the farthest. The objects were made iso-illuminant by converting colors from RGB to HSV–color space, where *Value* component was kept same for all three objects. To study the combination of color with DoF blur, two cases were generated: monochromatic and colored. In the *colored* case three warm to cool colors were chosen for the three nearest to farthest objects respectively, where colors in order of decreasing warmth are red, yellowish-green and blue. In the monochromatic case, a neutral color like gray was chosen for all three objects. The effect of object separation on decision response time and ordinal depth perception was evaluated by varying distance of objects in x–direction. The four test cases used in validation are shown in Fig. 2 (row 1).

Experiment 2: The purpose of the second experiment was to study the effect of occlusion cue, which is strongest to give ordinal information [8], on DoF blur, which lacks it. It is also reported in literature that occlusion asserts depth information and can be used to disambiguate other depth cues [7]. On the other hand, DoF blur is expected to complement weakness of occlusion cue in determining quantitative depth information.

The experiment was conducted in four sets. In two of the sets, DoF blur was combined with color cue and in another sets the color cue was missing.

3.4   Experimental Task

In the study, 11 young volunteers participated. All had either corrected-to-normal or normal vision. Volunteers were students, with some of them familiar with medical imaging or augmented reality, but none of them was fully aware about the purpose of the study. Images were shown to them on a computer monitor. Between images, randomly black blank screen was displayed for 5 s. Images shown contained only one of the objects in focus in different experimental setups. The images were shown in random order. Volunteers were asked to decide the depth order of the three objects shown in Fig. 2. Subjects were asked to press the stop button to stop time as soon as decision was taken and then the depth order was noted. All volunteers were aware that the time was being noted but no restriction on time limit was imposed.

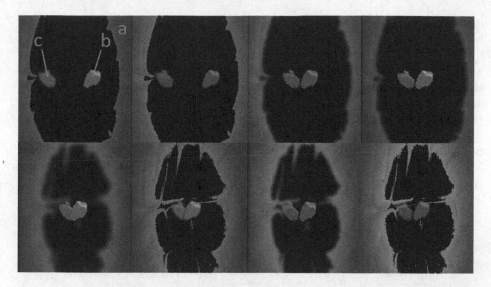

Fig. 2. (*Top row, left to right*) Sample images of four test cases: BCS, BMS, BMC and BCC. In all figures, labeled *a*, *b* and *c* are outer, middle and innermost surfaces, respectively. (*bottom row*) Sample video frames from experiment 2. (*left to right*) Blur + Color + Occlusion with surface *b* in focus, Blur + Color + Occlusion with surface *a* in focus, Blur + Monochrome + Occlusion with surface *b* in focus and Blur + Monochrome + Occlusion with surface *b* in focus, respectively (Color figure online)

In the second experiment, subjects were shown videos, in which they were allowed to freely change the focus themselves using keyboard buttons. This was done to mimic the real time DoF blur, like in a normal microscope, and to see its effect on decision making and response time. In the same experiment, users' comments were noted, while performing tasks according to Think Aloud Protocol. The discussions about DoF blur as possible depth cue were conducted with all the volunteers to make them familiar with what they were expected to see.

4   Results

4.1   Experiment 1

The effect of DoF blur was evaluated with color cue. The same combination was also evaluated by varying object distance in x-direction between objects *b* and *c* [Fig. 2 (top left)] i.e. objects were either close or separated in x–direction. Thus, four cases were evaluated in total i.e. Blur + Monochromatic + Separated (BMS), Blur + Monochromatic + Close (BMC), Blur + Colored + Close (BCC) and Blur + Colored + Separated (BCS). It should be noted here that the mean response time in the current study is the time taken by subjects to take final decision about depth order. Mean response times of all four cases came out to be 6.400 s, 5.475 s, 4.856 s and 5.029 s with standard errors (SE): 0.749 s, 0.638 s, 0.440 s and 0.462 s, respectively. While median values were 5.910 s, 4.435 s, 4.335 s and 4.280 s, respectively. The results are also shown in Fig. 3(A). The response times of DoF blur with color cue are nearly half of the DoF blur with no color cue. Also, it can be noticed that closer objects (Green Bar) have relatively less response time than the objects which were separated in x–direction (Blue Bar).

The mean correctness studied in the current work is the mean of the total number of times the subjects guessed the depth order of a surface correctly. Mean correctness of various surfaces was calculated in above mentioned four combinations, results of which are given in Table 1 and are shown in Fig. 3(B).

Table 1. Mean correctness of perceived ordinal depths of objects

	Surface c (s)	SE (s)	Surface b (s)	SE (s)	Surface a (s)	SE (s)
BMS	0.381	0.032	0.571	0.054	0.452	0.066
BMC	0.429	0.065	0.560	0.051	0.500	0.058
BCC	0.429	0.062	0.595	0.071	0.500	0.068
BCS	0.452	0.056	0.738	0.039	0.476	0.058

As can be seen in Fig. 3(B), mean correctness was highest for the middle surface b, then for the nearest surface a and lowest for the farthest surface c in all the cases. Also, as can be noticed, the mean correctness was almost the same in BMC and BCC combinations. The mean correctness for middle surface b was the highest in Blur + Colored + Separated case.

Probability of surface a (nearest in experiment) being perceived as the closest or the farthest in all the cases was also evaluated. The results are given in Fig. 3(C). Apart from Blur + Colored + Close case, in all of the cases probability of surface a being far and near was almost the same. In Blur + Colored + Close case the probability of surface a being the nearest was the highest which complies with reality too.

4.2   Experiment 2

In experiment 2, only perceived relative depths between different objects were asked from subjects, the results of which are shown in Fig. 3(D). The system was interactive and evaluation was done on all four cases like experiment 1. The results were in relative units on a scale from 1 to 10, where 1 meant the nearest (screen) and 10 meant the farthest (object c). The mean distances between objects a and b for BMS, BMC, BCC and BCS are 4.214, 4.458, 4.142 and 4.383 with standard deviation (SD): 1.329, 1.726, 1.698 and 1.332, respectively. While the mean distances between objects b and c are 1.714, 0.916, 1.250 and 1.666 with SD: 0.702, 0.790, 0.343 and 0.660, respectively [Fig. 3(D)].

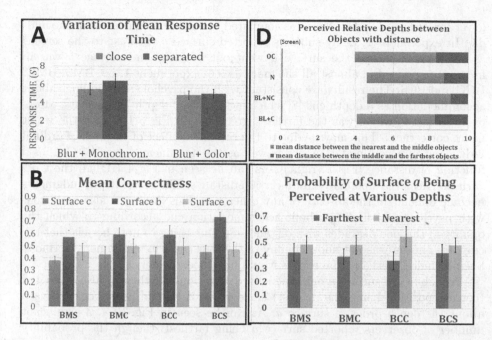

Fig. 3. (A) Mean response time (B) Mean correctness of Blur + Monochrom + Separated (BMS), Blur + Monochrome + Close (BMC), Blur + Colored + Close (BCC) and .Blur + Colored + Separated (BCS) cases (C) Probability of surface *a* being perceived as nearest or farthest (D) Perceived relative depths between different objects in experiment 2. OC, N, BL + NC, BL + C are blur + occlusion, no blur + color, blur + monochrome and blur + color. Note: In all graphs, error bars show standard error of mean (SEM) (Color figure online)

5 Discussion

In experiment 1, as can be seen in Fig. 3(A), the graph clearly shows the advantage of adding different colors to the objects when used with DoF blur. The response times decreased as compared to monochromatic sets. Therefore, color cue helped participants in taking quick decisions about depth order. Also in experiment 2, where the task was to evaluate relative depth perception between various objects, subjects responded quite quickly in presence of color cue. As a part of Think Aloud Protocol, almost all subjects reported that the addition of colors helped them to take quick decisions about relative depth. These results were similar to the findings of experiments of Nissen and Pokorny [12] where simple reaction times were affected by different wavelengths. Similar results were also reported by Breitmeyer and Breier [13]. Therefore it cannot be concluded if colors really affected perceptual judgments of subjects, but it might have influenced the response time.

Mean correctness of all surfaces, (the nearest, the middle and the farthest) in all the four cases in experiment 1 was evaluated. The mean correctness was lower for surface a and surface c as compared to surface b which was in the middle. In experiment 1, many subjects reported surface a (nearest to the screen) as the farthest, when the surface a went out of focus and surface b was in focus. It happened in almost all the four cases of experiment 1, i.e. BMS, BMC, BCC and BCS. The results are consistent with the psychological findings about accommodation as a depth cue [8] which lacks ordinal depth judgements. Moreover, surface c which was the farthest [green bar in Fig. 3(B)] gave the worst mean correctness. This may be due to the combined effect of the lack of ordinal judgement in accommodation cue as well as the non-linear nature of CoC as a function of distance [Fig. 1 (right)]. As can be seen in Fig. 1 (right), the CoC variation achieves a plateau after a certain distance. Therefore, depth judgments become difficult in the absence of any other cue. This finding is also consistent with psychological findings about accommodation cue according to which the quality of this cue degrades with distance [8]. One thing to note here is that the cue of occlusion was not added in any of the four cases in experiment 1. Had it been included, perhaps, the results would have been better.

Probability of surface a being perceived at various depths was also evaluated (correct position being the nearest) since most of the subjects were confused about the depth order of surface a. As can be seen in Fig. 3(C), a significant number of observers reported surface a being farthest, though the probability of its being near is still higher. This again can be due to inherent property of accommodation cue which lacks depth-order information.

In experiment 2, users reported general likeness for interacting freely with system to change DoF to estimate relative depths. Almost all the users remarked the ease to take depth judgments when system was interactive as compared to experiment 1, where images were still. The results of judgments about relative depths between different objects were rather interesting. In almost all four cases, i.e. Blur + Color, Blur + Monochromatic, No Blur + Color, Blur + Occlusion, the perceived distance between surface b (middle) and surface c (furthest) was much less than distance perceived between surface a (nearest) and surface b (middle). The degradation in quality of depth judgments is almost consistent with the graph shown in Fig. 1 (right), showing the variation of CoC with depths. As the amount of CoC and hence the amount of blur decreased with depth, so did the judgment about how far the object could be. For example, between surfaces b and c, the difference in amount of blur was negligible. Therefore, in the absence of any other cue, the subjects perceived the objects at almost same depths.

6   Conclusion

In the current work, DoF blur, combined with occlusion and color cue was presented as a technique to determine quantitative depth information between various layers of anatomy. The lack of ordinal depth information in accommodation cue was complemented with cue of occlusion, which rarely fails in giving depth order information. On the other hand, occlusion cue's lack of quantitative depth information was supplemented with ability of accommodation cue to give near metric accuracy of depth. Our visual system uses DoF blur effect in microscopy, as it's naturally present in microscope while changing focus on different objects. Therefore, our technique is expected to enhance natural intuitive view of surgeon in microsurgical view. Also, we applied DoF blur for thin lens, which can be modified for any lens by changing various lens parameters.

The relative depth judgment was observed to decline with distance. This was as expected from DoF blur, where initially CoC diameter increases with distance but later achieves plateau. In order to get better perception of relative depth DoF can be complemented with relative depth cue, from which relative distances can be deduced from difference in sizes of almost same size objects. Presence of this cue in almost all scenarios makes this complementation plausible. Further, DoF blur can be applied in linear range of CoC variation which can be adjusted by adjusting lens parameters in CoC equation.

The current work has potential to be used in neurosurgery. It can be applied to angiography data, which lacks 3D depth information. Its suitability for angiography comes from the fact that angiography has spatial spread of vessel tree which lacks 3-D depth cues. Although, DoF blur has previously been used by Ropinski et al. [4] their application of blur was empirical and static. Their application of blur was based on the assumption about point of view of user. This can make the surgical scene hazy at unwanted points. As reported in [22] users don't prefer DoF blur effect if it's applied on a fixed point presuming user's viewpoint. On the contrary, in our application of DoF blur, users reported better sense of depth when they were allowed to interact with system to change focus. Although, interaction with system improved the sense of perception and comfort, it might not be feasible in aseptic conditions in real surgical settings. Therefore, in future, eye-tracking to control DoF blur can be studied intra-operatively. In literature eye-tracking has also been reported to enhance users' comfort giving better depth perception [23].

References

1. Azuma, R., Baillot, Y., Behringer, R., Feiner, S., Julier, S., MacIntyre, B.: Recent advances in augmented reality. IEEE Comput. Graph. Appl. **21**(6), 34–47 (2001)
2. Bajura, M., Fuchs, H., Ohbuchi, R.: Merging virtual objects with the real world: seeing ultrasound imagery within the patient. ACM SIGGRAPH Comput. Graph. **26**(2), 203–210. ACM(1992)
3. Krüger, J., Schneider, J., Westermann, R.: Clearview: an interactive context preserving hotspot visualization technique. IEEE Trans. Vis. Comput. Graph. **12**(5), 941–948 (2006)
4. Ropinski, Timo, Steinicke, Frank, Hinrichs, Klaus H.: Visually Supporting Depth Perception in Angiography Imaging. In: Butz, Andreas, Fisher, Brian, Krüger, Antonio, Olivier, Patrick (eds.) SG 2006. LNCS, vol. 4073, pp. 93–104. Springer, Heidelberg (2006)
5. Ware, C.: Information Visualization: Perception for Design. Elsevier, Amsterdam (2012)

6. Johnson, L.G., Edwards, P., Hawkes, D.: Surface transparency makes stereo overlays unpredictable: the implications for augmented reality. Stud. Health Technol. Inform. **94**, 131–136 (2003)

7. Landy, M.S., Maloney, L.T., Johnston, E.B., Young, M.: Measurement and modeling of depth cue combination: in defense of weak fusion. Vis. Res. **35**(3), 389–412 (1995)

8. Cutting, J., Vishton, P.: Perceiving layout and knowing distances. In: Perception of Space and Motion, pp. 69–117 (1995)

9. Sundet, J.: Effects of colour on perceived depth: review of experiments and evalutaion of theories. Scand. J. Psychol. **19**(1), 133–143 (1978)

10. Dixon, B.J., Daly, M.J., Chan, H., Vescan, A.D., Witterick, I.J., Irish, J.C.: Surgeons blinded by enhanced navigation: the effect of augmented reality on attention. Surg. Endosc. **27**(2), 454–461 (2013)

11. Bailey, R., Grimm, C., Davoli, C.: The effect of warm and cool object colors on depth ordering. In: Proceedings of the 3rd Symposium on Applied Perception in Graphics and Visualization, p. 161. ACM (2006)

12. Nissen, M.J., Pokorny, J.: Wavelength effects on simple reaction time. Percept. Psychophysics **22**(5), 457–462 (1977)

13. Breitmeyer, B.G., Breier, J.I.: Effects of background color on reaction time to stimuli varying in size and contrast: inferences about human M channels. Vision. Res. **34**(8), 1039–1045 (1994)

14. Potmesil, M., Chakravarty, I.: A lens and aperture camera model for synthetic image generation. ACM SIGGRAPH Comput. Graph. **15**(3), 297–305 (1981)

15. Kersten-Oertel, Marta, Drouin, Simon, Chen, Sean J.S., Collins, DLouis: Volume Visualization for Neurovascular Augmented Reality Surgery. In: Liao, Hongen, Linte, Cristian A., Masamune, Ken, Peters, Terry M., Zheng, Guoyan (eds.) MIAR 2013 and AE-CAI 2013. LNCS, vol. 8090, pp. 211–220. Springer, Heidelberg (2013)

16. Shuhaiber, J.H.: Augmented reality in surgery. Arch. Surg. **139**(2), 170–174 (2004)

17. Bichlmeier, C., Wimmer, F., Heining, S.M., Navab, N.: Contextual anatomic mimesis hybrid in-situ visualization method for improving multi-sensory depth perception in medical augmented reality. In: ISMAR, pp. 129–138 (2007)

18. Cleary, K., Peters, T.M.: Image-guided interventions: technology review and clinical applications. Ann. Rev. Biomed. Eng. **12**, 119–142 (2010)

19. Kersten-Oertel, M., Jannin, P., Collins, D.L.: The state of the art of visualization in mixed reality image guided surgery. Comput. Med. Imaging Graph. **37**(2), 98–112 (2013)

20. Roberts, D.W., Strohbehn, J.W., Hatch, J.F., Murray, W., Kettenberger, H.: A frameless stereotaxic integration of computerized tomographic imaging and the operating microscope. J. Neurosurg. **65**(4), 545–549 (1986)

21. Tedford Jr., W.H., Bergquist, S.L., Flynn, W.E.: The size-color illusion. J. Gen. Psychol. **97**(1), 145–149 (1977)

22. Hillaire, S., Lécuyer, A., Cozot, R., Casiez, G.: Depth-of-field blur effects for first-person navigation in virtual environments. In: Proceedings of the ACM Symposium on Virtual Reality Software and Technology, pp. 203–206 (2007)

23. Hillaire, S., Lécuyer, A., Cozot, R., Casiez, G.: Using an eye-tracking system to improve camera motions and depth-of-field blur effects in virtual environments. In: IEEE Virtual Reality Conference, pp. 47–50 (2008)

24. Arnheim, R.: Art and Visual Perception: A Psychology of the Creative Eye. Univ of California Press, Berkeley (1954)

25. Gilinsky, A.S.: Perceived size and distance in visual space. Psychol. Rev. **58**(6), 460 (1951)

Augmented Reality for Neurosurgical Guidance: An Objective Comparison of Planning Interface Modalities

Ryan Armstrong[1(✉)], Trinette Wright[1], Sandrine de Ribaupierre[2], and Roy Eagleson[3]

[1] Biomedical Engineering Graduate Program,
The University of Western Ontario, London, Canada
rarmst2@uwo.ca

[2] Clinical Neurological Sciences, The University of Western Ontario, London, Canada

[3] Electrical and Computer Engineering,
The University of Western Ontario, London, Canada

Abstract. Numerous augmented reality image guidance tools have been evaluated under specific clinical criteria, but there is a lack of investigation into the broad effect on targeting ability and perception. In this paper, we evaluated performance of 18 subjects on a targeting task modeling ventriculostomy trajectory planning. Users targeted ellipsoids within a mannequin head using both an augmented reality interface and a traditional slice-based interface for planning. Users were significantly more accurate by several measures using augmented reality guidance, but were seen to have significant targeting bias; depth was underestimated by users with low targeting success. Our results further demonstrate the need for superior depth cues in augmented reality implementations while providing a framework for objective evaluation of augmented reality interfaces.

Keywords: Augmented reality · Ventriculostomy · Surgical simulation · Neurosurgery · Human performance

1 Introduction

Augmented reality (AR) technologies are gaining traction in the medical domain as tools for image guidance [1–5], preoperative planning [6], and training [7–10]. Although translation of these technologies from the research stage to clinical settings has been slow, numerous technologies have been demonstrated to be effective for improving surgical proficiency compared to traditional techniques [1,3,4,10]. While these platform-specific validation studies are providing converging evidence of clinical worth, there is a need for further evaluation of the specific ways that these augmented perceptual cues affect performance in terms of speed and accuracy.

In this paper, we describe the evaluation of a mobile AR interface in comparison to a traditional preoperative planning approach using 2D views sampled from orthogonal slices from a volumetric image modality. This paper will examine

© Springer International Publishing Switzerland 2016
G. Zheng et al. (Eds.): MIAR 2016, LNCS 9805, pp. 233–243, 2016.
DOI: 10.1007/978-3-319-43775-0_21

low-level targeting performance as a complement to high-level metrics involving patient outcomes and procedure-specific tasks. To examine these characteristics in a controlled environment, we specified a number of abstract tasks involving the targeting of ellipsoids of various sizes and shapes, displayed using a commercial neurosurgical simulator. The tasks model ventriculostomies - common neurosurgical procedures that requrie precise targeting of subsurface anatomy that is occluded to the surgeon. By providing a non-anatomical context, medical knowledge was not a prerequisite for performance of the tasks. As such, the tasks were entirely visuospatial in nature.

A total of 18 subjects were recruited to participate in the user study. Each user completed 30 tasks with the AR and 30 tasks with a traditional slice-based interface. Numerous measures of accuracy were derived in order to fully characterize user performance in both scenarios.

2   Methodology

2.1   Augmented Reality Interface

There are numerous approaches to AR implementation. Generally, systems are divided into the display and tracking components. The display is used to visually merge the virtual information onto the physical scene and present it intuitively to the user. These range from, projectors [5,12] and external monitors [13] to head mounted displays [2,6]. Tracking involves using references in the physical and virtual scenes in order to register the two into a single space. Optical [14], image-based markers [15], and now physical features [16] are all commonly employed to localize physical landmarks.

In our approach, we used a consumer-grade tablet computer as it provides a mobile and cost-effective all-in-one platform for computation, tracking, and display. The initial implementation of our AR system is described in Kramers et al. [17], but no user study was performed. The current application was implemented using Unity with the Vuforia augmented reality toolkit, rather than native Android development. We deployed it onto a Samsung Galaxy Tab S^{TM}, but the cross-platform nature allows for deployment onto other Android^{TM} and iOS^{TM} devices. Tracking utilizes the tablet's built-in camera to track image-based markers using Vuforia^{TM}. Vuforia^{TM} offers a number of trackable primitives and, although the implementation is closed source, it offers tools to optimize the robustness of image-based markers. Generally, images with a large number of asymmetric, high contrast points and corners are preferred. What the toolkit doesn't account for is the distance at which the marker must be tracked. For example, a marker image can be optimized for a large number of trackable points, but it would perform poorly at a long distance where those points cannot be resolved by the device camera. Our implementation made use of Vuforia's^{TM} cuboid primitive to facilitate tracking from a wide workspace. The image markers were then optimized for the application through an iterative trial-and-error approach. The final cuboid was affixed to the frame of sturdy eye glasses, seen in Fig. 1.

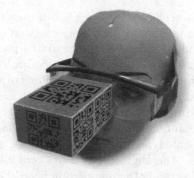

Fig. 1. The image-based cuboid marker has 4 trackable sides, allowing for a flexible workspace. As our platform's mannequin head is not fully supine, the apparatus is affixed.

2.2   Simulation Platform

An existing commercial surgical simulation platform was used as the foundation for simulated tasks. The NeuroTouch is a neurosurgical simulator that offers a number of modules for various procedures [18]. The simulator consists of a computer platform with a physical mannequin head and a haptic device that offers mechanical tracking. While other comprehensive neurosurgical simulators exist namely the ImmersiveTouch [19] the physical mannequin head is necessitated to provide the appropriate test-bed for our augmented reality interface. For the study, the image marker glasses were affixed to the mannequin. The physical and virtual spaces were registered using a graphical mesh of the mannequin head to align the two scenes identically using each ear helix and the nasion as anatomical landmarks. To provide visual feedback for registration accuracy as well as an additional depth cue, the graphical mannequin head mesh was overlaid on the physical head in the renderings with adjustable transparency.

Our user task is constructed around the NeuroTouch's burr hole selection task, which is typically used to test a surgeon's ability to localize a catheter tip within the ventricles for a range of ventriculostomy procedures. Ventriculostomies generally require a precise trajectory into the anterior horn of the lateral ventricles. Rather than target virtual anatomical features within the mannequin head, we constructed our module with a number of virtual ellipsoid targets of various shape, size and position within the mannequin head. This approach models the perceptual challenge of traditional ventriculostomies; surgeons must target a relatively small anatomical feature without sight of the feature inside the head and along a specific trajectory to avoid damaging eloquent tissue. Ellipsoids are well suited for 3D targeting tasks as they are a basic geometrical shape that can be used to specify a target which has a location as well as an orientation. The long axis allows us to specify the unique trajectory vector. Where the orientation of a sphere is indistinguishable, an ellipsoid's orientation is uniquely described by the vector of its longest axis (assuming that a longest axis exists on a given ellipsoid). As such, our targeting tasks were created in such a way as to permit a single ideal trajectory in each case. In total, 30 ellipsoids were created and positioned in the head in a pseudorandom approach. One of the limitations on ellipsoid position and orientation was imposed by the mechanical haptic device that acts as the input for trajectory selection; since the tool has a constrained workspace, all the ellipsoids were positioned in a way that they can be targeted by the device.

Each task involved planning, targeting and feedback. The planning stage utilized either the augmented reality guidance tool or a slice-based interface implemented in 3D Slicer. The augmented reality tool allowed the user to view the ellipsoids rendered directly on the mannequin head. The tablet could be held directly or mounted to a deformable spine to allow for hands-free operation. A stereoscopic display was not employed, so depth cues were largely gathered using cues from movement. Movement was constrained by the need to keep the image-based marker in the field of view of the device, but this still permits a rather large range of configurations in the approach. The alternative planning approach made use of a slice-based interface. Using this interface, users were able to view axial slices showing the intersection of the mannequin head and the current ellipsoid with each plane, which users could explore freely. Following the planning stage, users performed targeting. Targeting involved placing the tip of the mechanically tracked tool onto the mannequin head and indicating the chosen trajectory with its orientation. All targeting approaches originated from the right side as is standard for ventriculostomy procedures. Though the mechanically tracked arm limited tool range of motion, all ellipsoids were oriented to provide an accessible targeting path. A foot pedal was used for final selection of the trajectory. Though a haptic device was used, no haptic feedback was given as our task is a visuospatial abstraction of surgical procedures simulated by the platform. Finally, feedback was given after each task. The open-source 3D modeqiqqling software Blender was used for rendering feedback. In the feedback stage, the user's trajectory was rendered alongside a mesh of the mannequin head and views from 2 camera sources were shown. All components of the module were implemented on the NeuroTouch computer and automation between stages was achieved using AutoHotKey, which is an operating system level scripting program to automate tasks. This automation was necessitated because the NeuroTouch itself is a closed source system. Figure 2 displays screenshots of the planning and feedback stages.

2.3   User Study

The user study involved the recruitment of 18 subjects with no experience in the medical domain beyond basic anatomical knowledge. There was an even gender split and a single subject was left hand dominant. Subjects were randomly assigned to 2 groups; the first group completed all 30 tasks with the slice-based interface and then completed 30 tasks with the AR system, and the second group completed the AR component first followed by the slice-based interface. All users were first allowed time to become accustomed to the haptic tool. For each task, the position on the mannequin, the direction of the trajectory and

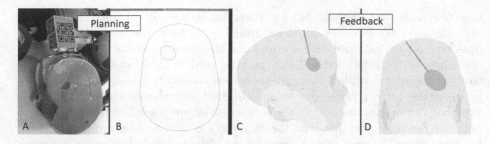

Fig. 2. *A.* Screenshot taken from the augmented reality tool during the planning stage. *B.* Screenshot taken from Slicer 3D during the slice-based planning stage. *C.* Screenshot from feedback stage showing right sagittal view. The user's trajectory is rendered green. *D.* Screenshot from feedback stage showing anterior coronal view. (Color figure online)

the time of completion were all recorded. Video was recorded of the tool space in order to examine how users interact with the different approaches. Participation time never exceeded an hour our subjects experienced minimal fatigue and maintained their enthusiastic motivation. Instructions were given in the form of a video tutorial and users were tasked to target the ellipsoids quickly and accurately. No additional instructions were given concerning specific techniques to approach each problem, permitting uninhibited learning and natural development of technique. Feedback was collected from each user following the tasks, but no formal questionnaire was administered. A user is shown using the AR interface with the system in Fig. 3.

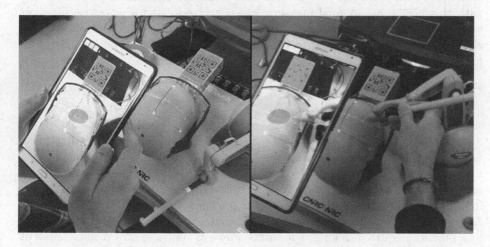

Fig. 3. A user guides their trajectory using the AR interface

2.4   Analysis

Analysis of user trajectories required development of objective metrics of performance. Bourdel et al. examined AR performance for a conceptually similar targeting task, but analysis did not cover broad metrics to fully characterize performance [20]. We considered the time of the task, the angle of deviation from the longest axis (rotational error) and the distance of the trajectory from the ellipsoid (translational error). The time and angle of deviation are relatively straightforward, but there are numerous candidate measures for the error between the correct trajectory to the ellipsoid and the user's trajectory. We explored various approaches. In the simplest case, we take the shortest distance between the trajectory line and the ellipsoid's centroid. This measure is valid for trajectories internal and external to the ellipsoid. In addition to the overall distance, we measured the distance in each Cartesian coordinate in order to examine targeting bias. The closest distance of the line to the surface was also considered, but this measure is only relevant when the trajectory does not enter the ellipsoid. The engagement is a measure that has been employed to evaluate ventriculostomy trajectories [21] and was adapted to ellipsoids in this study. The engagement is the length of the line segment that passes through the ellipsoid, which results in a value of 0 for trajectories that do not intersect the target. We adapted this measure as relative engagement, which takes the ratio of the engagement relative to the length of the target ellipsoid's longest axis. This allows for direct comparison of performance between ellipsoid cases. An additional relative measure is the relative distance from the centroid. To calculate this distance, we construct a line using the centroid and the closest point on the trajectory and we determine the distance from the centroid to the point on the ellipsoid that this new line intersects, which we term the inner distance. We calculate the relative distance by dividing the shortest distance from the centroid to the trajectory with this new value. A final measure was conceived using a piecewise function to penalize error in distance to a greater extent when trajectories are outside the target ellipsoid compared to those inside. The function is described by the following equation:

$$f(x) = \begin{cases} \frac{Distance\ from\ Center}{Inner\ Distance} & \text{Trajectory intersects} \\ ln(Distance\ from\ Surface + e) & \text{No intersection} \end{cases} \quad (1)$$

Inside the ellipsoid, a linear measure for error in position does not grow as largely as the logarithmic function outside. The function is continuous as a trajectory precisely on the surface of the ellipsoid will yield the same value on each side of the piecewise function. This function was derived to model the risk in clinical environments with a particular focus on ventriculostomy procedures. A small misplacement of the catheter in a ventriculostomy will likely still result in a functioning drain as long as it enters a lateral ventricle [22]. A minor miss of the ventricle will result in a non-functional drain and necessitate a second pass, but may not result in additional injury [23]. However, a trajectory and placement of the catheter that deviates significantly from standard clinical approaches can lead to severe injury in the patient [24]. A number of measures for trajectories internal and external to the ellipsoids are depicted in Fig. 4.

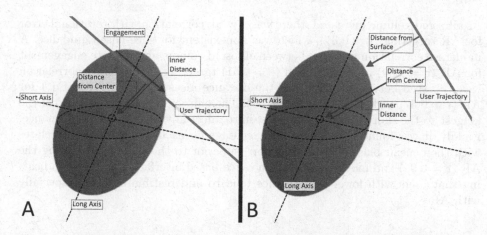

Fig. 4. *A*. Measures for a trajectory that intersect the ellipsoid *B*. Measures for targets that do not intersect the ellipsoid.

3   Results

Tables 1 and 2 compare various measures from all users using the AR interface compared to the slice-based interface. Significance was evaluated between means using the t-test.

There was no significant difference in time taken between interfaces. Over the order of cases, a weak learning curve was observed for rotational error ($r = -0.36$ for slice-based and $r = -0.23$ for AR) and there was a weak-moderate reduction in the task completion time ($r = -0.46$ for slice-based and $r = -0.59$ for AR).

Table 1. Mean values from all users for each modality for the percentage of intersecting trajectories, the deviation in the angle from the ellipsoid orientation and the relative engagement.

	Hit %	Angle error (degrees)	Relative engagement
Augmented mean:	0.59 ± 0.49	20.84 ± 17.03	$0.41 + 0.38$
Slice-based mean:	0.35 ± 0.47	28.03 ± 20.56	0.21 ± 0.31
Significance:	Yes ($p < 0.05$)	Yes ($p < 0.05$)	Yes ($p < 0.05$)

Table 2. Mean values for measures examining translational error. Positive X is towards the right side of the mannequin head, positive Y is towards the anterior and positive Z is towards the superior direction.

	Translation error (Eq. 1)	X Bias (mm)	Y Bias (mm)	Z Bias (mm)
Augmented mean:	1.45 ± 1.18	-5.72 ± 11.54	-1.09 ± 14.14	11.69 ± 15.67
Slice-based mean:	2.01 ± 1.18	-5.10 ± 12.57	-16.91 ± 16.53	9.40 ± 16.17
Significance:	Yes ($p < 0.05$)	No	Yes ($p < 0.05$)	Yes ($p < 0.05$)

As ellipsoid volume increased, there was a weak correlation with rotational error for AR targeting (r = 0.37), which was nonexistent for slice-based guidance. A moderate correlation was seen between ellipsoid volume and relative engagement for AR (r = 0.60) and slice-based (r = 0.61) targeting. A moderate correlation was also seen between volume and the distance measure presented in Eq. 1 for AR (r = 0.57) and slice-based (r = 0.60). The ellipsoid eccentricity (ratio of the longest to the shortest axis) was not seen to affect any measure of performance. Finally, it was found that mean hit percentage for each user strongly correlates with their mean bias in the Z direction (superior to the mannequin) using the AR (r = 0.96) and moderately with the slice-based interface (r = 0.71), indicating that users with lower performance tend to underestimate depth, especially with AR.

4 Discussion

By nearly all measures, AR guidance showed superior accuracy compared to the use of a traditional slice-based interface. No strong learning effects were seen, likely due to the nature of the experiment; it was relatively short and all tasks were performed in a single block session. Of particular interest was the examination of bias. Differences between approaches were seen in the Y and Z directions, which correspond to the posterior-anterior and inferior-superior planes in the mannequin, respectively. In the Z direction, large bias was seen with both approaches, but the bias is most prevalent among user with low hit ratios. Users who consistently miss the target using the AR guidance are nearly always underestimating the depth by choosing a trajectory that crosses the ellipsoid on the superior side. Difficulty estimating depth using augmented reality displays is a well-documented and investigated issue [24,25]. Similar to most implementations, our device is hindered by the problem of occlusion and lighting discrepancies. Additionally, our approach uses monoscopic rendering, necessitating strategic use of the tool to obtain depth cues from motion - a use that may not be intuitive to all users. While this is a pervasive problem, numerous consumer products aim to remedy the shortcomings, such as the Microsoft Hololens[TM] which will be released to market later this year and will be a target platform of our future work. In the Y direction, little bias was seen using AR compared to a strong bias towards the anterior using the slice-based approach. This phenomena warrants further investigation into the perceptual qualities of slice-based interfaces in the absence of anatomical structures to act as landmarks. Although no formal survey was administered, user feedback indicated that the constraints imposed by the mechanical haptic device impeded tool movement. Future work will involve improvements to the tracking and display of our AR system including targeting modern head-mounted platforms. Additionally, while our tracking system and registration is effective for our static mannequin, a more robust system is desired for translation to a clinical environment. An approach that tracks facial features is desirable, but these techniques have yet to prove robust. AR systems with as little as 2 mm of registration error have been noted to cause drastic performance degredation [25]. A free-hand tracking system will be incorporated into future revisions.

5   Conclusion

In this paper, we presented an approach to objectively evaluate targetting using various interface modalities. We found that our AR interface was more intuitive and resulted in more accurate targeting using numerous metrics, but caused users to underestimate target depth. While the AR tracking used was suitable for the static mannequin, a more robust approach is desirable for clinical applications. We hope that our evaluation approach can be adapted to additional environments and AR platforms as a standard for objective analysis of user performance.

Acknowledgments. The authors wish to ackowledge the assistance of Cody Bartel, Hunter Andrin, Ishan Tikku, Rebecca Whitney, Nimrita Bassi, and Sabrina Ren.

References

1. Ungi, T., Yeo, C.T., Paweena, U., McGraw, R.C., Fichtinger, G., et al.: Augmented reality needle guidance improves facet joint injection training. In: SPIE Medical Imaging, p. 79642E (2011)
2. Sauer, F., Khamene, A., Bascle, B., Rubino, G.J.: A head-mounted display system for augmented reality image guidance: towards clinical evaluation for iMRI-guided neurosurgery. In: Proceedings of the 4th International Conference on Medical Image Computing and Computer-Assisted Intervention, pp. 707–716 (2001)
3. Rosenthal, M., State, A., Lee, J., Hirota, G., Ackerman, J., Keller, K., Pisano, E.D., Jiroutek, M., Muller, K., Fuchs, H.: Augmented reality guidance for needle biopsies: an initial randomized, controlled trial in phantoms. Med. Image Anal. **6**, 313–320 (2002)
4. Chu, M.W., Moore, J., Peters, T., Bainbridge, D., McCarty, D., Guiraudon, G.M., Wedlake, C., Lang, P., Rajchl, M., Currie, M.E., et al.: Augmented reality image guidance improves navigation for beating heart mitral valve repair. Innov.: Technol. Tech. Cardiothorac. Vasc. Surg. **7**, 274–281 (2012)
5. Krempien, R., Hoppe, H., Kahrs, L., Daeuber, S., Schorr, O., Eggers, G., Bischof, M., Munter, M.W., Debus, J., Harms, W.: Projector-based augmented reality for intuitive intraoperative guidance in image-guided 3D interstitial brachytherapy. Int. J. Radiat. Oncol.* Biol.* Phys. **70**, 944–952 (2008)
6. Abhari, K., Baxter, J.S.H., Chen, E.S., Khan, A.R., Wedlake, C., Peters, T.M., de Ribaupierre, S., Eagleson, R.: Use of a mixed-reality system to improve the planning of brain tumour resections: preliminary results. In: Linte, C.A., Chen, E.C.S., Berger, M.-O., Mooro, J.T., Holmes III, D.R. (eds.) AE-CAI 2012. LNCS, vol. 7815, pp. 55–66. Springer, Heidelberg (2013)
7. Luciano, C., Banerjee, P., Lemole, G., Charbel, F., Charbel, F.: Second generation haptic ventriculostomy simulator using the ImmersiveTouch™ system. Stud. Health Technol. Inform. **119**, 343 (2005)

8. Leblanc, F., Champagne, B.J., Augestad, K.M., Neary, P.C., Senagore, A.J., Ellis, C.N., Delaney, C.P., Group, C.S.T.: A comparison of human cadaver and augmented reality simulator models for straight laparoscopic colorectal skills acquisition training. J. Am. Coll. Surg. **211**, 250–255 (2010)

9. Botden, S.M., Buzink, S.N., Schijven, M.P., Jakimowicz, J.J.: Augmented versus virtual reality laparoscopic simulation: what is the difference? World J. Surg. **31**, 764–772 (2007)

10. Lahanas, V., Loukas, C., Smailis, N., Georgiou, E.: A novel augmented reality simulator for skills assessment in minimal invasive surgery. Surg. Endosc. **29**, 2224–2234 (2015)

11. Mller, M., Rassweiler, M.-C., Klein, J., Seitel, A., Gondan, M., Baumhauer, M., Teber, D., Rassweiler, J.J., Meinzer, H.-P., Maier-Hein, L.: Mobile augmented reality for computer-assisted percutaneous nephrolithotomy. Int. J. Comput. Assist. Radiol. Surg. **8**, 663–675 (2013)

12. Fritz, J., Paweena, U., Ungi, T., Flammang, A.J., Kathuria, S., Fichtinger, G., Iordachita, I.I., Carrino, J.A., et al.: MR-guided vertebroplasty with augmented reality image overlay navigation. Cardiovasc. Interv. Radiol. **37**, 1589–1596 (2014)

13. Lpez-Mir, F., Naranjo, V., Fuertes, J.J., Alcaiz, M., Bueno, J., Pareja, E.: Design and validation of an augmented reality system for laparoscopic surgery in a real environment. Biomed. Res. Int. **2013** (2013). Article ID 758491

14. Sielhorst, T., Feuerstein, M., Navab, N.: Advanced medical displays: a literature review of augmented reality. J. Disp. Technol. **4**, 451–467 (2008)

15. Kramers, M., Armstrong, R., Bakhshmand, S.M., Fenster, A., de Ribaupierre, S., Eagleson, R.: Evaluation of a mobile augmented reality application for image guidance of neurosurgical interventions. Stud. Health. Technol. Inform. **196**, 204–208 (2014)

16. Suenaga, H., Tran, H.H., Liao, H., Masamune, K., Dohi, T., Hoshi, K., Takato, T.: Vision-based markerless registration using stereo vision and an augmented reality surgical navigation system: a pilot study. BMC Med. Imaging **15**, 51 (2015)

17. Kramers, M., Armstrong, R., Bakhshmand, S.M., Fenster, A., de Ribaupierre, S., Eagleson, R.: A mobile augmented reality application for image guidance of neurosurgical interventions. Am. J. Biomed. Eng. **3**, 169–174 (2013)

18. Delorme, S., Laroche, D., DiRaddo, R., Del Maestro, R.F.: NeuroTouch: a physics-based virtual simulator for cranial microneurosurgery training. Neurosurgery **71**, ons32–ons42 (2012)

19. Luciano, C., Banerjee, P., Florea, L., Dawe, G.: Design of the ImmersiveTouch[TM]: a high-performance haptic augmented virtual reality system. In: Proceedings of the 11th International Conference on Human-Computer Interaction, Las Vegas, Nevada (2005)

20. Bourdel, N., Collins, T., Pizarro, D., Bartoli, A., Da Ines, D., Perreira, B., Canis, M.: Augmented reality in gynecologic surgery: evaluation of potential benefits for myomectomy in an experimental uterine model. Surg. Endosc., 1–6 (2016)

21. Muirhead, W.R., Basu, S.: Trajectories for frontal external ventricular drain placement: virtual cannulation of adults with acute hydrocephalus. Br. J. Neurosurg. **26**, 710–716 (2012)

22. Kakarla, U.K., Chang, S.W., Theodore, N., Spetzler, R.F., Kim, L.J.: Safetyand accuracy of bedside external ventricular drain placement. Neurosurgery **63**, ONS162–ONS167 (2008)

23. Hsieh, C.-T., Chen, G.-J., Ma, H.-I., Chang, C.-F., Cheng, C.-M., Su, Y.-H., Ju, D.-T., Hsia, C.-C., Chen, Y.-H., Wu, H.-Y., Liu, M.-Y.: The misplacement of external ventricular drain by freehand method in emergent neurosurgery. Acta Neurol. Belg. 111, 22–28 (2011)
24. Berning, M., Kleinert, D., Riedel, T., Beigl, M.: A study of depth perception in hand-held augmented reality using autostereoscopic displays. In: 2014 IEEE International Symposium on Mixed and Augmented Reality (ISMAR), pp. 93–98 (2014)
25. Lee, C.-G., Oakley, I., Ryu, J.: Exploring the impact of visual-haptic registration accuracy in augmented reality. In: Isokoski, P., Springare, J. (eds.) EuroHaptics 2012, Part II. LNCS, vol. 7283, pp. 85–90. Springer, Heidelberg (2012)

Medical Image Analysis

Adaptive Mean Shift Based Hemodynamic Brain Parcellation in fMRI

Mohanad Albughdadi[✉], Lotfi Chaari, and Jean-Yves Tourneret

IRIT, INP-ENSEEIHT, University of Toulouse, Toulouse, France
{mohanad.albughdadi,lotfi.chaari,jean-yves.tourneret}@enseeiht.fr

Abstract. One of the remaining challenges in event-related fMRI is to discriminate between the vascular response and the neural activity in the BOLD signal. This discrimination is done by identifying the hemodynamic territories which differ in their underlying dynamics. In the literature, many approaches have been proposed to estimate these underlying dynamics, which is also known as Hemodynamic Response Function (HRF). However, most of the proposed approaches depend on a prior information regarding the shape of the parcels (territories) and their number. In this paper, we propose a novel approach which relies on the adaptive mean shift algorithm for the parcellation of the brain. A variational inference is used to estimate the unknown variables while the mean shift is embedded within a variational expectation maximization (VEM) framework to allow for estimating the parcellation and the HRF profiles without having any prior information about the number of the parcels or their shape. Results on synthetic data confirms the ability of the proposed approach to estimate accurate HRF estimates and number of parcels. It also manages to discriminate between voxels in different parcels especially at the borders between these parcels. In real data experiment, the proposed approach manages to recover HRF estimates close to the canonical shape in the bilateral occipital cortex.

1 Introduction

Functional magnetic resonance imaging (fMRI) is a powerful non-invasive imagining technique to indirectly measure neural activity from the blood-oxygen-level dependent (BOLD) signal [1]. fMRI data analysis relies on two main task; the detection of activation in brain areas after a given stimulus and the estimation of the underlying dynamics of the brain which is also called as the hemodynamic response function (HRF). Many attempts to describe the link between stimuli and the induced BOLD signal have been proposed. The basic model is the so-called general linear model (GLM). In this model, the link between the stimuli and the induced BOLD signal is modelled as a convolution between the HRF and the binary stimulus sequence. However, this model considers a fixed HRF shape [2,3]. Many extensions have been proposed to account for the variability of the

The authors would like to thank Dr. Philippe Ciuciu for providing them with the real data used for validation.

G. Zheng et al. (Eds.): MIAR 2016, LNCS 9805, pp. 247–258, 2016.
DOI: 10.1007/978-3-319-43775-0_22

HRF by using more regressors [4–6] which leads to less reliability in the detection task. Other approaches depending on physiologically-informed non-linear models (like the Balloon model) have been used to recover the hemodynamics in brain areas where activation has already been detected [5,7,8]. However, these approaches are computationally intensive for a whole brain analysis and the presence of noise causes some identifiability issues.

The detection of the evoked activity and the estimation of the dynamics have been mainly addressed as two separate tasks while each of them depends on the other. A precise localization of activations depends on a reliable HRF estimate, while a robust HRF shape is only achievable in brain regions eliciting task-related activity [9]. In this context, the joint detection estimation (JDE) model performs both tasks simultaneously [10–12]. In the JDE model, a single HRF shape is considered for a specific parcel (group of voxels). Although the JDE model jointly detects the evoked activity within the brain and estimates the HRF, it still requires a prior parcellation of the brain into functionally homogeneous regions. This challenge motivated the development of the joint parcellation detection estimation (JPDE) model [13,14] that performs online parcellation along with the detection and estimation tasks by setting voxels that share the same HRF pattern in the same HRF group (parcel). The JPDE model can be inferred using the VEM algorithm. However, this model still requires manual settings of the number of parcels. Indeed, carefully setting the true number of parcels is important for such a model which allows decomposing the brain into homogeneous regions from a functional point of view. Since the parcellation is based on the hemodynamic properties, it is supposed to change with the experiment type. Since a given voxel is supposed to respond differently for each stimulus, the number of parcels can therefore change with the experimental paradigm. For this reason, setting at once the number of parcels could not solve the model selection issue for the JPDE. To overcome this issue, a model selection procedure was proposed in [15] to select the optimum number of parcels. This procedure depends mainly on free energy calculations where the model that maximizes the free energy is the best fit for the data. The limitation of this procedure arises from the fact that it needs to be run for each candidate model which can be time consuming especially if no prior information exists about the number of parcels. The standard JPDE model has been adopted in a Bayesian non-parametric approach [16] by making use of the Dirichlet process mixtures model combined with a hidden Markov random field to automatically infer the number of parcels and their shapes simultaneously with the estimation and detection tasks.

In this paper, a new approach relying on the adaptive mean shift is proposed to estimate the number of parcels online from the fMRI data. The novelty in this approach lies in replacing the Bayesian non-parametric with the mean shift which implies a significant reduction in the computational cost associated with estimating the interaction parameter of the hidden Markov random field of the model proposed in [16]. More precisely, we propose to embed the adaptive mean shift algorithm (which is a common clustering algorithm) within the variational inference framework associated with the JPDE model to estimate the parcels and their corresponding HRF profiles.

The rest of the paper is organized as follows. The JPDE model is summarized in Sect. 2. The adaptive mean shift (AMS) algorithm is illustrated in Sect. 3. The inference strategy of the AMS-JPDE (for adaptive mean shift with JPDE model) model is described in Sect. 4 along with the use of the AMS algorithm within the VEM framework. Experimental validation on synthetic and real fMRI data is presented in Sect. 5. Finally, conclusion and future work are drawn in Sect. 6.

2   The JPDE Model

The adopted JPDE model is the one proposed in [13,14]. Let $\mathcal{P}$ be the set of voxels (J voxels) and $\boldsymbol{y}_j \in \mathbb{R}^N$ the fMRI time series for the voxel j at times $\{t_n, \ n = 1, \ldots, N\}$, where $t_n = n\,TR$, N is the number of scans and TR is the repetition time. The BOLD time series is denoted as $\boldsymbol{Y} = \{\boldsymbol{y}_j, j \in \mathcal{P}\}$. M different experimental conditions are considered. The model assumes that the HRFs are voxel-dependent and the whole set is denoted as $\boldsymbol{H} = \{\boldsymbol{h}_j, j \in \mathcal{P}\}$ with $\boldsymbol{h}_j \in \mathbb{R}^D$. Each $\boldsymbol{h}_j$ is associated with one among K considered HRF groups (parcels). A set of hidden variables $\boldsymbol{z} = \{z_j, j \in \mathcal{P}\}$ is used to encode these groups where $z_j \in \{1, \ldots, K\}$ and $\boldsymbol{z}$ follows a K-class Potts model with interaction parameter β_z to account for spatial connexity. In the group $\#k$ and voxel $\#j$, the HRF $\boldsymbol{h}_j$ is a stochastic perturbation of an HRF pattern $\bar{\boldsymbol{h}}_k$ such that $\boldsymbol{h}_j \sim \mathcal{N}(\bar{\boldsymbol{h}}_k, \nu_k \boldsymbol{I}_D)$, where ν_k is a parameter which controls the stochastic perturbations around $\bar{\boldsymbol{h}}_k$ and $\boldsymbol{I}_D$ is the identity matrix of size $D \times D$. Smooth HRF patterns are forced by assigning them the prior $\bar{\boldsymbol{h}}_k \sim \mathcal{N}(0, \sigma_h^2 \boldsymbol{R})$ where $\boldsymbol{R} = (\Delta t)^4 (\boldsymbol{D}_2^t \boldsymbol{D}_2)^{-1}$, $\Delta t < TR$ is the sampling period of the unknown HRFs and $\boldsymbol{D}_2$ is the second order finite difference matrix. The following observation model is considered

$$\forall j \in \mathcal{P}, \quad \boldsymbol{y}_j = \sum_{m=1}^M a_j^m \boldsymbol{X}_m \boldsymbol{h}_j + \boldsymbol{P}\boldsymbol{\ell}_j + \boldsymbol{\varepsilon}_j, \tag{1}$$

where the low frequency drifts are denoted by $\boldsymbol{P}\boldsymbol{\ell}_j$ and $\boldsymbol{X}_m = \{x_m^{n-d\Delta t}, n = 1, \ldots, N, d = 0, \ldots, D-1\}$ is a binary matrix that provides information on the stimulus occurrences for the mth experimental condition. The neural response levels (NRL) are denoted by $\boldsymbol{A} = \{\boldsymbol{a}^m, m = 1, \ldots, M\}$ with $\boldsymbol{a}^m = \{a_j^m, j \in \mathcal{P}\}$. The amplitudes $\boldsymbol{a}^m$'s follow spatial Gaussian mixtures defined by a set of parameters $\boldsymbol{\theta}_a$ and governed by binary Markov fields. More specifically, each NRL is assigned to one of the activation classes encoded by the variables $\boldsymbol{Q} = \{\boldsymbol{q}^m, m = 1, \ldots, M\}$ where $\boldsymbol{q}^m = \{q_j^m, j \in \mathcal{P}\}$ is a binary Markov field with interaction parameter β_m distributed according to an exponential distribution with parameter λ_m. Two classes are considered; ($q_j^m = 1$) if voxel j is activated by condition $\#m$ and ($q_j^m = 0$) otherwise. An additive Gaussian noise $\boldsymbol{\varepsilon}_j$ is considered with covariance matrix $\boldsymbol{\Gamma}_j^{-1}$. The set of all parameters is denoted as $\boldsymbol{\Theta} = \{\boldsymbol{L}, \boldsymbol{\Gamma}, \boldsymbol{\theta}_a, \boldsymbol{\nu}, \boldsymbol{\lambda}, \sigma_h^2, \bar{\boldsymbol{h}}, \boldsymbol{\beta}, \beta_z\}$ where $\boldsymbol{\Gamma} = \{\boldsymbol{\Gamma}_j, j \in \mathcal{P}\}$, $\boldsymbol{\nu} = \{\nu_k, k = 1, \ldots, K\}$, $\boldsymbol{\beta} = \{\beta_m, m = 1, \ldots, M\}$ and $\bar{\boldsymbol{h}} = (\bar{\boldsymbol{h}}_k)_{1 \leq k \leq K}$. More details about the meaning of these parameters are available in [13,14].

A variational approach was proposed in [13,14] to approximate the posterior of the JPDE model as the product of simple distributions. More precisely, the posterior of the JPDE model was approximated as

$$\tilde{p}(A, H, Q, z \,|\, Y) = \tilde{p}_A(A)\tilde{p}_H(H)\tilde{p}_Q(Q)\tilde{p}_z(z). \tag{2}$$

The inference was carried out in two parts: the expectation step which was divided into four main steps to compute approximate posteriors of the variables $\{A, H, Q, z\}$, and the maximization step to estimate the unknown parameters. The interested reader can refer to [13,14] for further details.

3   Adaptive Mean Shift Algorithm

Mean shift is a feature space analysis algorithm which has been widely used for computer vision tasks. Feature space analysis is used to reduce the data to sets of significant features which is also known as clustering or classification. This algorithm is a robust clustering technique which does not require setting the number of clusters. It is an iterative algorithm that estimates the modes of a multivariate distribution underlying the feature space. The number of clusters is obtained automatically by estimating centres of these clusters [17]. Dense regions presented in the feature space correspond to the modes (local maxima) of the probability density function (pdf) of the observed data. Each data point is associated with the nearby peak of the pdf. The mean shift defines a window (kernel) around each data point and then computes its mean. The center of the window is shifted to the mean in an iterative procedure until convergence. The mean shift algorithm relies on kernel density estimation which is a nonparametric approach to estimate the pdf of a random variable. Akin to [18], with a kernel K, each $h_j \in \mathbb{R}^D$ is associated with a bandwidth value w_j that defines the radius of the kernel. Since the set $H = \{h_j, j \in \mathcal{P}\}$ is not available, we will use the set of HRF estimates $m_H = \{m_{H_j}, j = 1, \ldots, J\}$ as in [13,14]. The kernel density estimator at point m_{H_x} can be defined as

$$\hat{f}_K(m_{H_x}) = \frac{1}{J} \sum_{j=1}^{J} \frac{1}{w_j^D} k\left(\left\|\frac{m_{H_x} - m_{H_j}}{w_j}\right\|_2^2\right), \tag{3}$$

where $k(\mathbf{x})$ is the profile of the spherically symmetric kernel K satisfying

$$K(\mathbf{x}) = c_{k,D} k(\|\mathbf{x}\|_2^2) > 0; \quad \|\mathbf{x}\|_2 \leq 1. \tag{4}$$

The normalization constant $c_{k,D}$ ensures that the kernel $K(\mathbf{x})$ integrates to one. Whenever the derivative of the kernel profile $k(\mathbf{x})$ exists, we can define a function $g(\mathbf{x}) = -k'(\mathbf{x})$. Using $g(\mathbf{x})$ as a profile, a kernel $G(\mathbf{x})$ can be defined as $G(\mathbf{x}) = c_{g,D}g(\|\mathbf{x}\|_2^2)$. Applying the gradient to (3), we can obtain the following result (see [17] for more details)

$$S_G(m_{H_x}) = C\frac{\hat{\nabla} f_K(m_{H_x})}{\hat{f}_G(m_{H_x})}, \tag{5}$$

where $\hat{\nabla} f_K(\mathbf{x})$ is the gradient density estimator. In (5), C is a positive constant and $S_G(\boldsymbol{m}_{H_x})$ is the mean shift vector which can be rewritten as

$$S_G(\boldsymbol{m}_{H_x}) = \frac{\sum\limits_{j=1}^{J} \frac{1}{w_j^{D+2}} \boldsymbol{m}_{H_j} g\left(\left\|\frac{\boldsymbol{m}_{H_x}-\boldsymbol{m}_{H_j}}{w_j}\right\|_2^2\right)}{\sum\limits_{j=1}^{J} \frac{1}{w_j^{D+2}} g\left(\left\|\frac{\boldsymbol{m}_{H_x}-\boldsymbol{m}_{H_j}}{w_j}\right\|_2^2\right)} - \boldsymbol{m}_{H_x}. \tag{6}$$

The mean shift vector will always move toward the maximum increase of the density [17]. This is due to the fact that at location $\boldsymbol{m}_{H_x}$, the weighted mean of the data points with kernel G is proportional to the normalized density gradient estimate with kernel K (see (5)). The stationary points obtained via a gradient ascent method represent the modes of the density function and all the points associated with the same stationary point belong to the same cluster. Let us define $\{\boldsymbol{B}_l\}_{l=1,2,\ldots}$ as the sequence of successive locations of kernel G. Using (6), we can write

$$B_{l+1} = \frac{\sum\limits_{j=1}^{J} \frac{1}{w_j^{D+2}} \boldsymbol{m}_{H_j} g\left(\left\|\frac{\boldsymbol{m}_{H_l}-\boldsymbol{m}_{H_j}}{w_j}\right\|_2^2\right)}{\sum\limits_{j=1}^{J} \frac{1}{w_j^{D+2}} g\left(\left\|\frac{\boldsymbol{m}_{H_l}-\boldsymbol{m}_{H_j}}{w_j}\right\|_2^2\right)} \quad l = 1, 2, \ldots. \tag{7}$$

Equation (7) is one of the properties of the mean shift: it is nothing but a hill climbing iterative procedure until the density gradient vanishes. After the convergence of this iterative procedure, we will obtain the local maxima of the density (modes). To overcome the problem of setting an optimal global bandwidth, w_j is estimated using an ℓ_1 norm as in [18]. Assuming that $\boldsymbol{m}_{H_{j,k}}$ is the k-nearest neighbour of the point $\boldsymbol{m}_{H_j}$, the bandwidth associated with $\boldsymbol{m}_{H_j}$ can be computed as follows

$$w_j = \left\|\boldsymbol{m}_{H_j} - \boldsymbol{m}_{H_{j,k}}\right\|_1. \tag{8}$$

After convergence of this procedure, the estimated modes are the HRF estimates of the parcels (see [17] for more details). The practical algorithm for mode detection can be summarized in two main steps; (1) More precisely, we propose to embed the adaptive mean shift algorithm (which is a common clustering algorithm) within the variational inference frameworrun the AMS algorithm to find stationary points of $\hat{f}_K$; (2) keep only the local maxima of these points.

4   AMS Within the VEM Framework of the JPDE Model

More precisely, we propose to embed the adaptive mean shift algorithm (which is a common clustering algorithm) within the variational inference framework. The AMS-JPDE model relies on the VEM algorithm for inference as in the standard JPDE model. However, modifications have to be carried out to embed the AMS algorithm within the VEM framework. The hierarchy of the classical JPDE model is slightly modified: no spatial prior is imposed over the HRF group assignment labels z. The posterior distribution in (2) is factorized as a product of pdfs of the missing variables yielding four different expectation steps (VE-A, VE-H, VE-Z and VE-Q). The pdfs of A, H and Q resulting from the variational Bayesian framework denoted as $\tilde{p}_A(A)$, $\tilde{p}_H(H)$ and $\tilde{p}_Q(Q)$, respectively have been determined in [13,14]. The determination of $\tilde{p}_z(z)$ associated with the proposed adaptive mean shift algorithm is detailed in this section.

The VE-Z step is obtained by neglecting the term that comes from the spatial prior over the labels z. As a consequence $\tilde{p}_{z_j}$ can be rewritten as follows

$$\tilde{p}_{z_j}^{(r)}(k) \propto \mathcal{N}\left(m_{H_j}^{(r)}; \bar{h}_k^{(r-1)}, \bar{\Sigma}_k^{(r-1)}\right),$$

$$\propto \exp\left(-\left(m_{H_j}^{(r)} - \bar{h}_k^{(r-1)}\right)^t \bar{\Sigma}_k^{-1}\left(m_{H_j}^{(r)} - \bar{h}_k^{(r-1)}\right)\right), \qquad (9)$$

where $\bar{h} = \left(\bar{h}_k^{(r-1)}\right)_{1 \le k \le K}$ are the modes of the parcels (HRF patterns) obtained by the AMS algorithm in the maximization step at iteration $(r-1)$. After completing the expectation step, the proposed VEM algorithm proceeds in the maximization step to compute the parameters. The corresponding M-step for the AMS-JPDE model can be rewritten as

$$\Theta^{(r)} = \arg\max_{\Theta}\left[\mathrm{E}_{\tilde{p}_A^{(r)}\tilde{p}_H^{(r)}}\left[\log p(Y \mid A, H; L, \Gamma)\right] + \mathrm{E}_{\tilde{p}_A^{(r)}\tilde{p}_Q^{(r)}}\left[\log p(A \mid Q; \mu, v)\right]\right.$$

$$\left. + \mathrm{E}_{\tilde{p}_Q^{(r)}}\left[\log p(Q; \beta)\right] + \mathrm{E}_{\tilde{p}_H^{(r)}\tilde{p}_z^{(r)}}\left[\log p(H \mid z; \bar{h}, \nu)\right]\right].$$

$$(10)$$

The term $\mathrm{E}_{\tilde{p}_H^{(r)}\tilde{p}_z^{(r)}}\left[\log p(H \mid z; \bar{h}, \nu)\right]$ is associated with the maximization of $\bar{h}$ and is replaced by the AMS algorithm (see Sect. 3 for more details). The maximization steps of the other parameters can be found in [13,14].

In the standard JPDE model, the smoothness of $\left(\bar{h}_k\right)_{1 \le k \le K}$ is favoured by controlling their second order derivatives with the following prior: $\bar{h}_k \sim \mathcal{N}\left(0, \sigma_h^2 R\right)$. In the AMS-JPDE model, we rely on a weighted least squares regularization for smoothness. A smooth $\bar{h}_k$ that approximates the non-smooth one $\bar{h}_k^0$ (the output of the AMS algorithm) can be obtained by solving the following problem

$$\arg\min_{\bar{h}_k} ||\bar{h}_k^0 - \bar{h}_k||_2^2 + \lambda_h ||D_2 \bar{h}_k||_2^2, \qquad (11)$$

where λ_h is a parameter to be fixed by the user and D_2 is the second order finite difference matrix. In the above expression, minimizing $||\bar{h}_k^0 - \bar{h}_k||_2^2$ forces the smooth $\bar{h}_k$ to be close to the non-smooth one $\bar{h}_k^0$. On the other hand, minimizing the term $||D_2 \bar{h}_k||_2^2$ favours the smoothness of $\bar{h}_k$. Straightforward computations lead to the following expression of $\bar{h}_k$ minimizing (11)

$$\bar{h}_k = \left(I_D + \lambda_h D_2^t D_2\right)^{-1} \bar{h}_k^0. \qquad (12)$$

Note that such a quadratic regularization is equivalent to fixing a Gaussian prior on $\bar{h}_k$ in the hierarchical Bayesian model.

5   Experimental Validation

To validate the AMS based parcellation with the JPDE model, we have performed numerical experiments on both synthetic and real data[1].

5.1   Synthetic fMRI Time Series

The proposed model was validated on four different experiments denoted as Exps. 1–4 and defined by different parcellation masks (see Fig. 1)[top row] to generate the BOLD signal according to (1). As regards the experimental conditions, we consider here two of them ($M = 2$) with 30 trials for each. The reference binary labels are shown in Fig. 2(left column). The NRLs are simulated from their prior conditionally to the activation labels Q as shown in Fig. 2(right column). Given these 20×20 binary labels, the NRLs were simulated as follows,

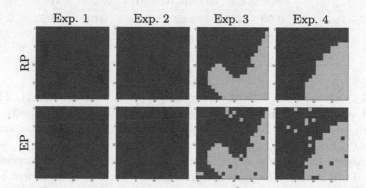

Fig. 1. Reference parcellations (RP) used for the 4 experiments and corresponding estimated parcellation (EP) (grid size = 20×20).

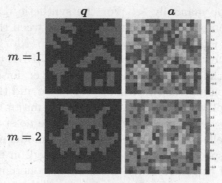

Fig. 2. Reference activation labels (left column) and reference NRLs (right column) for the two experimental conditions (grid size = 20×20).

---

[1] These experiments were implemented in Python within the framework offered by the Pyhrf software [19].

Table 1. Confusion matrices for Exps. 1 and 2. RP and EP refer to the reference and the estimated parcellations, respectively.

RP	EP			
	Parcel. 1		Parcel. 2	
	Exp. 1	Exp. 2	Exp. 1	Exp. 2
Parcel. 1	**0.98**	**0.98**	0.03	0.05
Parcel. 2	0.02	0.02	**0.97**	**0.95**

Table 2. Confusion matrices for Exps. 3 and 4. RP and EP refer to the reference and the estimated parcellations, respectively.

RP	EP					
	Parcel. 1		Parcel. 2		Parcel. 3	
	Exp. 3	Exp. 4	Exp. 3	Exp. 4	Exp. 3	Exp. 4
Parcel. 1	**0.93**	**0.94**	0.02	0.01	0.01	0.02
Parcel. 2	0.05	0.01	**0.96**	**0.96**	0.02	0.02
Parcel. 3	0.02	0.05	0.02	0.03	**0.97**	**0.96**

for $m = 0, 1$: $a_j^m \mid q_j^m = 0 \sim \mathcal{N}(0, 0.5)$ and $a_j^m \mid q_j^m = 1 \sim \mathcal{N}(3.2, 0.5)$. The inter stimuli interval and variance to generate the onsets of the trials were 3 s and 5 s, respectively. Finally, the fMRI time series $\boldsymbol{y}_j$ were generated according to (1) with $\Delta t = 0.5$ and $TR = 1$s.

We analyzed the generated fMRI time series for the four experiments using the AMS-JPDE model. The parcellation estimates for each experiment is shown in Fig. 1[bottom row]. It is worth noticing that for the AMS-JPDE, no prior initialization for the parcellation or truncation level for the maximum number of parcels is needed. The number of K-nearest neighbours (K_{NN}) is the only parameter that needs to be manually set. For the synthetic data experiments, we set $K_{NN} = 50$. The computed parcellation errors between the reference and the estimated parcellation is 2.25 %, 3.25 %, 4.5 % and 4.75 % for Exps. 1 to 4, respectively. These results show a good ability of the AMS-JPDE to recover the hemodynamic territories with low error probability. Moreover, for each experiment, we computed the confusion matrix between the reference and the estimated parcellation. The results displayed in Tables 1 and 2 show a major intersection between them. Although some voxels were misclassified (since no spatial constraints are imposed over the parcellation step), the AMS-JPDE model managed to establish a good parcellation especially for those voxels located on the borders between parcels. The results of the AMS-JPDE model were coherent with the results of the model selection procedure in [15] that calculates the free energy of different competing models each with K^ω parcels and $K^\omega = \omega + 1$, $\omega \in \{1, \ldots, 3\}$. The models maximizing the free energy are the best fit for the data. These optimal models lead to two parcels for Exp. 1 and 2 and three parcels for Exp. 3 and 4. Regarding the running time of the algorithm and considering Exp. 4 as an example, using the model selection procedure in [15] the accumulated time required to run the 3 competing models is around 35 min. On the other hand, the AMS-JPDE model takes less than 12 min. Thus, the computational time of the AMS-JPDE is reduced compared to free energy calculations of the competing models. Figure 3 shows the transformed voxel-dependent HRFs in 3-D representation using Principal Component Analysis (PCA) with the HRF groups labels for each experiment. We also explored the ability of the AMS-JPDE model to estimate the HRF profiles for the estimated parcels, as shown in Fig. 4. The modes of the parcels are the outputs of the AMS algorithm and here they represent the HRF estimate for each parcel. These results are close to the ground truth. The AMS-JPDE also managed to obtain a good performance in detecting the activation as in the JPDE model. The mean square error (MSE) was computed for each experimental condition in the four experiments. The average MSEs for the estimated NRLs and labels were 0.006 and 0.004, respectively.

5.2 Real Data

One experiment was conducted on real fMRI data to validate the AMS-JPDE model. The considered region of interest (ROI) is the bilateral occipital cortex. The fMRI data were collected using a gradient-echo EPI sequence (TE $= 30$ ms/TR $= 2.4$ s/thickness $= 3$ mm/FOV $= 192 \times 192$ mm^2, matrix size: 96×96) with a 3 T magnetic field during a localizer experiment. Sixty auditory, visual and motor stimuli were involved in the paradigm and defined in ten experimental conditions ($M = 10$). During the experiment, $N = 128$ scans were acquired and $\Delta t = 0.6$ s. The number of K-nearest neighbours was set to $K_{NN} = 50$. Running this experiment using the AMS-JPDE model, 3 parcels

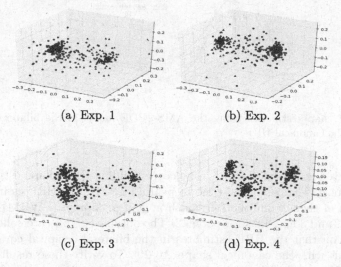

(a) Exp. 1   (b) Exp. 2

(c) Exp. 3   (d) Exp. 4

Fig. 3. Transformed voxel-dependent HRFs in 3-D representation using PCA with HRF groups labels.

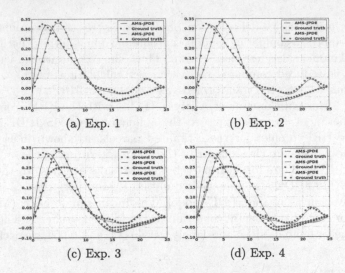

(a) Exp. 1   (b) Exp. 2

(c) Exp. 3   (d) Exp. 4

Fig. 4. HRF estimates for the synthetic data experiments.

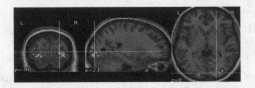

Fig. 5. The estimated parcellation in the bilateral occipital cortex.

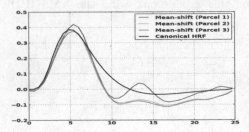

Fig. 6. HRF shape estimates using the AMS-JPDE model in the bilateral occipital cortex and the canonical HRF.

were estimated as shown in Fig. 5. The corresponding HRF shape estimates are shown in Fig. 6. The computed time to peak (TTP) for the HRF estimates was 5.4 s for all of them while the full width at half maximum (FWHM) was 4.2 s for parcels 1 and 3 and 4.8 s for parcel 2. The obtained results are coherent with the conclusion that the HRF estimates in the bilateral occipital cortex should be consistent with the canonical shape [16,20]. To verify these results, we also ran the JPDE model with the model selection procedure proposed in [15] on the same fMRI data using three candidate models with one, two and three parcels for initial parcellation. The candidate model maximizing the free energy was the one with three parcels and the reported value was -236604. This result is also coherent with our findings using the AMS-JPDE model.

6   Conclusion and Future Work

This paper proposed a new approach for automatic hemodynamic brain parcellation relying on the existing JPDE model and the adaptive mean shift algorithm yielding the so-called AMS-JPDE model. The AMS algorithm is used within the VEM framework of the JPDE model to formulate it as a non-parametric approach for model selection. In contrast with the standard JPDE model, the AMS-JPDE model requires no prior initialization for the parcellation as the HRF estimates are the modes obtained by the AMS algorithm of the underlying multivariate distribution of the voxel-dependent HRFs. Future work will focus on embedding spatial prior in the AMS algorithm to eliminate outlier voxels in the parcellation estimates and comparing the AMS-JPDE with less automated approaches as the one proposed in [21]. Future work will also cover more validations of the proposed model for different experimental paradigms and subjects.

References

1. Ogawa, S., Lee, T.-M., Kay, A.R., Tank, D.W.: Brain magnetic resonance imaging with contrast dependent on blood oxygenation. Proc. Natl. Acad. Sci. **87**(24), 9868–9872 (1990)
2. Friston, K.J., Holmes, A.P., Poline, J.-B., Grasby, P.J., Williams, S.C.R., Frackowiak, R.S.J., Turner, R.: Analysis of fMRI time-series revisited. Neuroimage **2**(1), 45–53 (1995)
3. Boynton, G.M., Engel, S.A., Glover, G.H., Heeger, D.J.: Linear systems analysis of functional magnetic resonance imaging in human v1. J. Neurosci. **16**(13), 4207–4221 (1996)
4. Glover, G.H.: Deconvolution of impulse response in event-related BOLD fMRI. Neuroimage **9**(4), 416–429 (1999)
5. Friston, K.J., Mechelli, A., Turner, R., Price, C.J.: Nonlinear responses in fMRI: the Balloon model, Volterra kernels, and other hemodynamics. Neuroimage **12**(4), 466–477 (2000)
6. Lindquist, M.A., Loh, J.M., Atlas, L.Y., Wager, T.D.: Modeling the hemodynamic response function in fMRI: efficiency, bias and mis-modeling. Neuroimage **45**(1), S187–S198 (2009)
7. Buxton, R.B., Frank, L.: A model for the coupling between cerebral blood flow and oxygen metabolism during neural stimulation. J. Cereb. Blood Flow Metab. **17**(1), 64–72 (1997)
8. Deneux, T., Faugeras, O.: Using nonlinear models in fMRI data analysis: model selection and activation detection. Neuroimage **32**(4), 1669–1689 (2006)
9. Ciuciu, P., Poline, J.B., Marrelec, G., Idier, J., Pallier, C., Benali, H.: Unsupervised robust non-parametric estimation of the hemodynamic response function for any fMRI experiment. IEEE Trans. Med. Imag. **22**(10), 1235–1251 (2003)

10. Makni, S., Idier, J., Vincent, T., Thirion, B., Dehaene-Lambertz, G., Ciuciu, P.: A fully Bayesian approach to the parcel-based detection-estimation of brain activity in fMRI. Neuroimage **41**(3), 941–969 (2008)
11. Vincent, T., Risser, L., Ciuciu, P.: Spatially adaptive mixture modeling for analysis of fMRI time series. IEEE Trans. Med. Imag. **29**(4), 1059–1074 (2010)
12. Chaari, L., Vincent, T., Forbes, F., Dojat, M., Ciuciu, P.: Fast joint detection-estimation of evoked brain activity in event-related fMRI using a variational approach. IEEE Trans. Med. Imaging **32**(5), 821–837 (2013)
13. Chaari, L., Forbes, F., Vincent, T., Ciuciu, P.: Hemodynamic-informed parcellation of fMRI data in a joint detection estimation framework. In: Ayache, N., Delingette, H., Golland, P., Mori, K. (eds.) MICCAI 2012, Part III. LNCS, vol. 7512, pp. 180–188. Springer, Heidelberg (2012)
14. Chaari, L., Badillo, S., Vincent, T., Dehaene-Lambertz, G., Forbes, F., Ciuciu, P.: Subject-level Joint Parcellation-Detection-Estimation in fMRI, January 2016. https://hal.inria.fr/hal-01255465/file/JPDE_CHAARI_submitted06012016.pdf
15. Albughdadi, M., Chaari, L., Forbes, F., Tourneret, J.-Y., Ciuciu, P.: Model selection for hemodynamic brain parcellation in fMRI. In: Proceedings of EUSIPCO, Lisbon, Portugal, pp. 31–35, September 2014
16. Albughdadi, M., Chaari, L., Tourneret, J.-Y., Forbes, F., Ciuciu, P.: Hemodynamic Brain Parcellation Using A Non-Parametric Bayesian Approach, February 2016. https://hal.inria.fr/hal-01275622/file/albugdhadi_paper.pdf
17. Comaniciu, D., Meer, P.: Mean shift: a robust approach toward feature space analysis. IEEE Trans. Pattern Anal. Mach. Intell. **24**(5), 603–619 (2002)
18. Georgescu, B., Shimshoni, I., Meer, P.: Mean shift based clustering in high dimensions: a texture classification example. In: Proceedings of ICCV, Nice, France, pp. 456–463. IEEE (2003)
19. Vincent, T., Badillo, S., Risser, L., Chaari, L., Bakhous, C., Forbes, F., Ciuciu, P.: Flexible multivariate hemodynamics fMRI data analyses and simulations with PyHRF. Front. Neurosci. **8**(67) (2014). doi:10.3389/fnins.2014.00067
20. Badillo, S., Vincent, T., Ciuciu, P.: Group-level impacts of within- and between-subject hemodynamic variability in fMRI. Neuroimage **82**, 433–448 (2013)
21. Badillo, S., Varoquaux, G., Ciuciu, P.: Hemodynamic estimation based on consensus clustering. In: Proceedings of PRNI, Philadelphia, USA, pp. 211–215, June 2013

Quantitative Analysis of 3D T1-Weighted Gadolinium (Gd) DCE-MRI with Different Repetition Times

Elijah D. Rockers[1], Maria B. Pascual[1], Sahil Bajaj[1],
Joseph C. Masdeu[1], and Zhong Xue[2(✉)]

[1] Department of Neurology, Nantz National Alzheimer Center,
Houston Methodist Neurological Institute, Houston, USA
[2] Houston Methodist Research Institute, Weill Cornell Medicine,
Houston, TX, USA
zxue@houstonmethodist.org

Abstract. Dynamic contrast-enhanced MRI (DCE-MRI) acquires T_1-weighted MRI scans before and after injection of an MRI contrast agent such as gadolinium (Gd). Gadolinium causes the relaxation time to decrease, resulting in higher MR image intensities after injection followed by a gradual decrease in image intensities during wash out. Gd does not pass the intact blood–brain barrier (BBB), thus its dynamics can be used to quantify pathology associated with BBB leaks. In current clinical practice, it is suggested to use the same pulse sequence for pre-injection T_1 calibration and Gd concentration calculation in the DCE image sequence based on the spoiled gradient recalled echo (SPGR) signal equation. A common method for T_1 estimation is using variable flip angle (VFA). However, when the parameters such as the repetition time (TR) for image acquisition could be tuned differently for T_1 estimation and DCE acquisition, the popular dcemriS4 software package that handles only a fixed TR often results in discrepancies in Gd concentration estimation. This paper reports a quick solution for calculating Gd concentrations when different TRs are used. First, the pre-injection T_1 map is calculated by using the Levenberg-Marquardt algorithm with VFA acquisition, then, because the TR used for DCE acquisition is different from the VFA TR, the equilibrium magnetization is updated with the TR for DCE, and the Gd concentration is calculated thereafter. In the experiments, we first simulated Gd concentration curves for different tissue types and generated the corresponding VFA and DCE image sequences and then used the proposed method to reconstruct the concentration. Comparing with the original simulated data allows us to validate the accuracy of the proposed computation. Further, we tested performance of the method by simulating different amounts of K^{trans} changes in a manually selected region of interest (ROI). The results showed that the new method can estimate Gd dynamics more accurately in the case where different TRs are used and be sensitive enough to detect slight K^{trans} changes in DCE-MRI.

Keywords: DCE-MRI · T_1 relaxation · Gd concentration · Pharmacokinetics

© Springer International Publishing Switzerland 2016
G. Zheng et al. (Eds.): MIAR 2016, LNCS 9805, pp. 259–268, 2016.
DOI: 10.1007/978-3-319-43775-0_23

1 Introduction

Dynamic contrast-enhanced (DCE) MRI has been widely used in many clinical studies for noninvasive detection and characterization of diseases [1]. For example, it can not only quantify pathologies of brain tumor associated with blood–brain barrier (BBB) leakage [2], but also study possible BBB disruption in aging, dementia, stroke and multiple sclerosis [3]. In acquiring DCE-MRI, a contrast agent (CA) such as gadolinium (Gd) is injected into the blood stream while acquiring a series of T_1-weighted MR images. CA concentration can be calculated from MR image intensities for quantitative pharmacokinetic analysis [4]. The injection of Gd results in T_1 relaxation time changes compared to the pre-injection T_1 (denoted as T_{10}). Therefore, DCE-MRI acquisition generally consists of two stages. The first stage is to estimate an intrinsic tissue T_1 map. This estimation can be done by acquiring images with variable flip angles. The second stage is to estimate the time varying $T_1(t)$ map sequence from the DCE-MRI sequence right before and after Gd injection.

To accurately estimate the pre-injection longitudinal relaxation time map T_{10}, the variable flip-angle (VFA) spoiled gradient recalled echo (SPGR) method provides high spatial resolution with relatively short acquisition times and is commonly used in basic and clinical research [5]. Specifically, by capturing T_1-weighted MR images at different flip angles, T_{10} can be calculated using the Levenberg-Marquardt algorithm based on the SPGR signal equation. Next, for computing the Gd concentration from the DCE-MRI image sequences, the same SPGR signal equation is employed to estimate the time varying $T_1(t)$ map sequences. In the dcemriS4 software [6], the CA.fast function can be used for this task.

However, in practice the parameters for image acquisition might have been tuned differently for T_1 calibration and for DCE acquisition stages. For example, in some of our clinical research data, different repetition times (TR) had been used. Because the equilibrium magnetization and T_{10} are estimated using one TR value, and the DCE acquisitions use another, the parameters estimated from the SPGR signal equation may generate discrepancies when applied to DCE. In this paper, we present a simple and practical solution for calculating Gd concentrations when different TRs are used for T_1 calibration and DCE acquisition.

The major steps remain the same as the dcemriS4 package. Specifically, first, the tissue T_{10} map is calculated by using the Levenberg-Marquardt algorithm with variable flip angles. Then, because the TR used for DCE acquisition is different the one used for T_{10} calibration, a new equilibrium magnetization map is calculated with the new TR, so that the SPGR signal equation can better fit the DCE image sequence. Then, the Gd concentration is calculated in a similar way.

In experiments, we first modified the dcemriS4 software package so that different TRs can be used for calculating Gd concentration from DCE-MRI image sequences. Then, we investigated the performance of the modification using simulated Gd concentration signals and different levels of K^{trans} changes in a manually marked ROI. After simulating Gd concentration curves for different brain tissues, we generated the DCE-MRI image sequences and then estimated the concentration curves using the proposed method. In this way, the estimation accuracy can be calculated.

For 3D DCE image series, spatially correlated Gaussian noises are added to the simulated DCE-MRI image sequences with predefined K^{trans} changes in a manual ROI. This allows us to compare two groups of DCE-MRI sequences, one with and another without K^{trans} changes. After simulating DCE-MRI sequences with different conditions and re-calculating K^{trans}, we use the SPM package to highlight group differences [7]. The experimental results showed that the new method can estimate Gd dynamics more accurately in the case of different TRs, and it is sensitive to K^{trans} changes in DCE-MRI.

2   Method

2.1   Estimation of T_1 from SPGR Images

In MR imaging, the T_1 relaxation time, or the spin-lattice relaxation time, measures how quickly the net magnetization vector recovers to its ground state along the direction of the main magnetic field B_0. Generally, the measured SPGR signal intensity can be defined as a function of the longitudinal relaxation time T_{10}, the repetition time TR, the flip angle θ, and the equilibrium longitudinal magnetization M_0 as,

$$S_0 = \frac{M_0(1 - \exp(-TR/T_{10}))\sin(\theta)}{1 - \exp(-TR/T_{10})\cos(\theta)}. \tag{1}$$

Variable flip angle acquisitions are commonly used to estimate the intrinsic relaxation time maps. Given a series of (N) flip angles $\theta_1, \ldots \theta_N$ and corresponding SPGR images $S_1, \ldots S_N$, with a fixed repetition time TR, the nonlinear least squares algorithm aims to estimate M_0 and T_{10} by minimizing the sum of squared errors between the left and right sides of Eq. (1) normalized/weighted by the expected signal standard deviation. The Levenberg-Marquardt algorithm is one such method for estimating M_0 and T_{10}. This can be achieved by using the M0.fast function in the dcemriS4 package.

2.2   Estimation of Gd Concentration from DCE-MRI Sequences

During DCE-MRI acquisition, a series of MRI images are captured while the contrast agent Gd is injected into the blood stream. Herein, we denote the DCE image sequence as I_t, with $t = 1, \ldots T$, and T is the number of DCE images captured. The first several (P) frames are pre-injection acquisitions, and the contrast agent injection starts from frame $P + 1$. Therefore, Eq. (1) can be directly used for calculating the dynamic $T_1(t)$ by simply modifying the equation to:

$$\frac{1}{T_1(t)} = \frac{-1}{TR} \ln\left[\frac{M_0 \sin(\theta) - I_t}{M_0 \sin(\theta) - I_t\cos(\theta)}\right]. \tag{2}$$

However, because of the multi-variable nature of the SPGR signal equation, the parameters estimated for one case may result in discrepancies when applied to another imaging case, particularly for new TR values. It has been suggested that the P

pre-injection frames of the DCE image sequences can be used to "normalize" the relaxation time sequences [8]. Thus, by replacing S_0 with the average of the first P pre-injection frames, the following equation is used:

$$I_t - S_0 = \frac{M_0(1 - \exp(-TR/T_1(t)))\sin(\theta)}{1 - \exp(-TR/T_1(t))\cos(\theta)} - \frac{M_0(1 - \exp(-TR/T_{10}))\sin(\theta)}{1 - \exp(-TR/T_{10})\cos(\theta)}, \quad (3)$$

where $S_0 = \text{average}(I_t, t = 1, \ldots P)$. Then, we can calculate the relaxation time by:

$$\frac{1}{T_1(t)} = \frac{-1}{TR}\ln\left[\frac{1 - (A + B)}{1 - \cos(\theta)(A + B)}\right], \quad (4)$$

where $A = \frac{I_t - S_0}{M_0 \sin(\theta)}$ and $B = \frac{1 - \exp\left(-\frac{TR}{T_{10}}\right)}{1 - \exp\left(-\frac{TR}{T_{10}}\right)\cos(\theta)}$. It has been assumed that the pulse

sequence for T_1 calibration and DCE acquisition is set to be the same during MRI scanning, i.e., TR remains the same in T_{10} estimation (Sect. 2.1) and Gd concentration computation (Sect. 2.2).

2.3 Improvement of Dynamic $T_1(t)$ Computation from DCE-MRI

In clinical practice, we found that the repetition time (TR) for T_1 estimation and DCE acquisition are often different. The effect is that the replacement of S_0 with the average of the pre-injection DCE images may result in discrepancies because the VFA images and DCE images have different TRs. Basically, denoting the new repetition time of DCE as TR_n, the parameters estimated in Sect. 2.1 will not hold during DCE concentration estimation because $S_0 \neq I_{\text{pre}} = \text{average}(I_t, t = 1, \ldots P)$ for the new flip angle θ_n of DCE, i.e.,

$$I_{\text{pre}} \neq \frac{M_0(1 - \exp(-TR/T_{10}))\sin(\theta_n)}{1 - \exp(-TR/T_{10})\cos(\theta_n)}. \quad (5)$$

As shown in Fig. 1, we optimized M_0 and T_{10} using four flip angles (2°, 7°, 18° and 25°) and tested the reconstructed SPGR images by using different TR and θ and computed the difference between the reconstructed images and the original captured images. When TR remains the same (top row), we can precisely reconstruct the SPGR images with different flip angles, while, when TR is different (bottom row), the reconstructed image demonstrated larger errors. The reason is not because the equilibrium magnetization and the intrinsic T_{10} maps are changed due to the acquisition parameter change, but because the original estimation of the multi-variate nonlinear equation (Eq. (1)) only applies to the original TR value.

To remedy this discrepancy we can use all the flip angles and TR values during T_1 calibration and DCE acquisition to estimate M_0 and T_{10} in Eq. (1). However, this requires more acquisitions at different combinations of flip angles and TR values. In practice, these extended multiple acquisitions may not be available.

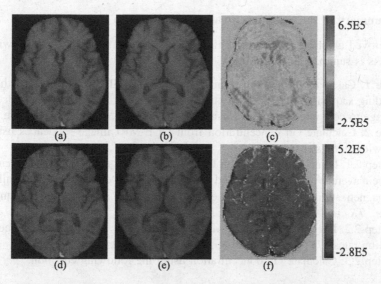

Fig. 1. Reconstructing SPGR images using the same T_{10} map with different TRs. Top: reconstruction using the same TR (5 ms) during T_1 calibration; (a) is the SPGR image captured using TR = 5, = 12°, and (b) is the reconstructed image using Eq. (1) with the same parameters. (c) shows the difference image between images (b) and (a). Bottom: reconstruction using different TR. (d) is the average of pre-injection DCE captured using TR = 3.14, $\theta = 10°$, (e) is the reconstructed MR image using Eq. (1), and (f) is the difference between images (e) and (d).

As mentioned in Introduction, the problem that we are often facing is that TR values may be different during T_1 calibration and DCE acquisition, and there is only one fixed TR and flip angle during DCE acquisition. Therefore, we can assume that the estimated T_{10} relaxation time map (an intrinsic property of tissues) is fixed and will estimate a new equilibrium magnetization map that better fits the new flip angle (θ_n) and the new TR, i.e., TR_n. Therefore, by solving

$$I_{\text{pre}} = \frac{M_n(1 - \exp(-TR_n/T_{10})) \sin(\theta_n)}{1 - \exp(-TR_n/T_{10}) \cos(\theta_n)}, \tag{6}$$

we get a new equilibrium magnetization map M_n for the new flip angle and new TR,

$$M_n = \frac{I_{\text{pre}}(1 - \exp(-TR_n/T_{10}) \cos(\theta_n))}{(1 - \exp(-TR_n/T_{10})) \sin(\theta_n)}. \tag{7}$$

Notice that although the real equilibrium magnetization has not been changed, we simply did not estimate it well particularly for the new TR value because of the lack of available TR and flip angles values during T_1 calibration in Sect. 2.1. Re-calculating M_n here makes the SPGR signal intensity equation better fits the new TR value for different flip angles. Finally, the new relaxation rates $1/T_1(t)$ can be calculated using Eq. (4), by applying the new parameters: M_n, TR_n, and θ_n.

2.4 Summary of the Gd Concentration Computation Algorithm

The improved algorithm for computing Gd Concentration from DCE-MRI with different TRs is summarized as follows:

- **Stage 1.** Calculate tissue relaxation T_{10} map. Input SPGR images S_i with corresponding acquisition TR and flip angles θ_i, $i = 1, \ldots, N$, and apply the dcemriS4 package to compute M_0 and T_{10} using the Levenberg-Marquardt algorithm.
- **Stage 2.** Calculate Gd concentration from DCE-MRI image sequences using the following three steps:
  - Step 2.1. Input the pre-injection DCE image frames $I_t, t = 1, \ldots P$, and calculate their average image as I_{pre}, and use Eq. (7) to calculate the new equilibrium magnetization map M_n using the new TR and flip angle for DCE acquisition, i.e., TR_n and θ_n.
  - Step 2.2. For the entire DCE-MRI sequence $I_t, t = 1, \ldots T$, calculate the relaxation rates $1/T_1(t)$ by replacing M_0 with M_n and θ with θ_n in Eq. (4).
  - Step 2.3. Calculate Gd concentration using the following equation:

$$C(t) = \frac{1}{\gamma} \left(\frac{1}{T_1(t)} - \frac{1}{T_{10}} \right), \tag{8}$$

where γ is the relaxivity of Gd, for which we assume an in-vitro value of $3.9[\text{mMol}]^{-1}s^{-1}$ [9]. The pharmacokinetic model used by dcemriS4 is the extended Tofts model [4] convolved with a population average of directly measured AIFs, modeled as a bi-exponential function [10]. This model can be used to determine K^{trans}, the transfer constant, which is a reflection of permeability, capillary surface area, and blood flow [11].

3 Experiments

3.1 Evaluation Using Simulated MR Signals

First, we evaluated the accuracy of the algorithm using simulated MR signals from Gd concentration curves. Specifically, after a bolus injection of dose D (mmol/kg), given the values of the transfer constant K^{trans}, the rate constant k_{ep}, we can use the following equation to simulate the Gd concentration curve [4]:

$$C(t) = DK^{trans} \sum_{i=1}^{2} a_i [\exp(-k_{ep}t) - exp(-m_i t)]/[m_i - k_{ep}], \tag{9}$$

where $a_1 = 3.99$ kg/liter, $a_2 = 4.78$ kg/liter, $m_1 = 0.144$/min, and $m_2 = 0.0111$/min Subsequently, the relaxation rate $R_1(t) = 1/T_1(t)$ can be obtained from Eq. (8), and the corresponding MR signal $S(t)$ can be calculated using Eq. (1). Then, temporally correlated Gaussian noises are added to the simulated MR signals. By setting the typical mean values of K^{trans} to 0.119, 0.071, 0.034 for CSF, GM, and WM, and those of k_{ep} to 0.480, 0.534, and 0.457, respectively, we simulated the concentration curves of

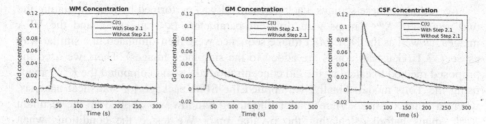

Fig. 2. The original and the reconstructed Gd concentration signals. Blue: original simulated concentration; red: reconstructed concentration using our method (with Step 2.1); green: original method (without Step 2.1). (Color figure online)

different tissues shown as blue curves in Fig. 2. These blue curves were used to generate MR signals, and the proposed algorithm (the method with Step 2.1 included) and the original algorithm (without Step 2.1) were used to reconstruct these concentration signals. We used TR = 3.14 ms, and $\theta = 10°$ for DCE, which are different than those used for simulating the flip angle MR signals (TR = 5 ms, and $\theta = 2°, 7°$, $18°, 27°$). After reconstruction, the recovered green curves were vertically shifted. For conveniently comparing their shapes, we shifted them back so the pre-injection concentration is zero. It can be seen from Fig. 2 that the green curves cannot fully recover the contrast of the original $C(t)$. Quantitatively, the areas under the curves (AUC) for red ones have small difference from the blue ones: 0.3 %, 0.8 %, and 4.0 %, and those for the green curves are more different from the blue curves: 45.0 %, 45.1 %, and 42.2 %, for CSF, GM, and WM, respectively.

3.2 Application in Gd DCE-MRI Analysis

We applied the proposed algorithm in pre-processing of DCE-MRI datasets by simulating K^{trans} change. Because of lack of ground truth for DCE-MRI images, first, we generated simulated DCE-MRI datasets from a segmented image using realistic K^{trans} and k_{ep} parameters for different tissue types, including WM, GM, and CSF. Then, K^{trans} and k_{ep} are subject to a spatially correlated Gaussian distribution for different tissue types, and a manually selected region of interest (ROI) was used to simulate the "abnormal" region, wherein the mean values of K^{trans} and k_{ep} are set differently.

The detailed simulation steps are as follows. First, we set the mean values of K^{trans} and k_{ep} for different tissues according to the segmented MR image, then, the standard deviation (std) of K^{trans} is set to x% of the mean values. In this way we generated the K^{trans} map for every voxel in the segmented MR image and spatially smoothed it with a $3 \times 3 \times 3$ window. A group of 10 K^{trans} maps are generated to act as the control group. Another study group was generated in a similar way, and additionally the K^{trans} values within the manual ROI (see Fig. 3) were shifted, and the shifting parameter is subject to a Gaussian distribution $N(m, \delta)$, with m as y% of the K^{trans} mean, and δ the prescribed std for m. In summary, x% reflects the variability of K^{trans} for each tissue type, and y% is the amount of relative changes of K^{trans} to simulate the abnormality within ROI. In the simulation, we kept k_{ep} unchanged as the desired mean values of different tissue types.

According to these settings, each experiment was performed by first simulating the two groups of K^{trans} maps with different parameters (x% and y%), and the VFA images, as well as the DCE-MRI image sequence were then simulated in a similar way as Sect. 3.1 (Gaussian noises are added to the simulated images). Then, we used the proposed method to calculate the Gd concentration maps and computed the K^{trans} maps using the Tofts model. Finally, we applied the SPM package for statistical analysis, where a 7mm × 7mm × 7mm spatial smoothing window was applied on the resultant K^{trans} maps before calculating the p-value map. We tested the conditions when x% = 10 % and 20 %, and y% = 1 %,...7 %, respectively. Figure 3(a) shows the segmented image used as the template image for the simulation, and the brown region is the manually picked abnormal region. In the subsequent images in Fig. 3, we show the $-log(p)$ maps when x% = 10 % and y% = 1 %,...5 %. It can be seen that at the variability level of 10 % (std of K^{trans} is 10 % of its mean), the method can catch the shape of the abnormal ROI when the different between control and abnormal is 4 % ~ 5 %.

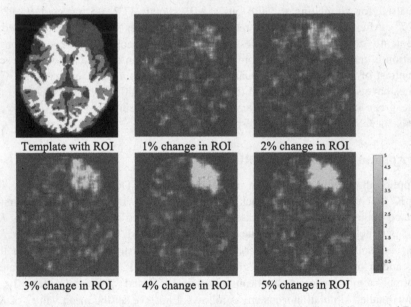

| Template with ROI | 1% change in ROI | 2% change in ROI |

| 3% change in ROI | 4% change in ROI | 5% change in ROI |

Fig. 3. Group comparison of K^{trans} change in ROI. The segmented image with a manual ROI is used to simulate the K^{trans} maps of two groups, one with and another without K^{trans} shifts in the ROI. The $-log(p)$ maps show group differences for different amount of shifts by applying SPM on the reconstructed K^{trans} maps.

Figure 4 plots the mean and std of the p-values within the ROI for two different K^{trans} variability levels: x % = 10 % and 20 %. It can be seen that as more variability appears in K^{trans} for the tissues, the minimal change that can be detected has been increased. Notice that these experiments have not incorporated image registration errors in the simulation. In real cases, the sensitivity for detecting permeability between groups could also be affected by image registration errors.

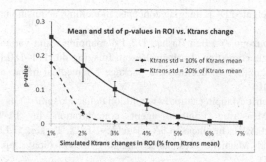

Fig. 4. The mean and std of p-values within the ROI under different simulation conditions.

Finally, it is worth noting that the objective of this paper is to evaluate the proposed method on simulated Gd concentrations to show that concentration maps can be estimated more accurately, particularly when the repetition time is different for T_1 calibration and DCE acquisition. In our recent study [12], the proposed method was applied to analyze real DCE-MRI imaging data for quantifying group differences of Gd dynamics between young and old healthy adults.

4 Conclusion

This paper presents a simple yet effective solution for calculating Gd concentrations when different TRs are used during T1 calibration and DCE acquisition. We showed that due to the limited number of VFA acquisitions during baseline calibration, the SPGR signal equation, as a multi-variate nonlinear function, has not been calibrated well enough to account for different TR values. To remedy this shortcoming, we first used the Levenberg-Marquardt method to estimate the intrinsic T_1 relaxation time from different flip angle acquisition, and then recalculate the equilibrium magnetization map using the pre-injection DCE images acquired with a new TR and new flip angle. The modified SPGR signal equation is thus tuned to the new TR and flip angle and can better represent the DCE image sequences. Gd concentration dynamics are then calculated. In experiments with simulated DCE-MRI, we showed that the new method can generate more accurate concentration maps, and hence improve the quantitative analysis of DCE-MRI for human brain BBB analysis.

References

1. Tofts, P.: Quantitative MRI of the Brain: Measuring Changes Caused by Disease. Wiley, Hoboken (2005)
2. O'Connor, J.P., Jackson, A., Parker, G.J., Jayson, G.C.: DCE-MRI biomarkers in the clinical evaluation of antiangiogenic and vascular disrupting agents. Br. J. Cancer **96**, 189–195 (2007)
3. Sourbron, S., Ingrisch, M., Siefert, A., Reiser, M., Herrmann, K.: Quantification of cerebral blood flow, cerebral blood volume, and blood–brain-barrier leakage with DCE-MRI. Magn. Reson. Med. **62**, 205–217 (2009)

4. Tofts, P.S.: T1-weighted DCE imaging concepts: modelling, acquisition and analysis. Signal **500**, 400 (2010)

5. Liberman, G., Louzoun, Y., Ben Bashat, D.: T-1 mapping using variable flip angle SPGR data with flip angle correction. J. Magn. Reson. Imaging **40**, 171–180 (2014)

6. Whitcher, B., Schmid, V.J.: dcemriS4: a package for medical image analysis. R package version 0.40 (2010)

7. Statistical Parametric Mapping. http://www.fil.ion.ucl.ac.uk/spm/

8. Parker, G.J.: Measuring contrast agent concentration in T1-weighted dynamic contrast-enhanced MRI. In: Jackson, A., Buckley, D.L., Parker, G.J.M. (eds.) Dynamic Contrast-Enhanced Magnetic Resonance Imaging in Oncology, pp. 69–79. Springer, Heidelberg (2005)

9. Kanal, E., Maravilla, K., Rowley, H.: Gadolinium contrast agents for CNS imaging: current concepts and clinical evidence. Am. J. Neuroradiol. **35**, 2215–2226 (2014)

10. Fritz-Hansen, T., Rostrup, E., Larsson, H.B., Søndergaard, L., Ring, P., Henriksen, O.: Measurement of the arterial concentration of Gd-DTPA using MRI: a step toward quantitative perfusion imaging. Magn. Reson. Med. **36**, 225–231 (1996)

11. Cuenod, C.A., Balvay, D.: Perfusion and vascular permeability: basic concepts and measurement in DCE-CT and DCE-MRI. Diagn. Interv. Imaging **94**, 1187–1204 (2013)

12. Pascual, B., Rockers, E., Bajaj, S., Anderson, J., Xue, Z., Karmonik, C., Masdeu, J.: Regional kinetics of [^{18}F]AV-1451 uptake and Gadolinium concentration in young and older subjects. In: Abstract in 10th Human Amyloid Imaging, Miami, FL, p. 170, 13–15 January 2016

Cascade Registration of Micro CT Volumes Taken in Multiple Resolutions

Kai Nagara[1(✉)], Hirohisa Oda[1], Shota Nakamura[2], Masahiro Oda[1],
Hirotoshi Homma[3], Hirotsugu Takabatake[4], Masaki Mori[3], Hiroshi Natori[5],
Daniel Rueckert[6], and Kensaku Mori[1,7]

[1] Graduate School of Information Science, Nagoya University, Nagoya, Japan
knagara@mori.m.is.nagoya-u.ac.jp
[2] Graduate School of Medicine, Nagoya University, Nagoya, Japan
[3] Sapporo-Kosei General Hospital, Sapporo, Japan
[4] Sapporo Minami-sanjo Hospital, Sapporo, Japan
[5] Keiwa-kai Nishioka Hospital, Nagoya, Japan
[6] Department of Computing, Imperial College London, London, UK
[7] Information and Communications, Nagoya University, Nagoya, Japan

Abstract. In this paper, we present a preliminary report of a multi-scale registration method between micro-focus X-ray CT (micro CT) volumes taken in different scales. 3D fine structures of target objects can be observed on micro CT volumes, which are difficult to observe on clinical CT volumes. Micro CT scanners can scan specimens in various resolutions. In their high resolution volumes, ultra fine structures of specimens can be observed, while scanned areas are limited to very small. On the other hand, in low resolution volumes, large areas can be captured, while fine structures of specimens are difficult to observe. The fusion volume of the high and low resolution volumes will have benefits of both. Because the difference of resolutions between the high and low resolution volumes may vary greatly, an intermediate resolution volume is required for successful fusion of volumes. To perform such volume fusion, a cascade multi-resolution registration technique is required. To register micro CT volumes that have quite different resolutions, we employ a cascade co-registration technique. In the cascade co-registration process, intermediate resolution volumes are used in a registration process of the high and low resolution volumes. In the registration between two volumes, we apply two steps registration techniques. In the first step, a block division is used to register two resolution volumes. Afterward, we estimate the fine spatial positions relating the registered two volumes using the Powell method. The registration result can be used to generate a fusion volume of the high and low resolution volumes.

1 Introduction

In medical imaging fields, it is important to understand anatomical structures to achieve better clinical outcomes based on computerized processing of the medical volumes. For example, organ region extraction from medical images has

© Springer International Publishing Switzerland 2016
G. Zheng et al. (Eds.): MIAR 2016, LNCS 9805, pp. 269–280, 2016.
DOI: 10.1007/978-3-319-43775-0_24

been investigated by many researchers for images taken by clinical X-ray CT or MR scanner [1,3,8]. Most of these scanners provide 1000 μm (1 mm) scale images. In the pathological imaging filed, images of HE-stained specimens taken by a microscope (10 μm scale) are utilized. These images enable us to depict cell-level anatomical structures and are being utilized for making definitive diagnosis. Although these pathological images can capture precise structure of micro-level anatomy, two dimensional imaging are commonly used. Three dimensional imaging is also performed for HE-stained specimen. However, these imaging are destructive inspection due to slice-by-slice imaging using very sharp cutting knife called microtome.

Micro-focus X-ray CT (micro CT) scanners enable us to take precise volumetric images of specimens in very high resolution in comparison with the clinical X-ray CT scanners. Micro CT scanners can take volumetric images (volumes) in the range of 50 μm to 1 μm. It enables us to depict semi-micro anatomical structure in non-destructive way [13]. For example, micro CT volumes of inflated fixed lung specimens taken in 10 μm resolution can depict clearly the alveoli regions, terminal bronchial regions, as well as the interlobular septa. Such structures cannot be observed on conventional clinical X-ray CT volumes.

Although micro CT scanners can take very high resolution volumetric images of specimens, global structures are difficult to be observed on such volumes of micro-level resolutions. One solution to overcome this problem would be to co-register the volumetric images of mm-level resolution and μm-level resolutions. In some micro CT scanning devices, it is possible to take volumetric images in different resolutions by moving the scanning table. The resolution can be changed in degree of ten times. The most coarse resolution and the finest resolution can cover FOV's of $5 \times 5 \times 2.5$ cm and $5 \times 5 \times 2.5$ mm respectively. If we could co-register the coarse and the fine resolution volumetric images, it would help us to understand macro and micro structures simultaneously. In case of lung cancer, lungs are partially resected during the lung cancer surgery. Resected lung specimen can then be scanned by a micro CT scanner after the fixation process. As the pre-operative CT scans are also available for such cases, the co-registration of clinical CT volumes and micro CT volumes will assist to understand the correspondence of macro anatomical structures and micro anatomical structures.

To perform co-registration of clinical CT volumes and micro CT volumes, one must carefully consider the large resolution gap. While the typical clinical CT resolution is 0.625 to 1 mm per voxel, that of micro CT is 5 to 10 μm in the finest resolution. It is quite difficult to co-register these two volumetric images due to large difference in image resolution. As we mentioned above, most of the micro CT scanners can take volumetric images in different resolutions. If we take CT volumes of intermediate resolutions, the intermediate resolution volumes would become an interface of co-registration which enables us to co-register clinical CT and micro CT volumes.

Some researches related to micro CT have been proposed in the medical imaging fields. Three-dimensional visualization results of lung micro structures from micro CT volumes was reported by Watz et al. [13]. Anatomical structures analysis techniques from micro CT volumes have also been investigated [6,12]. In all related studies registration method between multi-modal single-modal images have been reported. A MR-CT registration method using the normalized mutual information [10] is proposed and utilized for many applications. Local patch-based entropy images have been proposed by [11]. In this method, each of the voxel values depends on the local structure. Furthermore, Heinrich et al. [4] propose MIND (modality independent neighborhood descriptor) as a similarity metric. To the best of our knowledge, in all related studies no registration method for micro CT volumes that have different resolutions have been proposed yet.

Registration between micro CT volumes that have different resolutions is difficult due to the following reasons: (1) the difference of resolutions between micro CT volumes is large, (2) region included in micro CT volumes may different (some parts in the volumes overlap and some parts not overlap), and (3) micro CT volumes have strong image noise. For the reasons mentioned above, previous registration techniques fail to register micro CT volumes.

This paper presents a method for cascade co-registration of volumetric images taken in different resolutions. We try to embed micro-structure information depicted on higher resolution CT volumes into the lower resolution CT volumes. Also we show a preliminary study on cascade co-registration of volumes taken by a micro CT scanner enabling scanning in different resolutions.

2 Registration Between Two Different Resolution Volumes

2.1 Overview

The proposed method performs a registration between two input volumes that have different resolutions. The method consists of the following steps: (1) volume similarization, (2) global registration, and (3) local registration. In the volume similarization step, the high resolution (high-reso.) input volume is processed so that to make it similar to the low resolution (low-reso.) input volume. Thereafter, the global registration is performed by block division to estimate roughly their matching position, finally the local registration is performed to compute precisely the matching positions. A transformation matrix that transforms the high-reso. volume to matching position on the low-reso. volume is calculated by these processes.

2.2 Volume Similarization

We perform the volume similarization for making the high-reso. input volume H similar to the low-reso. input volume L. To suppress the noise on the volumes, we apply an $M \times M \times M$ median filter to both H and L to obtain the smoothed volumes H_{med} and L_{med}, respectively. For removing small structures appear in the high-reso. input volume, we apply the Gaussian smoothing filter to H_{med} with the standard deviation σ μm. The result is denoted by $H_{Gaussian}$. We perform a downscaling process an $H_{Gaussian}$ by linear interpolation so that both $H_{Gaussian}$ and L have the same resolution. The resulting volume is called as $H_{downscale}$.

2.3   Global Registration

The global registration roughly estimates the transformation (including translation and scaling) between the high-reso. and low-reso. volumes. The high-reso. volume is transformed to a matched position on the low-reso. volume. We simply utilize the template matching by using the block division technique [7]. The block division technique is robust for small resolution change and noise. Especially, the block division technique is robust for shielding of parts in volumes. Shielding of parts are observed in many micro CT volume pairs of registration target. The block division technique performs registration ignoring small shielding of parts in volumes.

We divide $H_{\text{downscale}}$ into $D \times D \times D$ blocks in a reticular pattern along the x, y, and z axes. We call each block as *block-template* $B_{n,m,l}$ ($0 \le n < D, 0 \le m < D, 0 \le l < D$). The size of each block-template $w_B \times h_B \times d_B$ is computed as

$$\begin{cases} w_B = w_H/D, \\ h_B = h_H/D, \\ d_B = d_H/D, \end{cases} \tag{1}$$

where w_H, h_H, d_H are the size of $H_{\text{downscale}}$.

Then we perform registration between each $B_{n,m,l}$ and L_{med}. The optimal translation parameter $\hat{\mathbf{t}}_{n,m,l}$ of the translation vector $\mathbf{t}_{n,m,l}$, describing the translation to each axis of block-template $B_{n,m,l}$, is obtained by

$$\hat{\mathbf{t}}_{n,m,l} = \arg \max_{\mathbf{t}_{n,m,l}} R_{\text{NCC}}(B_{n,m,l}, \mathbf{t}_{n,m,l}). \tag{2}$$

We use the normalized cross correlation (NCC) [2] as the metric to measure volume similarity. The term R_{NCC} calculates NCC value as

$$R_{\text{NCC}}(B_{n,m,l}, \mathbf{t}_{n,m,l}) =$$
$$\frac{\displaystyle\sum_{\mathbf{b} \in B_{n,m,l}} (L_{\text{med}}(\mathbf{b} + \mathbf{t}_{n,m,l}) - \mu_L)(B_{n,m,l}(\mathbf{b}) - \mu_B)}{\sqrt{\displaystyle\sum_{\mathbf{b} \in B_{n,m,l}} (L_{\text{med}}(\mathbf{b} + \mathbf{t}_{n,m,l}) - \mu_L)^2} \sqrt{\displaystyle\sum_{\mathbf{b} \in B_{n,m,l}} (B_{n,m,l}(\mathbf{b}) - \mu_B)^2}}, \tag{3}$$

where μ_L and μ_B are the mean value of L_{med} and $B_{n,m,l}$.

Then, we perform a voting process to estimate a transformation parameter (including translation and scaling) of the entire volume $H_{\text{downscale}}$. The translation $\mathbf{l}_{n,m,l}$ from the center point $\mathbf{b}_{n,m,l}$ of $B_{n,m,l}$ by $\hat{\mathbf{t}}_{n,m,l}$ is written as

$$\mathbf{l}_{n,m,l} = \mathbf{b}_{n,m,l} + \hat{\mathbf{t}}_{n,m,l}. \tag{4}$$

$\mathbf{l}_{n,m,l}$ is the translation of $B_{n,m,l}$ to a corresponding position on the low-reso. volume. Also, the translation of $B_{n,m,l}$ to a corresponding position on the high-res. volume is

$$\mathbf{h}_{n,m,l} = (w_B n, h_B m, d_B l)^T + \mathbf{b}_{n,m,l}. \tag{5}$$

We introduce a set of scaling parameters a_c $(c = 1, \ldots, C)$, which is calculated by

$$a_c = a_{min} + a_{step} \cdot c. \tag{6}$$

The scaling is applied to the high-reso. volume. One scaling parameter is selected from $a_1, \ldots, a_C$ by the voting process explained below. The translation between the low-reso. volume and the high-reso. volume is

$$\mathbf{t}_{c,n,m,l} = \mathbf{l}_{n,m,l} - a_c \mathbf{h}_{n,m,l}. \tag{7}$$

Considering the scaling parameters a_c and translation parameters $\mathbf{t}_{c,n,m,l}$, a voting parameter $\mathbf{p}_{c,n,m,l}$ is then defined as

$$\mathbf{p}_{c,n,m,l} = (a_c, \mathbf{t}_{c,n,m,l}). \tag{8}$$

We calculate voting parameters of all block-templates and vote them to a four-dimensional voting space V. V has the bin-width of $(b_a, \mathbf{b}_t) = (b_a, (b_x, b_y, b_z)^T)$. From the voting result, the parameter that has the maximum number of votes is

$$\hat{\mathbf{p}}_{\text{coarse}} = (\hat{a}_{\text{coarse}}, \hat{\mathbf{t}}_{\text{coarse}}) = \underset{\mathbf{p}_{c,n,m,l}}{\arg \max} V(\mathbf{p}_{c,n,m,l}), \tag{9}$$

where $V(\mathbf{p}_{c,n,m,l})$ is a vote number about $\mathbf{p}_{c,n,m,l}$. As a result, the transformation vector (including translation and scaling) from the high-reso. volume to the low-reso. volume can be obtained which has been denoted by $\hat{\mathbf{p}}_{\text{coarse}}$.

2.4   Local Registration

We perform the local registration here. To this ends, the transformation parameters obtained in the global registration, $\hat{\mathbf{p}}_{\text{coarse}}$, is used as initial value of this local registration. A rigid transformation matrix A is defined as

$$H_{\text{reg}}^{(n)} = A(H_{\text{Gaussian}}, \mathbf{p}_{\text{fine}}^{(n)}) = \mathbf{S}^{(n)} \mathbf{R}^{(n)} H_{\text{Gaussian}} + \mathbf{t}^{(n)}, \tag{10}$$

where $\mathbf{p}_{\text{fine}}^{(n)}$ is the nine-dimensional rigid transformation vector that contains the scaling, rotation, and translation of each axis. n is the iteration number of the optimal parameter searching performed by using the Powell method [9]. The initial parameters of affine registration are defined by using the global registration results.

$$\mathbf{S}^{(0)} = \hat{a}_{\text{coarse}} \mathbf{E} \tag{11}$$
$$\mathbf{R}^{(0)} = \mathbf{E} \tag{12}$$
$$\mathbf{t}^{(0)} = \hat{\mathbf{t}}_{\text{coarse}} \tag{13}$$

where $\mathbf{E}$ is identity matrix.

We compute the optimal parameter by using the Powell method [9]. We used the Powell method to find the optimal parameter $\hat{\mathbf{p}}_{\text{fine}}$ that maximizes the NCC similarity measure R'_{NCC}. The iteration of finding the optimal parameter halts when the difference of the similarity from the previous iteration step is smaller than t_{powell}. The NCC similarity measure is described as

$$
R'_{NCC}(\mathbf{p}^{(n)}_{\text{fine}}) =
$$
$$
\frac{\sum_{\mathbf{h} \in H^{(n)}_{\text{reg}}} (L_{\text{med}}(\mathbf{h}) - \mu'_L)(H^{(n)}_{\text{reg}}(\mathbf{h}) - \mu_H)}{\sqrt{\sum_{\mathbf{h} \in H^{(n)}_{\text{reg}}} (L_{\text{med}}(\mathbf{h}) - \mu'_L)^2} \sqrt{\sum_{\mathbf{h} \in H^{(n)}_{\text{reg}}} (H^{(n)}_{\text{reg}}(\mathbf{h}) - \mu_H)^2}} \tag{14}
$$

where μ_H and μ'_L are the mean value of $H^{(n)}_{\text{reg}}$ and L_{med}.

We create the local registration result volume $\hat{H}_{\text{reg}}$ by using the rigid transformation with the optimal parameters as

$$
\hat{H}_{\text{reg}} = A(H_{\text{med}}, \hat{\mathbf{p}}_{\text{fine}}). \tag{15}
$$

The high-reso. volume H_{med} is transformed to a position on the low-reso. volume, where these volumes match. The transformation result of the high-reso. volume is called $\hat{H}_{\text{reg}}$.

3   Cascade Co-registration

We introduce the cascade co-registration as a registration technique for two volumes having large image resolution gap between them. In the cascade co-registration, we prepare some intermediate resolution volumes of them, and we compute parameter of each set of two volumes which have small resolution gap step by step. The resolution of micro CT volumes can be easily and physically changed in degree of more than five times at the scanning time (changing X-ray optic system). Our registration method described in Sect. 2 cannot register two volumes in such case. Therefore, We propose the cascade co-registration, the registration method between volumes of no less than three different resolutions. The permutation of the input volumes is written as $P = \{I_0, \cdots, I_i, I_j, \cdots, I_N\}$ $(0 \leq i < j \leq N)$. Note that P is sorted in ascending order of the voxel size. $N+1$ is the total number of the input volumes. The transformation matrix $H_{0,N}$ between I_0 and I_N is written as

$$
H_{0,N} = H_{0,1} H_{1,2} \ldots H_{N-1,N}, \tag{16}
$$

with the transformation matrices $H_{i,j}$ between neighboring volumes in P. These transformation matrices $H_{i,j}$ are calculated by using the registration method described in Sect. 2. Using the cascade co-registration, we can register two volumes even if they have a large resolution gap.

4   Experiments

We performed two different of experiments to evaluate (1) the registration accuracy of the proposed registration method in Sect. 2 and (2) evaluate the proposed cascade co-registration method in Sect. 3. We used one micro CT volume for experiment (1) and four micro CT volumes for experiment (2). The parameter settings of the method were: $M = 3, D = 7, a_{\min} = 0.7, a_{\text{step}} = 0001, C = 500, b_a = 0.05, b_x = 10, b_y = 10, b_z = 10$, and $t_{\text{powell}} = 0.001$.

4.1 Registration Between Two Different Resolution Volumes

To evaluate registration accuracy of the registration method between volumes having two different resolutions, we applied the method to micro CT volumes.

Micro CT Volume Specification. We used a micro CT volume of a formalin-fixed inflated lung specimen that was scanned by a micro CT scanner (SMX-90CT Plus, Shimadzu Inc., Kyoto, Japan). The specimen was fixed by the Heitzman method [5] and scanned at 90 kV of the X-ray tube voltage and 110 μA of the tube current. The original volume size was $1024 \times 1024 \times 1081$ voxels and the volume resolution was $10.21 \times 10.21 \times 10.21$ μm/voxel. We generated a high and a low resolution volumes from the original volume as described below. The high-reso. volume was generated by cropping small regions from the original volume. The high-reso. volume image size was $341 \times 341 \times 360$ voxels and its volume resolution was $10.21 \times 10.21 \times 10.21$ μm/voxel. The low-reso. volume was generated by downsampling the original volume. The low-reso. volume size was $341 \times 341 \times 360$ voxels and its volume resolution was $30.62 \times 30.62 \times 30.62$ μm/voxel. We used the artificially generated volumes to evaluate accuracy of the registration method because the ground truth transformation matrix between the high- and low-reso. volumes are known. Examples of the volumes are shown in Fig. 1. These artificially generated volumes were quite similar to real micro CT volumes taken in the corresponding resolutions.

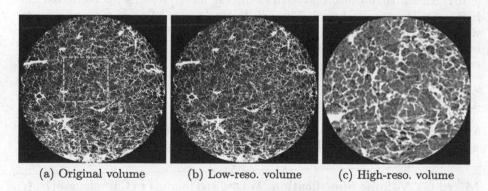

(a) Original volume   (b) Low-reso. volume   (c) High-reso. volume

Fig. 1. Examples of volumes used in the experiment. Transverse slices are shown here.

Experimental Results. The registration result of the high- and low-reso. volumes was shown in Fig. 2. Figure 2(a) is one slice of the original volume. Figure 2(b) shows the registration result by the proposed method. In this figure, registered high-reso. volume was overlaid on the original volume. This figure

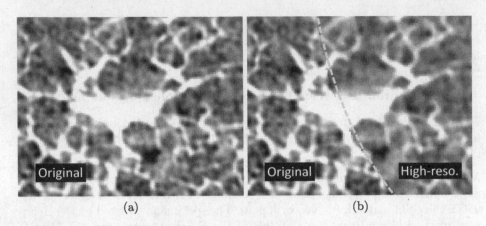

(a)   (b)

Fig. 2. Registration results of the proposed method. (a) The original volume and (b) registered high-reso. volume overlaid on the original volume. The border between original and high-reso. volumes has been indicated by a yellow broken line. (Color figure online)

Table 1. Registration errors of the proposed method.

Process	SAD/V	NCC	DCP (voxels)
None	3.401×10^3	0.0884	734.8
Global registration	3.904×10^2	0.8645	1.733
Local registration	2.495×10^2	0.9493	0.9723

clearly shows that the proposed registration method correctly registered the high- and low-reso. volumes. The registration errors of the proposed method were shown in Table 1. We computed the sum of absolute difference per number of voxels (SAD/V), normalize cross-correlation (NCC), and the distance between center points (DCP) as the evaluation criteria.

4.2   Cascade Co-registration

We have tested the performance of the proposed cascade co-registration method using micro CT volumes taken in various resolutions.

Micro CT Volume Specification. We utilized four micro CT volumes $\{I_0, I_1, I_2, I_3\}$ with different resolutions. Their specifications and sample images are shown in Table 2 and Fig. 3. First we computed the transformation matrices $\{H_{0,1}, H_{1,2}, H_{2,3}\}$ between the micro CT volumes. By using them, we computed $H_{1,4}$, $H_{2,4}$, $H_{3,4}$ and obtained the registration result.

Table 2. Specifications of micro CT volumes.

	Size (voxels)	Resolution (μm/voxel)
I_0	$1024 \times 1024 \times 501$	$7.18 \times 7.18 \times 7.18$
I_1	$1024 \times 1024 \times 497$	$11.60 \times 11.60 \times 11.60$
I_2	$1024 \times 1024 \times 532$	$17.70 \times 17.70 \times 17.70$
I_3	$1024 \times 1024 \times 545$	$30.06 \times 30.06 \times 30.06$

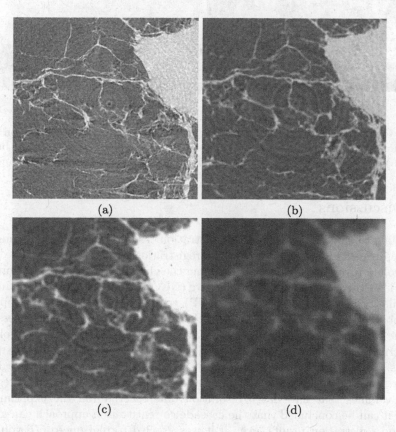

(a)   (b)

(c)   (d)

Fig. 3. Example of slice images of micro CT volumes used in the cascade co-registration experiment. Resolutions of the micro CT volumes were (a) 7.18 (pixel/μm), (b) 11.60 (pixel/μm), (c) 17.70 (pixel/μm), and (d) 30.06 (pixel/μm).

Experimental Results. The cascade co-registration result is shown in Fig. 4. In figure, higher resolution volumes were overlaid on lower resolution volumes. The area near the center of Fig. 4(a) was enlarged and shown in Fig. 4(b). From these figures, we can see that the cascade co-registration method correctly registered many volumes that have different resolutions.

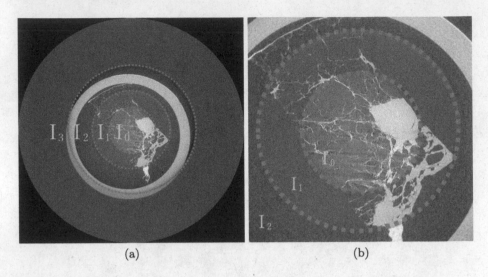

(a)   (b)

Fig. 4. Cascade co-registration result. Higher resolution volumes were overlaid on lower resolution volumes. Borders between different volumes were indicated by red broken lines. (a) is overall, (b) is enlarged image of the center of (a). (Color figure online)

5   Discussions

According to the Table 1, accurate registration results were obtained using the two-step registration framework. In the registration process between two different resolution volumes, two steps including the global and local registrations are utilized. In Table 1, the similarity measure (NCC) was greatly increased and the dissimilarity measures (SAD/V and DCP) were greatly decreased by applying the global registration. This means that the global registration could successfully find the corresponding position of the high-reso. volume in the low-reso. volume. Furthermore, the global registration result was refined by the local registration process. Quite accurate registration result was obtained by the two step registration process. We also proposed the cascade co-registration approach to register image volumes that have large resolution differences. From the experimental result, it can be concluded that the cascade co-registration approach can generate good registration results, even if it was applied to real micro CT volumes. This result showed the cascade co-registration approach is practically applicable to real images. In our registration methods, we assume that there is no large differences in rotation angle between volumes. We applied the proposed registration method to micro CT volumes which are taken with translation and scaling transformations of samples. However, in real situations, samples such as lung specimens may rotate before each volume acquisition. Consideration of rotation transformations between registration target volumes is necessary for practical use of the proposed methods. Furthermore, non-rigid deformation is needed to be introduced for volume registration of soft tissues. Soft tissues change its shapes and positions easily in the period of two different scale volume acquiring. We need to consider not only rotation but also non-rigid deformation of samples for registrations. We will introduce rotation and non-rigid deformation in our registration method to improve the applicability.

6   Conclusion

In this work, we proposed the two-step multi-scale registration method between micro CT volumes taken in different resolutions. The global registration utilizing the block division and the local registration utilizing the Powell method is combined to register the high-resolution volume to low-resolution volume. Furthermore, we proposed the cascade co-registration method to register micro CT volumes that have quite different resolutions. The experimental results showed that the proposed method can generate accurate registration results.

Future work includes registration between volumes that have rotation and non-rigid transformations. Also, comparison with other methods and adding further quantitative evaluation results are necessary. Moreover, applying the proposed method to other image modalities such as clinical CT and MR and application of the proposed method to pathological research such as tumor structure analysis are also one of our future work.

Acknowledgments. Parts of this research were supported by the MEXT, the JSPS KAKENHI Grant Numbers 25242047, 26108006, and the Kayamori Foundation of Informational Science Advancement.

References

1. Boykov, Y., Jolly, M.-P.: Interactive organ segmentation using graph cuts. In: Delp, S.L., DiGoia, A.M., Jaramaz, B. (eds.) MICCAI 2000. LNCS, vol. 1935, pp. 276–286. Springer, Heidelberg (2000)
2. Bracewell, R.: The Fourier Transform and Its Applications, 2nd edn. Mcgraw-Hill College, Pennsylvania (1986)
3. Campadelli, P., Pratissoli, S., Casiraghi, E., Lombardi, G.: Automatic abdominal organ segmentation from CT images. ELCVIA: Electron. Lett. Comput. Vis. Image Anal. **8**(1), 1–14 (2009)
4. Heinrich, M.P., Jenkinson, M., Bhushan, M., Matin, T., Gleeson, F.V., Brady, S.M., Schnabel, J.A.: Mind: modality independent neighbourhood descriptor for multi-modal deformable registration. Med. Image Anal. **16**(7), 1423–1435 (2012). Special Issue on the 2011 Conference on Medical Image Computing and Computer Assisted Intervention
5. Heitzman, E.R.: The Lung: Radiologic-Pathologic Correlations, 2nd edn. Mosby-Year Book, Maryland Heights (1984)
6. Kawata, Y., Niki, N., Umetani, K., Nakano, Y., Ohmatsu, H., Moriyama, N., Itoh, H.: Stochastic tracking of small pulmonary vessels in human lung alveolar walls using synchrotron radiation micro CT images. SPIE Med. Imaging **8672**, 867211-1–867211-8 (2013)

7. Mitani, K., Saji, H.: Robust template matching by using variable size block division. In: Sumi, K. (ed.) Optomechatronic Technologies 2005, vol. 6051, pp. 60510X–60510X-8. International Society for Optics and Photonics, December 2005

8. Okada, T., Linguraru, M.G., Yoshida, Y., Hori, M., Summers, R.M., Chen, Y.-W., Tomiyama, N., Sato, Y.: Abdominal multi-organ segmentation of CT images based on hierarchical spatial modeling of organ interrelations. In: Sakas, G., Linguraru, M.G., Yoshida, H. (eds.) Abdominal Imaging. LNCS, vol. 7029, pp. 173–180. Springer, Heidelberg (2012)

9. Powell, M.J.D.: An efficient method for finding the minimum of a function of several variables without calculating derivatives. Comput. J. 7(2), 155–162 (1964)

10. Rueckert, D., Sonoda, L.I., Hayes, C., Hill, D.L., Leach, M.O., Hawkes, D.J.: Nonrigid registration using free-form deformations: application to breast MR images. IEEE Trans. Med. Imaging 18(8), 712–721 (1999)

11. Wachinger, C., Navab, N.: Entropy and Laplacian images: structural representations for multi-modal registration. Med. Image Anal. 16(1), 1–17 (2012)

12. Wan, S.Y., Kiraly, A.P., Ritman, E.L., Higgins, W.E.: Extraction of the hepatic vasculature in rats using 3-D micro-CT images. IEEE Trans. Med. Imaging 19(9), 964–971 (2000)

13. Watz, H., Breithecker, A., Rau, W.S., Kriete, A.: Micro-CT of the human lung: imaging of alveoli and virtual endoscopy of an alveolar duct in a normal lung and in a lung with centrilobular emphysema-initial observations. Radiology 236(3), 1053–1058 (2005)

3D Vessel Segmentation Using Random Walker with Oriented Flux Analysis and Direction Coherence

Qing Zhang[1,2] and Albert C.S. Chung[1(✉)]

[1] Lo Kwee-Seong Medical Image Analysis Laboratory,
Department of Computer Science and Engineering,
The Hong Kong University of Science and Technology, Kowloon, Hong Kong
achung@cse.ust.hk
[2] Department of Electronic and Computer Engineering,
The Hong Kong University of Science and Technology, Kowloon, Hong Kong

Abstract. Accurate 3D vessel segmentation remains challenging due to varying intensity contrast, high noise level, topological complexity and large extension area. In this paper, we propose an efficient graph-based method for 3D vessel segmentation with the help of oriented flux analysis and direction coherence, which work both in the graph construction and energy function formulation. To address the shrinking problem and seed sensitivity in conventional graph-based methods, new metrics based on hand-draft features are designed to encode vessel-dedicated information as prior probability into the optimization framework and to guide the segmentation towards elongated structures. Optimal vessel segmentation results can then be obtained with the random walker implementation efficiently. For evaluation, the proposed method is compared with classical random walker and region growing. We also conduct the comparison with a Hessian-enhanced graph-based method by providing the same graph construction and optimization strategy. The results demonstrate that our method performs better on both synthetic and real images and has higher robustness when the noise level increases.

1 Introduction

Vascular disease is one of the most serious health problems around the world. Taking coronary artery disease (CAD) as an example, which happens when plaque builds up inside vessels, it threatens millions of people's life in the United States. For disease diagnosis and therapy planning, an accurate and efficient segmentation of target vessel structure from complex clinic datasets is extremely important. Therefore, vessel segmentation has attracted much attention in recent years and various useful techniques [13] have been proposed to address this problem.

Some of the existing methods extract vessel-specific features by filtering [3,6,8,10,12,14–17] and measure the vesselness of each voxel for the purpose of vessel enhancement. Hessian matrix [8,10] and gradient flux [3,6,10] are two widely used low-level local structure detectors, which exploit second-order and

© Springer International Publishing Switzerland 2016
G. Zheng et al. (Eds.): MIAR 2016, LNCS 9805, pp. 281–291, 2016.
DOI: 10.1007/978-3-319-43775-0_25

first-order information of the images respectively. Hessian matrix is obtained by convolving the image with the second order derivatives of Gaussian functions at multiple scales. Therefore, its response can be heavily affected by intensity fluctuation and nearby tissues. Flux measures quantify the gradient flow through some predefined enclosed local regions, such as circular cross-sections and spheres. The major drawback of flux-based techniques is the lack of directional information. Recently, a flux-based anisotropy descriptor, termed Optimally Oriented Flux (OOF) [3,12], is proposed for vasculature centerline tracking, which turns out to address the aforementioned issues. OOF computes the gradient flux through multi-scale local spheres and takes the vessel directionality into consideration by projecting the flux along some optimal axes before the integral (see Fig. 1a). Since the evaluation of OOF is localized at the sphere boundaries, the response is robust against the disturbance from adjacent structures and thus more sensitive to small vessels with low contrast in comparison to Hessian-based analysis. However, OOF response is no longer reliable when it encounters bifurcations, which is common in vascular structures. The magnitude of OOF suffers a suddenly fall at the bifurcations and the estimated direction is unpredictable, leading to discontinuities in tracking and segmentation results.

Besides the local structure extracting techniques, to enforce global consistency, graph-based segmenting schemes [4,7,9], such as graph cuts, random walker, power watershed and their extensions, have been gaining in popularity recently for vascular structures segmentation [2,11,18] because of their straightforward implementation and global optimal solution. However, for segmenting elongate shapes, general graph-based methods suffer from shrinking problem (Graph cuts) and seed sensitivity (Random walker). Small vessels and distal parts will be ignored due to the low intensity contrast, indistinguishable boundary and large extension area.

To combine the advantages and alleviate the limitations of both methods, in this paper, we construct novel metrics by extending the OOF descriptor proposed in [12] and incorporate them into a graph-based optimization framework for 3D vessel segmentation. The contribution of the proposed method is threefold: (i) With the help of oriented flux analysis and direction coherence, reliable prior vesselness probability is encoded in a graph-based method to guide the segmentation towards elongated solutions, which is evaluated to be beneficial for vessel extraction; (ii) The new energy function (Eq. 6) can be optimized efficiently with the random walker implementation; (iii) Through carefully metric design and graph construction, bifurcations do not require extra consideration in the proposed method.

2   Methodology

In this section, a novel graph-based optimization framework is proposed for 3D vessel segmentation. First, vessel-dedicated metrics are constructed based on oriented flux analysis and direction coherence. Then, with the help of new measures, we propose an enhanced random walker framework for vessel segmentation, through which both prior vesselness probability and directional information

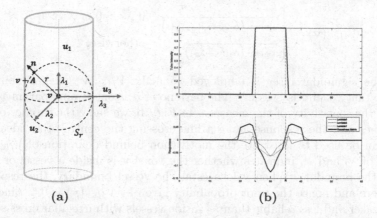

(a)   (b)

Fig. 1. Illustrations of oriented flux. (a) Geometric model; (b) response profiles.

can be embedded to guide the labeling procedure. Carefully graph settings and optimization strategy are also included.

2.1 Oriented Flux Analysis

The aim of oriented flux analysis is to construct a confidence measure which is able to estimate the probability that a voxel locates inside the vessel. Without loss of generality, hereafter we assume that the vessels are brighter than the background.

Given an image volume of interest, for each voxel $\mathbf{v}$, the normalized outward oriented flux along the direction $\hat{\rho}$ is defined as follows,

$$f(\mathbf{v}; r, \hat{\rho}) = \frac{1}{4\pi r^2} \int_{\partial S_r} \left((\mathbf{g}(\mathbf{v} + \mathbf{A}) \cdot \hat{\rho}) \hat{\rho} \right) \cdot \hat{n} dS . \tag{1}$$

Here S_r is a local sphere centered at $\mathbf{v}$ with radius r, $\mathbf{g}(\cdot)$ is the gradient vector on ∂S_r, $\hat{n}$ is the corresponding outward unit normal (Fig. 1a). The idea behind optimal orientations is to decompose the flux along some principle directions that are closely related to local structures of the volume. Equation 1 can be further expressed in the matrix form $\hat{\rho}^T \mathbf{Q_{r,v}} \hat{\rho}$, where $\mathbf{Q_{r,v}}$ is referred to as the oriented flux matrix. Through the eigenvalue analysis of $\mathbf{Q_{r,v}}$, optimal directions and corresponding flux contributions can be captured simultaneously [12].

The extracted pairs of eigenvalues and eigenvectors are denoted as $\lambda_i(\mathbf{v}; r)$ and $\mathbf{u}_i(\mathbf{v}; r)$, where $i \in [1, 2, 3]$, and $|\lambda_1(\cdot)| \leq |\lambda_2(\cdot)| \leq |\lambda_3(\cdot)|$. If the voxel $\mathbf{v}$ locates inside the vessel, the eigenvectors $\mathbf{u}_2, \mathbf{u}_3$ lie in the perpendicular plane of the vessel direction and $\mathbf{u}_1$ goes along the estimated local direction. When $\mathbf{v}$ is on the centerline with radius r equal to the exact radius of the vessel, Eq. 1 achieves the optimal value along the direction $\mathbf{u}_3$, see Fig. 1a, b.

Partly inspired by [8,12], we design a new vesselness metric based on oriented flux analysis, which takes into account the magnitude and polarity of all the eigenvalues. It is defined as follows,

$$V_{flux}(\mathbf{v}) = \begin{cases} \dfrac{1}{1+\exp\left(\alpha\cdot 2\cdot\max(\lambda_2,\lambda_3)\right)} & \text{if } \lambda_2 > 0 \text{ or } \lambda_3 > 0 ; \\[3mm] \dfrac{1}{1+\exp\left(\alpha\cdot(\lambda_3+\lambda_2)\right)} & \text{otherwise}, \end{cases} \qquad (2)$$

where the sigmoidal filter is employed to make $V_{flux}(\mathbf{v})$ as probability-like response that voxel $\mathbf{v}$ is "vessel". The parameter α is one tuning parameter that controls the sensitivity of the measure. In Fig. 1b, we show the profiles of three eigenvalues and the response along a line crossing the centre of an ideal tube, which can be used to illustrate the motivation behind definition of V_{flux}. The polarity of λ_2 and λ_3 indicates whether the voxel $\mathbf{v}$ is inside a vessel or closely outside the boundary. When $\mathbf{v}$ locates at the vessel boundary, the response is nearly zero and hence the prior probability given by $V_{flux}(\mathbf{v})$ is 0.5. Since λ_2 is much weaker and less reliable than λ_3 inside vessels with irregular cross-sections and outside the vessels, which is also illustrated in [16], we replace $(\lambda_3+\lambda_2)$ with $\max(\lambda_2,\lambda_3)$ in V_{flux} when they may have opposite polarities. As such, with the help of sigmoidal filter, V_{flux} can provide good prior vesselness probability for each voxel $\mathbf{v}$.

To suppress the low-contrast background regions without vessels, we further remove the voxels by setting the value of V_{flux} to 0 when the magnitude sum of three eigenvalues is less than one threshold τ. Multi-scale analysis is exploited by evaluating V_{flux} with a range of radii to deal with vessels in various sizes. Different from the detector defined in [12], where the geometric mean of λ_2 and λ_3 is used for vessel detection, V_{flux} proposed in this paper considers all the eigenvalues and the sigmoidal filter is incorporated to provide the probability of voxel $\mathbf{v}$ being "vessel".

2.2   Direction Coherence Enforcement

Inside a possible vascular structure, $\mathbf{u}_1(\mathbf{v})$ indicates the local direction along the vessel. Since the orientation of blood vessels change smoothly, the directional information extracted from oriented flux analysis can be employed to enforce the orientation coherence between neighborhood voxels by computing the angular discrepancy,

$$A(\mathbf{v}_i,\mathbf{v}_j) = \frac{2}{\pi}\arccos\left(\frac{|\mathbf{u}_1(\mathbf{v}_i)\cdot\mathbf{u}_1(\mathbf{v}_j)|}{|\mathbf{u}_1(\mathbf{v}_i)|\cdot|\mathbf{u}_1(\mathbf{v}_j)|}\right), \qquad (3)$$

where the range of $A(\mathbf{v}_i,\mathbf{v}_j)$ is restricted to $[0,1]$ and a high value represents good orientation coherence between neighboring voxels. We propose a Gaussian-like penalty function to enforce the direction coherence,

$$P_{dir}(\mathbf{v}_i,\mathbf{v}_j) = \gamma\cdot\exp(-A(\mathbf{v}_i,\mathbf{v}_j)^2), \qquad (4)$$

where the parameter γ controls the sensitivity of the measure.

Consisting of V_{flux} and P_{dir}, the new metrics are designed from the extension of OOF descriptor and extract as much vessel-dedicated features as possible with the final purpose of benefiting vessel segmentation. Different from the detector proposed in [12], V_{flux} and P_{dir} take into account all the eigenvalues and estimated direction eigenvector, transfer them into probability-like estimation and penalty multiplier, which then can be encoded in a graph-based segmentation framework as cost functions. Although eigenvalue decomposition and analysis are widely used in intensity-related Hessian matrix, the proposed metrics are novel extensions from one new flux-based anisotropic descriptor OOF. Inheriting all the superior features from OOF [12], the new metrics are thus more robust against noise and sensitive to small vessels. It is noted that this is also quite different from the work of [16], which considers multi-directional projections instead of two for enhancing the detection of elongated structures with irregular boundaries.

2.3   Graph Construction and Random Walker Implementation

In this section, a graph-based optimization framework is proposed for vessel segmentation, where new vessel-dedicated metrics work both in the graph construction and energy function formulation. With the random walker implementation [9], optimal segmentation results can be obtained efficiently.

Given an undirected weighted graph $G_0 = (V_0, E_0)$ constructed from the volume with predefined seed points, in the segmentation framework proposed by authors of [9], the objective function in the form of combinatorial Dirichlet problem is defined as follows,

$$x = \arg\min_x(\frac{1}{2}x^T Lx) = \arg\min_x \sum_{e_{ij} \in E_0} w_{ij}(x_i - x_j)^2,$$

$$\text{s.t.}\quad x(v_V) = 1, x(v_B) = 0,$$

(5)

where L is the combinatorial Laplacian matrix, w_{ij} represents the non-negative weight assigned to the edge e_{ij} spanning neighboring voxels v_i and v_j, v_V and v_B are the foreground and background seeds respectively. For two-phase partition problems, x_i indicates the probability that voxel v_i first arrives the foreground seed. Equation 5 can then be solved efficiently with conjugate gradient method.

For 3D vessel segmentation, to encode the new metrics constructed from oriented flux analysis and direction coherence, we modify the energy function from Eq. 5,

$$x = \arg\min_x \sum_{e_{ij} \in E_0} w_{ij} \cdot c_{ij} \cdot (x_i - x_j)^2 + \sum_{v_i \in V_f} \left(w_{Vi} \cdot (x_i - 1)^2 + w_{Bi} \cdot (x_i - 0)^2\right),$$

$$\text{s.t.}\quad x(v_V) = 1, x(v_B) = 0.$$

(6)

Here $V_f = V_0 \setminus \{v_F, v_B\}$, the weight w_{ij} enforces neighborhood intensity affinity, which is defined using Gaussian function,

$$w_{ij} = \exp(-\beta \cdot (I(\mathbf{v}_i) - I(\mathbf{v}_j))^2),$$

(7)

where β is one tuning parameter. The weights w_{Vi} and w_{Bi} for label competition terms in Eq. 6 act as prior "vessel" and "background" indicators, which are defined as follows,

$$w_{Vi} = V_{flux}(\mathbf{v}_i), \quad w_{Bi} = 1 - V_{flux}(\mathbf{v}_i).$$

(8)

All weights are restricted in the range of $[0, 1]$. The multiplier c_{ij} given by $P_{dir}(\mathbf{v}_i, \mathbf{v}_j)$ penalizes the neighborhood direction dissimilarity. The output x is a vector indicating the probability that each voxel $\mathbf{v}_i$ starting from current position first reaches the vessel seed instead of the background seed. Hard labeling results can be obtained according to x.

Algorithm 1. Graph Construction and Random Walker Optimization

---

Input: Image Volume I, Seeds v_F and v_B
1: Conduct oriented flux filtering for the whole volume I.
2: Build 3D 6-connected lattice $G_0 = (V_0, E_0)$.
3: **for** $e_{ij} \in E_0$ **do**
4:    Calculate c_{ij} and w_{ij} with Equation 4 and Equation 7.
5:    Assign weights $(c_{ij} \cdot w_{ij})$ to e_{ij}.
6: **end for**
7: Build label competition graph $G_f = (V_0, E_f)$.
8: **for** $v_i \in V_f$ **do**
9:    Assign w_{Vi} to $e_{Vi} \in E_f$, which connects v_i and v_F.
10:   Assign w_{Bi} to $e_{Bi} \in E_f$, which connects v_i and v_B.
11: **end for**
12: $G = (V_0, E_0 \cup E_f)$.
13: Random walker algorithm for optimization.
Output: Probability vector x.

For random walker implementation, a new graph is constructed by merging the 3D lattice G_0 with the label competition graph G_f (see Algorithm 1). In particular, direct edges between all voxels and seeds are appended in addition to the 6-connected lattice connections used in G_0. We give a brief proof that Eq. 6 can be optimized by random walker algorithm.

Proof: Since $x(v_V) = 1$, $x(v_B) = 0$, the label competition terms in Eq. 6 can be reformulated as

$$\sum_{v_i \in V_f} \left(w_{Vi} \cdot (x_i - x(v_V))^2 + w_{Bi} \cdot (x_i - x(v_B))^2 \right). \tag{9}$$

Then the graph G_f can be constructed with the help of v_V and v_B without adding extra graph nodes (see Algorithm 1). And we have

$$\sum_{v_i \in V_f} \left(w_{Vi} \cdot (x_i - 1)^2 + w_{Bi} \cdot (x_i - 0)^2 \right) = \sum_{e_{ij} \in E_f} w_{ij}(x_i - x_j)^2. \tag{10}$$

After merging G_0 and G_f, the Eq. 6 is finally expressed as its equivalent random walker model,

$$x = \arg\min_x \sum_{e_{ij} \in E} w_{ij}(x_i - x_j)^2, \tag{11}$$

$$\text{s.t.} \quad x(v_V) = 1, x(v_B) = 0,$$

which can be optimized using the random walker algorithm proposed in [9].

To summarize, Algorithm 1 describes each step of the proposed vessel segmentation framework.

3   Experiments

For evaluation, experiments have been carried out on both synthetic images and clinic images. The results of proposed method were compared with some closely related segmentation techniques, classical random walker [9], region growing [1] and a Hessian-enhanced [8] graph-based method with the same graph construction and optimization strategy.

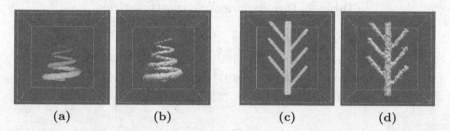

Fig. 2. Evaluation on synthetic images. (a) Synthetic spiral; (b) segmentation results ($\sigma^2 = 0.2$); (c) synthetic tree; (d) Segmentation results ($\sigma^2 = 0.3$).

The first group of experiments were conducted on synthetic spiral (Fig. 2a) and synthetic tree (Fig. 2c). The two synthetic images are carefully designed to simulate different challenges for segmenting real vessel structures, which are described in Sect. 1. For the synthetic spiral, both structure intensity and inner radius are decreased gradually from the value 1 to value 0.5 and 4 voxel to 1 voxel respectively. For the synthetic tree, the structure intensity is set to value 1. The radius of trunk is set to 4 voxel and the radii of branches are set to 2 voxel. The background intensity is set to value 0 in both synthetic images. The size of images are $80 * 80 * 80$ voxels. Additional Gaussian noise with different variance σ^2 were used to generate a set of noisy synthetic images for validation. Only one vessel seed near the root and one background seed around are provided in all the synthetic experiments.

The numerical results on synthetic images for method comparison are listed in Tables 1 and 2. Here Dice Coefficient (DC) is employed to measure the segmentation accuracy. As can be seen in the tables, with the help of new graph construction and energy function, the enhanced framework can provide accurate and stable segmentation results when the noise level increases, while the performance of other approaches drops rapidly. Figure 2b and 2d display the rendering results obtained with the proposed method on two synthetic images with noise variance $\sigma^2 = 0.2$ and $\sigma^2 = 0.3$ respectively. Although the original OOF response is unreliable at bifurcations, the incorporation of sigmoidal filter alleviates the drawback and global consistency enforced by graph-based framework considerately addresses this issue, as is shown in Fig. 2d. Bifurcations thus do not require extra consideration in the proposed method.

The classical random walker gives perfect segmenting results on synthetic images with no noise. However, the cost function of the method only enforces the

Table 1. Dice coefficient on synthetic spiral

Noise level (σ^2)	0	0.1	0.2	0.4	0.5
Proposed method	99.08 %	89.35 %	89.32 %	85.49 %	82.30 %
Random walker	100 %	30.11 %	18.91 %	12.68 %	8.40 %
RW with Hessian	99.80 %	9.98 %	9.15 %	8.55 %	8.28 %

Table 2. Dice coefficient on synthetic tree

Noise level (σ^2)	0	0.1	0.3	0.4	0.5
Proposed method	98.31 %	85.09 %	86.02 %	84.70 %	82.92 %
Random walker	100 %	26.41 %	24.53 %	16.56 %	8.94 %
RW with Hessian	98.00 %	8.73 %	7.84 %	7.65 %	7.49 %

intensity homogeneity between neighboring voxels. Besides, the random walker method suffers from seed sensitivity problem. Thus, the random intensity fluctuation in noisy images leads to unpredictable segmentation results. For Hessian-enhanced random walker, we only replaced oriented flux matrix in proposed method with Hessian matrix obtained using Frangi's filter [8] for fair comparison. The performance drops even faster when the noise level increases. Hessian matrix is calculated based on image intensity and Gaussian smoothing process with large scales exploited for removing noise will also erase vessel boundaries. Therefore, the proposed method is more robust against high level noise than Hessian-based method thanks to the superior properties introduced by the new metrics, as is presented in Tables 1 and 2. In the synthetic spiral segmentation results, the advantage of proposed method is more obvious, which indicates that our method is more sensitive to small vessels with lower intensity contrast.

The second group of experiments have been carried out on a set of clinic MRA images obtained from one open dataset [5]. Due to the lack of publicly available ground truth segmentation and the space limitation, we only present the rendering results for one of the segmentation ("Normal002") and compare the methods qualitatively. As is shown in Fig. 3a, given a small number of seed points (Five randomly selected vessel seeds with equal number of background seeds around are provided in this case), the proposed method can achieve promising segmentation results around the Circle of Willis with the help of new metrics and graph construction. It is noted that the vesselness map obtained from Eq. 2 can provide reliable estimation under high noise level and intensity fluctuation along the vessel. Since the classical random walker method failed to segment the vessels, the results are not presented here. For the Hessian-enhanced method, the results suffer a lot from the noisy environment and the bright boundary issue in MRA images (see Fig. 3b (top row)). We also conducted the experiments with region growing [1] by providing the same seed points. As is shown in Fig. 3b (second row), the region growing method stop growing early due to the

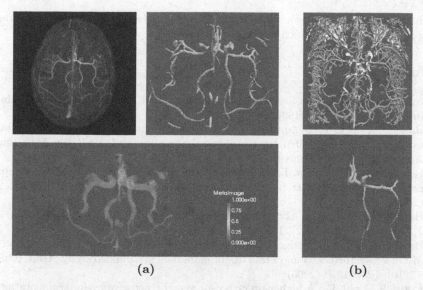

Fig. 3. Evaluation on MRA images. (a) MIP view of the sample MRA data, segmentation results and vesselness map of the proposed method; (b) comparison with Hessian-enhanced method (top row) and region growing (second row).

varying intensity contrast and indistinguishable boundary at the thin vessels, which result in the severe missing problem.

In all the experiments, we set β in Eq. 7 to 100. The parameter α for calculating oriented flux based metric was set to 10, γ for penalizing direction discrepancy was set to 5, τ for background suppression was set to 0.02. To cover the radius range of typical cerebral vessels, the scales for computing OOF (r in Eq. 1) were selected from 1 pixel to 4 pixels with a fix step of 0.5 pixel. For the sake of fairness, the graph constructed for classical random walker method is also a 6-connected lattice and β for calculating edge weights was set to 100. As for the parameters involved in Hessian-enhanced graph-based method, we set them to the same values used in our method.

4   Conclusion

In this paper, we propose an optimal graph-based method for 3D vessel segmentation. To incorporate the vessel-dedicated information into the segmenting framework and to guide the segmentation towards elongated structures, we exploit new metrics based on oriented flux analysis and direction coherence which are extended from optimally oriented flux descriptor. With the help of random walker implementation, optimal segmentation results can be obtained efficiently and bifurcations do not require extra consideration. The proposed method has been compared with some closely related techniques on both noisy synthetic and clinic images. Promising results demonstrate the effectiveness of our method in extracting vessel tree structures from noisy images.

Acknowlegdement. We would like to acknowledge the financial support of the Hong Kong Research Grants Council under grant 16203115.

References

1. Adams, R., Bischof, L.: Seeded region growing. IEEE Trans. Pattern Anal. Mach. Intell. **16**(6), 641–647 (1994)
2. Bauer, C., Pock, T., Sorantin, E., Bischof, H., Beichel, R.: Segmentation of interwoven 3D tubular tree structures utilizing shape priors and graph cuts. Med. Image Anal. **14**(2), 172–184 (2010)
3. Benmansour, F., Cohen, L.D.: Tubular structure segmentation based on minimal path method and anisotropic enhancement. Int. J. Comput. Vision **92**(2), 192–210 (2011)
4. Boykov, Y., Funka-Lea, G.: Graph cuts and efficient N-D image segmentation. Int. J. Comput. Vision **70**(2), 109–131 (2006)
5. Bullitt, E., Zeng, D., Gerig, G., Aylward, S., Joshi, S., Smith, J.K., Lin, W., Ewend, M.G.: Vessel tortuosity and brain tumor malignancy: a blinded study. Acad. Radiol. **12**(10), 1232–1240 (2005)
6. Cetin, S., Unal, G.: A higher-order tensor vessel tractography for segmentation of vascular structures. IEEE Trans. Med. Imaging **34**(10), 2172–2185 (2015)
7. Couprie, C., Grady, L., Najman, L., Talbot, H.: Power watershed: a unifying graph-based optimization framework. IEEE Trans. Pattern Anal. Mach. Intell. **33**(7), 1384–1399 (2011)
8. Frangi, A.F., Niessen, W.J., Vincken, K.L., Viergever, M.A.: Multiscale vessel enhancement filtering. In: Medical Image Computing and Computer-Assisted Intervention, pp. 130–137 (1998)
9. Grady, L.: Random walks for image segmentation. IEEE Trans. Pattern Anal. Mach. Intell. **28**(11), 1768–1783 (2006)
10. Jerman, T., Pernus, F., Likar, B., Spiclin, Z.: Enhancement of vascular structures in 3D and 2D angiographic images. IEEE Trans. Med. Imaging **PP**(99), 1–1 (2016)
11. Kitamura, Y., Li, Y., Ito, W., Ishikawa, H.: Coronary lumen and plaque segmentation from CTA using higher-order shape prior. In: Golland, P., Hata, N., Barillot, C., Hornegger, J., Howe, R. (eds.) MICCAI 2014, Part I. LNCS, vol. 8673, pp. 339–347. Springer, Heidelberg (2014)
12. Law, M.W.K., Chung, A.C.S.: Three dimensional curvilinear structure detection using optimally oriented flux. In: Forsyth, D., Torr, P., Zisserman, A. (eds.) ECCV 2008, Part IV. LNCS, vol. 5305, pp. 368–382. Springer, Heidelberg (2008)
13. Lesage, D., Angelini, E.D., Bloch, I., Funka-Lea, G.: A review of 3D vessel lumen segmentation techniques: models, features and extraction schemes. Med. Image Anal. **13**(6), 819–845 (2009)
14. Merveille, O., Talbot, H., Najman, L., Passat, N.: Tubular structure filtering by ranking orientation responses of path operators. In: Fleet, D., Pajdla, T., Schiele, B., Tuytelaars, T. (eds.) ECCV 2014, Part II. LNCS, vol. 8690, pp. 203–218. Springer, Heidelberg (2014)
15. Moreno, R., Smedby, Ö.: Gradient-based enhancement of tubular structures in medical images. Med. Image Anal. **26**(1), 19–29 (2015)
16. Turetken, E., Becker, C., Glowacki, P., Benmansour, F., Fua, P.: Detecting irregular curvilinear structures in gray scale and color imagery using multi-directional oriented flux. In: IEEE International Conference on Computer Vision, pp. 1553–1560 (2013)

17. Xiao, C., Staring, M., Wang, Y., Shamonin, D.P., Stoel, B.C.: Multiscale Bi-Gaussian filter for adjacent curvilinear structures detection with application to vasculature images. IEEE Trans. Image Process. **22**(1), 174–188 (2013)
18. Zhu, N., Chung, A.C.S.: Random walks with adaptive cylinder flux based connectivity for vessel segmentation. In: Mori, K., Sakuma, I., Sato, Y., Barillot, C., Navab, N. (eds.) MICCAI 2013, Part II. LNCS, vol. 8150, pp. 550–558. Springer, Heidelberg (2013)

Registration of CT and Ultrasound Images of the Spine with Neural Network and Orientation Code Mutual Information

Fang Chen[1], Dan Wu[2], and Hongen Liao[1(✉)]

[1] Department of Biomedical Engineering, School of Medicine,
Tsinghua University, Beijing, China
liao@tsinghua.edu.cn
[2] Department of Electronics, Tsinghua University, Beijing, China

Abstract. Pairwise registration of 2D ultrasound (US) and 3D computed tomography (CT) images can improve the efficiency and safety of image-guided anesthesia in spine surgery. However, accurate 2D US and 3D CT registration for multiple vertebras without an appropriate initial registration position is still a challenge, due to the difference of image modalities and missing bone structures in US image. This paper proposes a novel 2D US and 3D CT registration method, in which convolutional neural network (CNN) classification of US images is reported for the first time to achieve rough image registration. And a new orientation code mutual information metric is further applied to finish local registration refinement. By combining automatic rough registration with fine registration refinement, our algorithm achieves 2D US and 3D CT registration for multiple vertebras (L2-L4) without the requirement of an appropriate initial alignment. The accuracy of our algorithm is validated on 50 in vivo clinical US images dataset of multiple vertebras. And a mean target registration error of 2.3 mm is acquired, which is lower than the clinically acceptable accuracy 3.5 mm.

Keywords: Registration · Ultrasound · Neural network · Orientation code

1 Introduction

Anesthesia for spine surgery is a popular way to alleviate back pain by inserting a needle to target pain location and performing spines' local anesthesia. Image-guided surgical navigation provides surgeons with the information of target lesion and surrounding structures by using sophisticated medical imaging technology [1]. Anesthesia for spine surgery is also usually performed with the aid of image guidance. The early navigation method uses intraoperative 2D X-ray images, but causes repeated radiation exposure. To reduce radiation dose, US image-based navigation is developed due to its safety, portability, and low cost [2]. Although 2D ultrasound (US) is a promising alternative to the common X-ray image and can be used to directly visualize needle, poor image quality and restrictions to the imaging field limit its application. To improve image quality and US image-guided spine surgery, some researches introduce the combination of 2D US image with preoperative 3D computed tomography

© Springer International Publishing Switzerland 2016
G. Zheng et al. (Eds.): MIAR 2016, LNCS 9805, pp. 292–301, 2016.
DOI: 10.1007/978-3-319-43775-0_26

(CT) images [3]. However, 2D US-3D CT registration is difficult for the following reasons: (1) the representation of US image differs from CT image; (2) there are missing data in bone regions of US images, due to the reflection of ultrasound waves at tissue-bone interface.

Two general methods including feature-based and intensity-based approaches are proposed for registration between 3D CT and US images of the spine. Feature-based method is common based on anatomical structures and fiducial markers in CT and US images [4, 5]. Feature-based registration methods by thresholding segmentation of feature points [4] and special surface extraction [5] are used for lumbar vertebrae. However, these methods rely on segmentation preprocess with some manual operation. Intensity-based approaches for US-CT registration are also developed [6, 7]. Khallaghi *et al.* register 3D US images to a statistical shape model by optimizing the Linear Correlation of Linear Combinations metric [6], but just achieves the registration of only one L3 vertebra. A registration pipeline by simulating US images from re-sliced CT data is used to register 2D US and 3D CT images within the limited misalignment range of 0–20 mm [7]. In summary, due to difference of image modalities and missing bone structures in US image, accurate 2D US and 3D CT registration without manual segmentation or an appropriate initial alignment is still a challenge.

In this paper, we propose a novel registration algorithm of 2D US and 3D CT images for multiple vertebras (L2-L4) without an appropriate initial registration position. Firstly, our method uses convolutional neural network (CNN) to classify the US image and acquire rough registration result automatically. This step avoids the requirement of an appropriate initial alignment. Secondly, we apply a new orientation code mutual information (OCMI) metric to achieve local registration refinement. Considering missing bone structures in US image, OCMI metric makes full use the information of small portion of the bone which is coexisted in US and CT images. By integrating CNN rough registration with OCMI metric based local refinement, our method achieves precise registration of 2D US and 3D CT images of the spine.

2 Materials and Methods

The workflow of the proposed registration algorithm of 2D US and 3D CT images of the spine is shown in Fig. 1. Preoperative preparation of training data for CNN is the first step. In this step, according to basic scanning orientations of the US probe in spine surgery, US training images are manually classified into five standard scan scenarios. Then, we need to calculate registration transform between the US training image of every standard scan scenario and 3D CT image in advance. In the second step, CNN's architect is constructed, and by testing the CNN model, the 2D US image to be registered is classified automatically into a correct standard scan scenario. Our rough registration result is the calculated transform of the correct standard scan scenario in the first step. In the final step of local registration refinement, we define an OCMI metric. And by taking rough registration result as initialization, we execute Powell optimizer to find optimum value of OCMI metric and final registration transform.

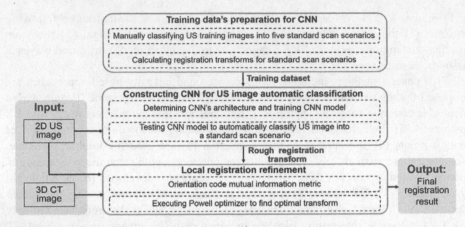

Fig. 1. The workflow of the proposed algorithm.

2.1 Training Data's Preparation for CNN

Five Standard Scan Scenarios. In 2D US image-guided spine surgery, there are five standard scan scenarios [2] including paramedian sagittal transverse (PST), paramedian

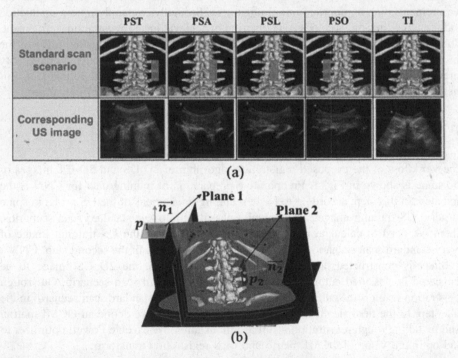

Fig. 2. Training data's preparation; (a) five standard scan scenarios; (b) transform calculation by creating a plane in a standard scan scenario. (Color figure online)

sagittal articular (PSA), paramedian sagittal laminar (PSL), paramedian sagittal oblique (PSO) and transverse interlaminar (TI) (Fig. 2(a)). To generate large amounts of training data, 500 in vivo 2D US images are manually classified into corresponding standard scan scenario with the help of an expert surgeon.

Calculating Registration Transform for a Standard Scan Scenario. A semi-automatic method is used to calculate registration transform between the US training image of every standard scan scenario and 3D CT image. The semi-automatic method is as follows: (1) in CT volume, we need to create a plane (plane 2 in Fig. 2(b)) which corresponds to a standard scan scenario shown in Fig. 2(a). The plane's size is the same as the US training image's size. The plane 2 is created by two points (red and green points in Fig. 2(b)) and a normal vector (vector $\vec{n_2}$). Two points are drawn by an expert surgeon in a standard scan scenario. And normal vector $\vec{n_2}$ is calculated according to it is perpendicular to the line which is determined by two drawn points. (2) The plane of US training image (plane 1) is placed on the upper left of the CT volume and by registering plane 1 and plane 2, we can calculate a rigid transform. This rigid transform is the registration transform of a standard scan scenario. In this way, the registration transforms of five standard scan scenarios are acquired and defined as $RT = \{T_1, T_2, T_3, T_4, T_5\}$.

2.2 Constructing CNN for US Image Classification

After finishing the preparation of training data, the CNN is constructed to classify an US image to be registered into a correct standard scan scenario. The CNN has been established as a powerful classifier for image recognition problem and in this paper, we use CaffeNet model [8]. The CaffeNet consists of five convolutional layers and three fully connected layers, and we replaced the final fully connected layer with a 5-neuron layer because our problem involves five categories of standard scan scenarios. The full neural network architecture used for our US image classification is shown in Fig. 3. The pre-trained Caffenet is performed with the open source Caffe CNN library [9]. By testing CaffeNet model, US image to be registered is classified into i th standard scan scenario. And corresponding transform T_i in RT is our rough registration result T^0.

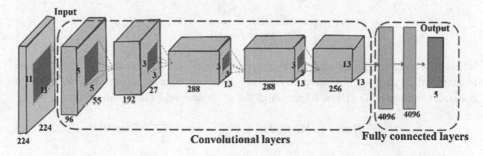

Fig. 3. Full neural network architecture used for our US image classification

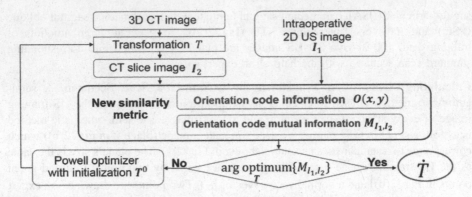

Fig. 4. The process of local registration refinement

2.3 Local Registration Refinement

Through CNN classification, a rough registration transform T^0 is acquired to be used as initial registration transform. Then OCMI metric based local registration refinement is applied to achieve final registration result $\dot{T}$. The process of local registration refinement is shown in Fig. 4. During local registration refinement, an appropriate registration metric is very important. Conventional mutual information (MI) is inappropriate for US and CT image registration of the spine, because it ignores the problem that CT image contains the complete structure of the spine while only a small portion of the bone appears in US images. So coexisted bone structures in US and CT images is limited. To make full use of the small portion of the bone which is coexisted in US and CT images, we integrate orientation code information with intensity information to achieve a new OCMI metric.

Orientation Code Information. For orientation code information, we first apply a process with phase-based 2D Gabor filter [10], to enhance bone construct in US image I_1 and CT images I_2. Then we calculate orientation code information $O(x, y)$ by using the similarity of gradient vectors in enhanced US and CT images.

Firstly, 2D Gabor filters in the frequency domain with different orientations and scales are defined as follows:

$$G(\omega, \theta) = exp\left[-\frac{(log(\omega/\omega_0))^2}{2 * (log(\kappa/\omega_0))^2} + (\theta - \theta_0)^2/(2\sigma_\theta^2)\right] \tag{1}$$

where κ is a scaling factor and ω_0 is center frequency, θ_0 is orientation of the filter, σ_θ is standard deviation of Gaussian function. We use 6 orientations and 4 scales to construct multiple 2D Gabor filters. And the even and odd Gabor filters are

$$M_{so}^e = real\left(FT^{-1}G(\omega, \theta)\right), \quad M_{so}^o = imag\left(FT^{-1}G(\omega, \theta)\right) \tag{2}$$

where FT^{-1} is the inverse Fourier transform. The even and odd Gabor filters are applied to convolve image $I(x, y)$ and acquire processed results $e_{so}(x, y)$, $o_{so}(x, y)$.

Secondly, to enhance image $I(x, y)$ and retain bone construct, e_{so} and o_{so} are used to get amplitude A_{so}, phase angle φ_{so} and phase deviation $\Delta\varphi_{so}$, as follows:

$$A_{so}(x,y) = \sqrt{e_{so}(x,y)^2 + O_{so}(x,y)^2}, \quad \varphi_{so}(x,y) = \operatorname{atan}\left(\frac{O_{so}(x,y)}{e_{so}(x,y)}\right) \tag{3}$$

$$\Delta\varphi_{so}(x,y) = \cos\left(\varphi_{so}(x,y) - \overline{\varphi_{so}(x,y)}\right) - \left|\sin\left(\varphi_{so}(x,y) - \overline{\varphi_{so}(x,y)}\right)\right| \tag{4}$$

where $\overline{\varphi_{so}}$ is the mean phase angle at orientation o. The enhanced image $I'(x, y)$ is acquired with amplitude A_{so} and phase deviation $\Delta\varphi_{so}$ by Eq. 5

$$I'(x,y) = \frac{\sum_s \sum_o (A_{so}(x,y) \cdot \Delta\varphi_{so}(x,y))}{\sum_s \sum_o A_{so}(x,y) + \varepsilon_0}, \tag{5}$$

ε_0 is a very small value. By above two steps, we can acquire enhanced image I'_1 of US image and enhanced image I'_2 of CT slice image I_2.

Finally, because in multimodal US and CT images, gradients of the bone structures have the same orientation, we calculate the normalized gradient vectors $\overrightarrow{V_1(x,y)}$ and $\overrightarrow{V_2(x,y)}$ at each pixel (x, y) in enhanced US image I'_1 and CT image I'_2 by convolving the image with the appropriate first derivatives of a Gaussian kernel of scale ε. The similarity of gradient vectors is our defined orientation code information $O(x, y)$, and it is calculated by Eq. 6

$$O(x,y)_{(x,y)\in\Omega} = \frac{cov\left(\overrightarrow{V_1(x,y)}, \overrightarrow{V_2(x,y)}\right)}{\sqrt{cov\left(\overrightarrow{V_1(x,y)}, \overrightarrow{V_1(x,y)}\right)} * \sqrt{cov\left(\overrightarrow{V_2(x,y)}, \overrightarrow{V_2(x,y)}\right)} + 1}{2}, \tag{6}$$

where $cov(,)$ is the covariance and Ω is the overlap region of images I'_1 and I'_2.

Orientation Code Mutual Information. To integrate orientation code information $O(x, y)$ with intensity information, a new probability density function p between US image and CT slice image is defined as

$$p(l,k) = \frac{1}{N} * \sum_{i=1}^{N} O(x_i, y_i) * S(I_1(x_i, y_i) - l, I_2(x_i, y_i) - k), \tag{7}$$

where (x_i, y_i) is the i th pixel in the overlap region of two images and N is the number of pixels; l, k are intensity values appearing in images I_1 and I_2, respectively. $S(,)$ is an indicator function and is defined as:

$$S(m,n) = \begin{cases} 1 & m = 0 \, or \, n = 0 \\ 0 & otherwise \end{cases} \tag{8}$$

After calculating probability density function p, the joint entropy H_{I_1,I_2} between US image I_1 and CT slice image I_2 is as follows:

$$H_{I_1,I_2} = \sum_{l,k} -p(l,k) * \log(p(l,k)) \tag{9}$$

Finally, the OCMI metric M_{I_1,I_2} between US and CT images I_1 and I_2 is

$$M_{I_1,I_2} = (H_{I_1} + H_{I_2})/H_{I_1,I_2}, \tag{10}$$

where H_{I_1} and H_{I_2} are the entropy of US and CT images respectively and they are calculated as same as the entropy of the image in traditional MI metric, H_{I_1,I_2} is our proposed joint entropy. In local registration refinement, we use Powell optimizer to find optimum value of OCMI metric and final registration transform $\dot{T}$.

3   Experiment and Results

3.1   Data Acquisition and Experiments

Our proposed registration algorithm was evaluated with dataset from in vivo human spine. The preoperative CT and intraoperative US dataset were collected at Beijing Tsinghua Changgung Hospital. The 3D CT image was captured with a CT scanner (Discovery CT750 HD, GE) and CT image was $512 \times 512 \times 463$ voxels with resolution 0.625 mm $\times$ 0.625 mm $\times$ 0.625 mm. Three vertebras (L2-L4) were scanned by an expert sonographer using Phillips SONOS 7500 US machine to collect 500 US images. The size of the 2D US images was 600×800 pixels with resolution 0.275 mm $\times$ 0.275 mm. Before US dataset collection, in order to minimize intervertebral motion between pre- and intraoperative spinal postures, intraoperative posture of patient was adjusted to be consistent with preoperative posture under the supervision of experienced doctor. Therefore, the intervertebral motion could be ignored. To evaluate the efficacy of the proposed registration, we performed two experiments. The first experiment was to quantitatively evaluate the CNN architecture for classification accuracy of US images. The rough registration transform T^0 was from US images classification result, so if the classification accuracy is high, correctness of T^0 will be guaranteed. The second experiment was to evaluate the precision of our registration algorithm and usefulness of OCMI metric.

3.2   CNN Classification of US Images

To quantitatively evaluate the CNN architecture for US images classification, we trained Caffenet model by using stochastic gradient descent with a batch size of 64, momentum of 0.9, weight decay of 0.0005, bias 0.1, a learning rate of 0.01, and max iteration 45000. There were 500 images of three vertebras (L2-L4) for training and 100 images for testing. Every standard scan scenario (defined in Sect. 2.1) contained 20 testing US images and there were totally 100 testing images for five standard scan

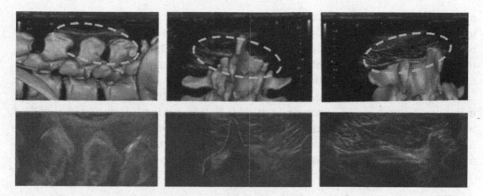

Fig. 5. Three examples of registration trials; first row: the corresponding position of registered 2D US image in 3D CT of the spine; second row: the enlarged views of the key region around bone edge (region of magenta dashed line in first row). (Color figure online)

Table 1. Results of 50 registration trials on in vivo US data.

Measurements	Using OCMI metric	Using traditional MI metric
TRE	2.3 ± 0.8 mm	5.9 ± 1.8 mm
Success rate	82.0 %	64.0 %

scenarios. These images were resized to 224×224 to fit the input layer of Caffenet model. Final classification accuracies of Caffenet for US images was 91.09 %. So by using CaffeNet, we could achieve high classification accuracy and ensure the correctness of rough registration transform T^0.

3.3 Registration of the US and CT Images of the Spine

During experiment, we performed 50 registration trials for in vivo clinical US image from multiple vertebras (L2-L4) and preoperative 3D CT image. The parameters constrained in our OCMI metric were set as follows: $\omega_0 = \frac{1}{18}$, $\theta_0 = \frac{\pi}{4}$, $\frac{\kappa}{\omega_0} = 0.50$, and $\sigma_\theta = \frac{\pi}{4}$. Our registration approaches were implemented in MATLAB and run on Intel (R) Core™ i7 with 16 GB RAM. Figure 5 showed three examples of registration results between 2D in vivo US images and CT images by using our method. In Fig. 5, bone edge in US image (red line) was registered with bone edge in CT image (yellow line). This result qualitatively confirm that our method successfully aligned 2D US and 3D CT slice images although CT image contained the complete structure of the spine while only a small portion of the bone appeared in US images.

To further finished quantitative evaluation of our registration results and validated usefulness of OCMI metric, an expert surgeon was asked to identify corresponding spine edge points on the US and corresponding CT images after registration. The average Euclidean distance between these edge points was chosen as a measure of the final target registration error (TRE). Furthermore, in US image guided spine surgery, the registration was considered successful if the TRE is less than 3.5 mm, which is the clinically accepted error. During experiment, the US-CT registration was performed by using either our registration method, or the method which used CNN rough registration and traditional MI metric based local refinement. Table 1 showed the results of 50 registration trials between in vivo US images from multiple vertebras (L2-L4) and 3D CT image. The method which used traditional MI metric, acquired TRE of 5.9 ± 1.8 mm. Comparatively, our proposed registration method acquired smaller TRE of 2.3 ± 0.8 mm. In addition, there were only nine of 50 registration trials failed to register correctly while using our method, so the success rate of 82.0 % was acquired. However, the method which used traditional MI metric, acquired low success rate of 64.0 %. These experimental results demonstrated that our registration was accurate, and the OCMI metric was more effective for local registration refinement than traditional MI.

4   Discussions and Conclusion

In this paper, we proposed a 2D US and 3D CT image registration algorithm by using CNN rough registration and OCMI metric for image-guided spine surgery. The proposed method is able to register 2D US and 3D CT images of multiple vertebrates (L2-L4), without an appropriate initial position of registration. In our method, CNN classification of US images is reported for the first time to achieve rough image registration and avoid initial alignment. Furthermore, new OCMI metric is applied which makes full use of the coexisted small portion of the bone in US and CT images by integrating the orientation with intensity information. The feasibility of our method is verified in vivo US images of human spine.

To improve generality of our algorithm, we will finish two improvements in the step of training data's preparation for CNN. (1) we will create a larger training database of US images to cover different appearances in the US images of patients; (2) we will replace pre-operative CT scans with a general statistical spine model, and calculate registration transform between the US training image of standard scan scenario and 3D spine model in advance. These two improvements ensure that the prepared training dataset and trained CNN is generally applicable for different patient in US-image-guided spine surgery. In conclusion, we developed a 2D US and 3D CT images registration method which firstly integrates popular CNN to registration pipeline and it has the potential to be applied to other image modalities and clinical applications.

Acknowledgments. This study was supported in part by National Natural Science Foundation of China (Grant No. 81427803, 61361160417, 81271735), Grant-in-Aid of Project 985, and Beijing Municipal Science & Technology Commission (Z151100003915079). The Authors would like to thank Mr. Zhe Zhao from Beijing Tsinghua Changgung Hospital for assistance in acquiring US and CT image data for this study.

References

1. Foley, K.T., Smith, M.M.: Image-guided spine surgery. Neurosurg. Clin. N. Am. **7**(2), 171–186 (1996)
2. Ortega-Romero, A., et al.: Ultrasound-guided interventional procedures for lumbar pain. Tech. Reg. Anesth. Pain Manag. **17**(3), 96–106 (2013)

3. Galiano, K., et al.: Ultrasound-guided and CT-navigation-assisted periradicular and facet joint injections in the lumbar and cervical spine: a new teaching tool to recognize the sonoanatomic pattern. Reg. Anesth. Pain Med. **32**(3), 254–257 (2007)
4. Rasoulian, A., Abolmaesumi, P., Mousavi, P.: Feature-based multibody rigid registration of CT and ultrasound images of lumbar spine. Med. Phys. **39**(6), 3154–3166 (2012)
5. Brounstein, A., Hacihaliloglu, I., Guy, P., Hodgson, A., Abugharbieh, R.: Towards real-time 3D US to CT bone image registration using phase and curvature feature based GMM matching. In: Fichtinger, G., Martel, A., Peters, T. (eds.) MICCAI 2011, Part I. LNCS, vol. 6891, pp. 235–242. Springer, Heidelberg (2011)
6. Khallaghi, S., et al.: Registration of a statistical shape model of the lumbar spine to 3D ultrasound images. In: Jiang, T., Navab, N., Pluim, J.P., Viergever, M.A. (eds.) MICCAI 2010, Part II. LNCS, vol. 6362, pp. 68–75. Springer, Heidelberg (2010)
7. Gill, S., Abolmaesumi, P., Fichtinger, G., et al.: Biomechanically constrained groupwise ultrasound to CT registration of the lumbar spine. Med. Image Anal. **16**(3), 662–674 (2012)
8. Jia, Y., Shelhamer, E., et al.: Caffe: convolutional architecture for fast feature embedding. In: Proceedings of the ACM International Conference on Multimedia, pp. 675–678. ACM (2014)
9. http://caffe.berkeleyvision.org/
10. Daugman, J.: Complete discrete 2D Gabor transform by neural networks for image analysis and compression. IEEE Trans. ASSP **36**(7), 1169–1179 (1988)

A New Statistical Image Analysis Approach and Its Application to Hippocampal Morphometry

Mark Inlow[1]($\boxtimes$), Shan Cong[2], Shannon L. Risacher[1], John West[1], Maher Rizkalla[2], Paul Salama[2], Andrew J. Saykin[1], Li Shen[1]($\boxtimes$), and for the ADNI

[1] Radiology and Imaging Sciences, Indiana University School of Medicine, Indianapolis, IN, USA
`minlow@iupui.edu,shenli@iu.edu`
[2] Electrical and Computer Engineering, Purdue University Indianapolis, Indianapolis, IN, USA

Abstract. In this work, we propose a novel and powerful image analysis framework for hippocampal morphometry in early mild cognitive impairment (EMCI), an early prodromal stage of Alzheimer's disease (AD). We create a hippocampal surface atlas with subfield information, model each hippocampus using the SPHARM technique, and register it to the atlas to extract surface deformation signals. We propose a new alternative to standard random field theory (RFT) and permutation image analysis methods, *Statistical Parametric Mapping (SPM) Distribution Analysis or SPM-DA*, to perform statistical shape analysis and compare its performance with that of RFT methods on both simulated and real hippocampal surface data. The major strengths of our framework are twofold: (a) SPM-DA provides potentially more powerful algorithms than standard RFT methods for detecting weak signals, and (b) the framework embraces the important hippocampal subfield information for improved biological interpretation. We demonstrate the effectiveness of our method via an application to an AD cohort, where an SPM-DA method detects meaningful hippocampal shape differences in EMCI that are undetected by standard RFT methods.

1 Introduction

The hippocampus plays an important role in learning and memory, and is a widely studied brain structure in Alzheimer's Disease (AD). Hippocampal measures extracted from magnetic resonance imaging (MRI) scans have been shown

This work was supported by NIH R01 LM011360, U01 AG024904, R01 AG19771, P30 AG10133, UL1 TR001108, R01 AG 042437, and R01 AG046171; DOD W81XWH-14-2-0151, W81XWH-13-1-0259, and W81XWH-12-2-0012; and NCAA 14132004. ADNI—Data used in preparation of this article were obtained from the Alzheimer's Disease Neuroimaging Initiative (ADNI) database (http://adni.loni.usc.edu/). As such, the investigators within the ADNI contributed to the design and implementation of ADNI and/or provided data but did not participate in analysis or writing of this report. A complete listing of ADNI investigators can be found at: http://adni.loni.usc.edu/wp-content/uploads/how_to_apply/ADNI_Acknowledgement_List.pdf.

© Springer International Publishing Switzerland 2016
G. Zheng et al. (Eds.): MIAR 2016, LNCS 9805, pp. 302–310, 2016.
DOI: 10.1007/978-3-319-43775-0_27

as effective biomarkers for detecting the status of AD or mild cognitive impairment (MCI, a prodromal stage of AD) [4,8,9,14]. Investigation of hippocampal morphometry as an early biomarker for detecting early MCI (EMCI) is a significant but yet under-explored topic. Cong et al. [2] studied this topic using random field theory [12,13] and surface-based morphometry, but identified no significant difference between healthy control (HC) and EMCI participants.

To bridge this gap, we propose a novel and powerful image analysis framework for hippocampal morphometry in EMCI. We create a hippocampal surface atlas with subfield information using the method described in [2]. We model each hippocampus using the SPHARM technique [7] and register it to the atlas for subsequent analyses. We propose analyzing the resulting data using a new approach, *Statistical Parametric Mapping (SPM) Distribution Analysis or SPM-DA*. SPM-DA methods can provide greater power by more fully exploiting SPM information than current random field theory (RFT) and permutation methods which only use information provided by SPM peaks and/or clusters. In addition, SPM-DA methods use permutation inference to allow the use of algorithms with mathematically intractable distributions and to avoid restrictive RFT assumptions which, if violated, can reduce power. Thus the major strengths of this work are twofold: (a) SPM-DA provides potentially more powerful algorithms than current RFT and permutation methods for detecting weak signals and (b) the work embraces, rather than ignores, the important hippocampal subfield information for improved interpretation of the identified pattern.

We compare the performance of RFT Peak and RFT Peak methods with that of a specific SPM-DA histogram method by analyzing simulated and real (Alzheimer's Disease Neuroimaging Initiative (ADNI) [10]) data. We also conduct a subfield analysis of the ADNI data to fully demonstrate the utility of our hippocampal morphometric analysis framework.

2 Materials and Methods

ADNI Data: The real data used in this study were downloaded from the ADNI database [10]. One goal of ADNI has been to test whether serial MRI, positron emission tomography, other biological markers, and clinical and neuropsychological assessment can be combined to measure the progression of MCI and early AD. For up-to-date information, see www.adni-info.org. We downloaded baseline 3T MRI scans of 172 HC, 267 early MCI (EMCI), and 140 late MCI (LMCI), along with demographic and diagnostic information.

Hippocampal Surface Modeling and Alignment: Hippocampal segmentation is conducted by FIRST [3], a surface registration and segmentation tool developed as part of the FMRIB Software Library (FSL). FreeSurfer is not used here since it tends to yield noisy hippocampal boundary not suitable for shape analysis [2]. Topology fix is performed on the binary segmentation results to make sure that each hippocampal surface has spherical topology. The SPHARM method [7] is used to model each surface. FreeSurfer is used for hippocampal subfield segmentation, because this function is unavailable in FIRST. Following [2], we create a hippocampal surface atlas labelled with five subfields: hippocampal tail, CA1, CA2-3, CA4-DG, and SUB (containing both presubiculum and subiculum). Each hippocampal surface is a SPHARM reconstruction registered to the atlas by aligning its first order ellipsoid. Surface signals are extracted as the deformation along the surface normal direction of the atlas.

RFT Surface Analysis: Using random field theory (RFT) implemented in SurfStat [12], the surface signals $N_{i,j}$ are analyzed using the regression model

$$N_{i,j} = \beta_0 + \beta_{1,j}I_i + \beta_{2,j}\text{age}_i + \beta_{3,j}\text{gender}_i + \epsilon_{i,j}, \ i = 1, \ldots, n, \ j = 1, \ldots, m$$

in which I_i is the group indicator, e.g., 1 if EMCI and 0 if HC, n is the number of subjects, m is the number of surface vertices. The SPM consisting of the t statistics for testing H_o: $\beta_{1,j} = 0$, $j = 1, \ldots, m$, is then analyzed using both peak amplitude and cluster size statistics as implemented by SurfStat [12,13].

SPM Distribution Analysis (SPM-DA): The SPM-DA method investigated here captures the information provided by the SPM statistics by estimating their distribution with a frequency histogram. The histogram bin boundaries are chosen so that each bin is equally likely under the null (permutation) distribution. The bin frequencies are then analyzed to detect departures from count uniformity. In these analyses two regression models are employed,

$$F_i = \beta_u x_{u,i} + \epsilon_i, \ i = 1, \ldots, n, \tag{1}$$
$$F_i = \beta_l x_{l,i} + \epsilon_i, \ i = 1, \ldots, n, \tag{2}$$

in which F_i denotes the frequency of the ith of $n = 12$ bins. For the first model in Eq. (1), we let $x'_u = (0,0,0,0,0,0,0,1,2,3,4,5)'$ be our predictor. Thus, the coefficient β_u will be positive when there is an overabundance of positive SPM statistics (right-tail values) indicating a positive relationship between image values and the predictor of interest. Similarly, for the second model in Eq. (2), we let $x'_l = (5,4,3,2,1,0,0,0,0,0,0,0)'$ be our predictor. Thus, the coefficient β_l will be positive when there is an overabundance of negative (left-tail) values indicating a negative relationship. Shown in Fig. 2 are a few examples of the Eq. (1) predictor data (i.e., the solid line) and the bin counts computed from the real hippocampal data (i.e., the "•" values).

To detect a relationship between the image and the predictor of interest generating the SPM, the following compositive hypotheses are tested:

$$H_0 : \beta_u \leq 0 \text{ and } \beta_l \leq 0 \text{ versus } H_1 : \beta_u > 0 \text{ or } \beta_l > 0.$$

Let $\hat{\beta}_u$ and $\hat{\beta}_l$ denote the least squares estimates of β_u and β_l from the unpermuted data. The corresponding one-sided p-values, $p_u = P(\beta_u \geq \hat{\beta}_u)$ and $p_l = P(\beta_l \geq \hat{\beta}_l)$, are combined using Bonferroni to get the p-value for testing H_0 vs. H_1, $p = 2\min(p_l, p_u)$. Simulation is used to compute p_u and p_l by randomly permuting the predictor (after it's orthogonalized with respect to covariates if they are present [11]) with respect to the surface data, recomputing the SPM, and

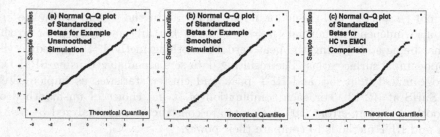

Fig. 1. Normal Q–Q plot of standardized betas for (a–b) example unsmoothed and smoothed simulations and (c) HC vs EMCI comparison.

then computing the corresponding permutation coefficient estimates $\hat{\beta}_u^*$ and $\hat{\beta}_l^*$. This process is repeated N times and then p_u is estimated by

$$p_u = (\# \text{ of } \hat{\beta}_u^* \text{'s} \geq \hat{\beta}_u)/N; \tag{3}$$

p_l is estimated similarly. The only requirement for p-values p_u and p_l to be valid is the usual permutation assumption of exchangeability. Exchangeability is satisfied much more readily than the stringent RFT assumptions [11].

If, in addition, the distributions of the permutation coefficient estimates $\hat{\beta}_u^*$ and $\hat{\beta}_l^*$ are normal, as will often be the case for large samples [6] (e.g., those shown in Fig. 1(a–b)) then p_u and p_l can be computed using the t distribution:

$$p_u = P\left(t_{N-1} \geq \frac{\hat{\beta}_u - \bar{X}}{S\sqrt{1 + 1/N}}\right) \tag{4}$$

in which $\bar{X}$ and S are the sample mean and sample standard deviation of the N $\hat{\beta}_u^*$'s. The factor $\sqrt{1 + 1/N}$ in the denominator is needed since $\text{Var}[\hat{\beta}_u - \bar{X}] = \sigma^2(1+1/N)$ under the null hypothesis. Using this approach small p-values can be accurately estimated with N as small as 30 or so. This procedure, implemented in R, is used to analyze the hippocampal surface normals and the simulated data described below. The results are compared with the SurfStat RFT results.

Simulation Studies: SPM-DA and RFT peak and cluster methods are compared using two simulation studies. For both studies random data on a hippocampal template surface with 652 vertices are generated for 72 subjects according to the model

$$S_{i,j} = \beta x_i + \epsilon_{i,j}, \ i = 1,\ldots,72, \ j = 1,\ldots,126,$$
$$= \epsilon_{i,j}, \ i = 1,\ldots,72, \ j = 127,\ldots,652,$$

in which $S_{i,j}$ represents the surface value at location j for subject i. Both studies simulate two-sample data with x_i equal to -1 for $i = 1,\ldots,36$ and 1 for $i = 37,\ldots,72$. Thus the signal, which extends across 126 contiguous locations, is constant with a magnitude determined by β. For both studies, values for β are 0, 1/12, 1/6, and 1/3. In the first study the random errors $\epsilon_{i,j}$ are independent normal ($\mu = 0, \sigma^2 = 1$) pseudorandom numbers. In the second study the $\epsilon_{i,j}$ are also independent normal ($\mu = 0, \sigma^2 = 1$) but are smoothed prior to the signal being added using the heat kernel smoothing method [1] applied to the hippocampal surface atlas. The resulting data sets are analyzed using SPM-DA (programmed in R [5]) and RFT peak and cluster statistics as implemented by SurfStat [12,13]. For each combination of β and choice of unsmoothed or smoothed random errors, 100 data sets are constructed and analyzed by SPM-DA and RFT methods to compare their power.

3   Results

In our simulation studies, the distributions of the permutation coefficient estimates by SPM-DA are always normal (see Fig. 1(a–b) for a couple of examples). Thus, p_u and p_l are computed using the fast approach of Eq. (4). However, in the real data study, the distributions of the permutation coefficient estimates are nonnormal (see Fig. 1(c) for one example). In this case, we compute p_u and p_l using Eq. (3) with $N = 10,000$ permutations.

Table 1. Simulation results: The number of rejections (out of 100 runs) at $\alpha = 0.05$ and 0.01 for the SPM-DA (SDA), RFT Peak (RFP), and RFT Cluster (RFC) methods.

Signal strength	Unsmoothed data						Smoothed data					
	$\alpha = 0.05$			$\alpha = 0.01$			$\alpha = 0.05$			$\alpha = 0.01$		
	SDA	RFP	RFC	SDA	RFP	RFC	SDA	RFP	RFC	SDA	RFP	RFC
0	5	1	0	1	0	0	3	2	0	0	1	0
1/12	92	7	1	65	3	0	83	10	0	60	3	0
1/6	100	57	6	100	17	5	100	47	51	100	17	43
1/3	100	100	5	100	100	5	100	100	49	100	100	44

Table 1 presents the results of our simulation studies by providing the number of rejections (out of 100 runs) of the SPM-DA, RFT Peak, and RFT Cluster methods for significance levels $\alpha = 0.05$ and 0.01. For the null (signal strength $= 0$) scenarios, all three methods have type I error rates at or below α. For all non-null scenarios the SPM-DA method dominates the RFT Cluster method, exhibiting substantially greater power at all signal strengths. It also dominates the RFT Peak method in all but the strongest signal case. In particular, its power is at least eight times greater than RFT Peak for the weakest signals.

Table 2 presents the results of analyzing the three hippocampal pairwise comparisons using the three methods. The SPM-DA method was the most powerful, detecting shape differences at level $\alpha = 0.01$ for all three comparisons in contrast to RFT Peak which detected two and RFT cluster which detected none. We believe that SPM-DA would yield smaller p-values than RFT Peak for the

Table 2. Statistical analysis results on real data using three approaches: SPM-DA, RFT Peak and RFT Cluster. P values are shown for pairwise comparison among three groups HC, EMCI and LMCI. N.S. indicates not significant. Note that 2E-04 is the smallest nonzero p value that can be obtained in our SPM-DA permutation tests.

Comparison	P from SPM-DA	Smallest P	
		RFT peak	RFT cluster
HC vs EMCI	9.20E-03	1.51E-01	N.S.
EMCI vs LMCI	<2E-04	9.46E-08	N.S.
HC vs LMCI	<2E-04	1.72E-08	N.S.

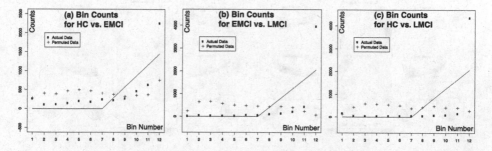

Fig. 2. Bin counts for (a) HC vs EMCI, (b) EMCI vs LMCI, and (c) HC vs LMCI. Our linear model in Eq. (1) aims to use the values on the solid line to predict the "+" values (for permuted data) or the "•" values (for real data). Note that the count scales on the y-axis are different across these three cases, and the significance of the group difference is driven mainly by the "•" value on the 12th bin in each case.

EMCI vs LMCI and HC vs LMCI comparisons if sufficient permutations, e.g. 10^9, were used. The encouraging fact that the SPM-DA method was able to detect HC vs EMCI shape differences demonstrates the promise of SPM-DA for detecting early biomarkers in AD studies.

Figure 2 shows the Eq. (1) predictor data (i.e., the solid line) and the bin counts generated by SPM-DA for each of the three comparisons. It is obvious that the shape differences were detected by the first regression model (see Eq. (1)) in each case. In other words, SPM-DA detected trends toward an overabundance of SPM values in the upper tail of the distribution, indicating hippocampal atrophy in EMCI compared with HC, in LMCI compared with EMCI, and in LMCI compared with HC.

Figure 3(b) shows the surface map of the SPM values for HC vs EMCI, where the red color indicates the atrophy region in EMCI compared with HC. For comparison, Fig. 3(a) shows the t-map of the SurfStat analysis (p-map not shown due to lack of signal). Although capturing a similar pattern, the RFT methods used by SurfStat cannot claim the group differences between HC and EMCI are significant. However, the RFT Peak method used by SurfStat was able to identify statistical shape differences between EMCI and LMCI (t-map

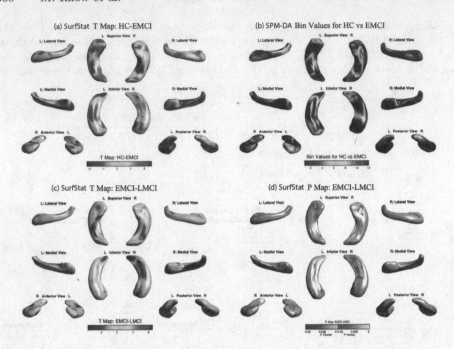

Fig. 3. (a) The SurfStat t-map of the diagnostic effect (HC-LMCI) on surface signals after removing the effects of age and gender. (b) The SPM-DA bin value map for the comparison of HC vs EMCI after removing effects of age and gender. (c–d) The SurfStat t-map and p-map of the diagnostic effect (EMCI-LMCI) on surface signals after removing the effects of age and gender.

Table 3. Comparison between RFT Peak and SPM-DA on the signal region size (i.e., number of vertices with $p < 0.05$ and number of vertices with bin value (bv) $= 12$ respectively) in each subfield. No data are shown for the RFT Cluster method, since no signals were identified in any RFT cluster analysis on real data.

Hemisphere		Left					Right				
Subfield		Tail	CA1	CA2-3	CA4-DG	SUB	Tail	CA1	CA2-3	CA4-DG	SUB
Total # of vertices		398	389	728	91	956	405	362	735	119	941
RFT Peak: # of vertices with $p < 0.05$	HC vs EMCI	0	0	0	0	0	0	0	0	0	0
	EMCI vs LMCI	48	15	39	0	92	15	0	49	3	351
	HC vs LMCI	64	92	204	27	501	94	116	184	28	450
SPM-DA: # of vertices with $bv = 12$	HC vs EMCI	87	113	260	85	572	128	273	263	80	393
	EMCI vs LMCI	291	389	441	49	896	242	295	450	97	805
	HC vs LMCI	283	389	507	91	914	278	362	509	117	903

and p-map shown in Fig. 3(c–d)) and between HC and LMCI (t-map and p-map similar to Fig. 3(c–d) and thus not shown).

Given that we have a surface atlas of hippocampal subfields, Table 3 shows the signal region size in each subfield according to RFT Peak and SPM-DA methods, i.e., number of vertices with $p < 0.05$ and number of vertices with bin value (bv) $= 12$ respectively. Below we summarize the amount of the subfield atrophy region detected by SPM-DA. (1) HC vs EMCI: EMCI demonstrated atrophy patterns compared with HC in 27 % of tail, 51 % of CA1, 36 % of CA2-3, 79 % of CA4-DG, and 51 % of SUB. (2) EMCI vs LMCI: LMCI demonstrated atrophy patterns compared with EMCI in 66 % of tail, 91 % of CA1, 61 % of CA2-3, 70 % of CA4-DG, and 90 % of SUB. (3) HC vs LMCI: LMCI demonstrated atrophy patterns compared with HC in 70 % of tail, 100 % of CA1, 69 % of CA2-3, 99 % of CA4-DG, and 98 % of SUB.

4   Discussion

We have proposed a novel and powerful image analysis approach, *Statistical Parametric Mapping (SPM) Distribution Analysis or SPM-DA*, and applied it to statistical shape analysis in hippocampal morphometry coupled with subfield information. We have compared its performance with that of standard random field theory (RFT) in surface-based morphometry. Our empirical studies on both simulated and real hippocampal data demonstrate that the SPM-DA method has greater power than either RFT Peak or RFT Cluster methods. Of particular importance to early MCI biomarker research, it has substantially greater power to detect weak signals, e.g., it was able to detect HC vs. EMCI differences undetected by RFT methods. These results provide proof of concept evidence for the core premise of SPM-DA, namely, that greater power can be achieved by more fully utilizing SPM distribution information. The specific method considered here used histograms to capture this information. Although this approach worked well in our proposed hippocampal morphometry analysis framework, one future direction is to explore other means of fully utilizing SPM distribution information. Given that SPM-DA is a generic approach, another future direction is to apply it to other image and/or shape analysis studies.

References

1. Chung, M.K., Robbins, S., et al.: Cortical thickness analysis in autism via heat kernel smoothing. Neuroimage **25**, 1256–1265 (2005)
2. Cong, S., Rizkalla, M., et al.: Surface-based morphometric analysis of hippocampal subfields in mild cognitive impairment and Alzheimer's disease. In: IEEE 58th International Midwest symposium on Circuits and Systems, MWSCAS 2015, pp. 813–816 (2015)
3. Patenaude, B., Smith, S.M., et al.: A Bayesian model of shape and appearance for subcortical brain segmentation. Neuroimage **56**(3), 907–922 (2011)

4. Pluta, J., Yushkevich, P., et al.: In vivo analysis of hippocampal subfield atrophy in mild cognitive impairment via semi-automatic segmentation of T2-weighted MRI. J. Alzheimer's Dis. **31**(1), 85–99 (2012)

5. R Core Team: R: A Language and Environment for Statistical Computing. R Foundation for Statistical Computing, Vienna (2015). https://www.R-project.org/

6. Sen, P.K., Singer, J.M.: Large Sample Methods in Statistics. An Introduction with Applications. Chapman & Hall, London (1993)

7. Shen, L., Farid, H., McPeek, M.A.: Modeling three-dimensional morphological structures using spherical harmonics. Evolution **63**(4), 1003–1016 (2009)

8. Shen, L., et al.: Comparison of manual and automated determination of hippocampal volumes in MCI and early AD. Brain Imaging Behav. **4**(1), 86–95 (2010)

9. Testa, C., Laakso, M.P., et al.: A comparison between the accuracy of voxel-based morphometry and hippocampal volumetry in Alzheimer's disease. J. Magn. Reson. Imaging **19**(3), 274–282 (2004)

10. Weiner, M.W., et al.: The Alzheimer's disease neuroimaging initiative: a review of papers published since its inception. Alzheimers Dement. **9**(5), e111–e194 (2013)

11. Winkler, A.M., Ridgway, G.R., Webster, M.A., Smith, S.M., Nichols, T.E.: Permutation inference for the general linear model. Neuroimage **92**, 381–97 (2014)

12. Worsley, K.J.: SurfStat. http://www.math.mcgill.ca/keith/surfstat

13. Worsley, K., et al.: A unified statistical approach for determining significant signals in images of cerebral activation. Hum. Brain Mapp. **4**, 58–73 (1996)

14. Yushkevich, P.A., Pluta, J.B., et al.: Automated volumetry and regional thickness analysis of hippocampal subfields and medial temporal cortical structures in mild cognitive impairment. Hum. Brain Mapp. **36**(1), 258–287 (2015)

Clustering of MRI Radiomics Features for Glioblastoma Multiforme: An Initial Study

Zhi-Cheng Li[1]([✉]), Qi-Hua Li[1], Bo-Lin Song[1], Yin-Sheng Chen[2],
Qiu-Chang Sun[1], Yao-Qin Xie[1], and Lei Wang[1]

[1] Shenzhen Institutes of Advanced Technology, Chinese Academy of Sciences,
Shenzhen, China
zc.li@siat.ac.cn
[2] Sun Yat-Sen University Cancer Center, Guangzhou, China

Abstract. This paper proposed a radiomics model from magnetic resonance imaging (MRI) for Glioblastoma Multiforme (GBM) patients. One challenge of radiomics study is to reduce the redundancy of the features. Totally 466 radiomics features were extracted from automatically segmented tumors from T1, T1 contrast, T2, and FLAIR MRIs. The consensus clustering method was used and 10 feature clusters were obtained. All clusters had a prognostic association with survival, where three clusters had a mean C-index ≥ 0.60. The medoid features in each clusters with highest C-index were selected as radiomics signature candidates. The maximum and mean C-indices of the medoids are 0.75 and 0.68. The results demonstrated that the clusters reduced the data redundancy as well as generated clinical relevant radiomics features.

Keywords: Radiomics · Automatic segmentation · Extraction · Clustering · Glioblastoma Multiforme

1 Introduction

Glioblastoma Multiforme (GBM), the most-frequent primary malignant brain tumor in adults, remains a big therapeutic challenge. The median survival time is only 12–14 months [1]. The poor prognosis is mainly due to the intratumor spatial and temporal heterogeneity [2], which poses clear barriers to target therapies based on invasive biopsy-based genomics, but provides unprecedented opportunities for medical imaging that captures a comprehensive view of the entire tumor in a non-invasive and repeatable way.

Z.-C. Li—This work was supported by the National Natural Science Foundation of China (No. 61571432), National High-Tech R&D Program of China for Young Scientist (863 program, No. 2015AA020933), National Basic Research Program of China (973 Program, No. 2015CB755500), Outstanding Young Scholar Program of Guangdong Province (2014TQ01R060), Shenzhen Basic Research Project (JCYJ20140417113430585), Shenzhen Kongque Overseas Innovation Program (KQCX20140521115045441), and Innovation Team Program in Guangdong Province (2011S013).

© Springer International Publishing Switzerland 2016
G. Zheng et al. (Eds.): MIAR 2016, LNCS 9805, pp. 311–319, 2016.
DOI: 10.1007/978-3-319-43775-0_28

To explore the correlation between imaging traits and underlying genetic characteristics, an emerging technique, radiomics, has been proposed [3]. Radiomics refers to a process explicitly designed to extract high-throughput quantitative imaging features from standard of care images, convert the features into minable data, and build predictive models relating image features to genomic patterns and clinical outcomes [4]. Recently, several radiomics studies were conducted in lung cancer, head & neck cancer and GBM [5–7]. Early evidence of the correlation with survival, mutant, molecular subtype, and gene expression has been reported. Up-to-date reviews on this area can be found in [4,8].

The most critical and challenging component in radiomics is the extraction of stable and non-redundant quantitative features from medical images. It involves three sequential steps: tumor segmentation, high-throughput feature extraction and feature selection. Several studies have shown that quantitative features extracted from expert manually-delineated tumor have prognostic value, although the reproducibility is contentious [6–9]. On the other hand, one recent work has validated that fully-automatic segmented MRI GBM can generate statistically comparable features, despite only four VASARI features were evaluated [10]. To our best, automatic segmentation has never been evaluated in a full radiomics model for GBM.

Radiomics requires a large amount of minable features, leading to a data redundancy problem as with any high-throughput data-mining field. Feature selection strategies are needed to reduce the redundancy and moreover avoid the over-fitting problem. To address this, a clustering method was incorporated in radiomics to provide reliable prognostic signatures for lung and head & neck cancer [11]. Based on the same patient data, a large panel of feature selection and machine learning classification methods were evaluated in terms of their predictive performance and stability [12]. To our knowledge, automatic and non-redundant radiomics model dedicated to GBM has not been yet reported. Compared with lung or head & neck cancers, further complications arise for establishing such an MRI radiomics model for GBM, as spatially explicit subregions (enhancing and non-enhancing core, necrosis, and edema) in multimodality MRIs (T1, T1 contrast, T2, and FLAIR) should be considered [13].

This paper proposes a complete MRI radiomics model for GBM. It comprises a fully-automatic supervised subregion segmentation, high-throughput features extraction, and consensus clustering-based feature selection. We report our initially evaluation of the radiomics clusters using 83 GBM patient data, in terms of their quantitative association with patient survival. The aim of this initial study is to validate the clinical relevance of the proposed radiomics clusters in GBM patients.

2   Methods

2.1   Automatic Tumor Segmentation

Each patient image dataset consists of T1, T1C, T2, and FLAIR modality. First, the four modalities are rigidly registered and undergo a skull-stripping process.

A median filter is used for boundaries smooth. Far each modality the voxel resolutions and histograms are normalized across all patients. Next, we use a supervised machine learning method to separate the images into five classes: normal brain, enhancing area, non-enhancing area, necrosis, and edema [13]. 23 low-level features are extracted for each voxel in each modalities, including 14 intensities (for each voxel and its 6 neighbours, and mean intensities of 7 3×3 block centered at the same 7 locations), 6 first-order textures (mean, variance, skewness, kurtosis, energy, entropy from small patches at each voxel) and location features. Therefore, for each voxel in all modalities we have 92 features in total. Note that these features are only used for segmentation purpose.

After the feature extraction, we use random forests to classify each voxel to one of the five classes. In this initial study we do not employ spatial regularization strategy in the classifier, therefore small false positive outliers may occur. Isolated regions containing less than 230 voxels are removed as false positive. A median filter is used to for boundaries smooth. Finally, all voxels surrounded by enhancing area are labeled as necrosis. A similar but more complicated methods can be found in work [14], where 219 features are used for classification. An in-house Matlab program was used for subregion classification.

2.2   High-Throughput Features Extraction

We define four groups of quantitative features as follows.

(1) Habitat shape features are defined to describe the three dimensional shape characteristics for the solid core, including volume, longest diameter, surface area, solidity, compactness, isoperimetric quotient, spherical disproportion, sphericity, surface to volume ratio, and eccentricity.
(2) Histogram-based first-order features that describe the distribution of the voxel intensities are calculated from the histogram of all subregions, including mean, median, maximum, minimum, range, RMS, energy, entropy, kurtosis, skewness, SD, and variance.
(3) Texture features that quantify the intratumor heterogeneity are calculated for all subregions, including gray level co-occurrence matrix (GLCM)-based second-order textures, and grey level run length matrix (GLRLM)-based, grey level size-zone matrix (GLSZM)-based, neighbourhood grey tone difference matrix (NGTDM)-based high-order textures [5, 7].

The detail of the radiomics features are shown in Table 1.

Note that isolated and connected abnormal regions less than 150 vexols are considered as false positive. Before calculating texture feature for each subregion, voxels with intensities out of the range $\mu \pm 3\sigma$ are not included in subsequent processing, where μ and σ are mean and standard deviation for that subregion. Then, the intensity range is quantified to R_q using equal-probability quantization method (R_q is set to 128 or 256). In the cases of multifocal or multicentric tumors, the features are averaged for each area. Due to the limited space, we cannot include detailed description of all features here. Totally 466 quantitative features are calculated using a Matlab program developed in our lab.

Table 1. Radiomics features used in the proposed model (to be continue in next page).

Group	Feature index	Feature name
Shape	1	Volume
	2	Size
	3	Surface area
	4	Solidity
	5	Compactness
	6	Isoperimetric quotient
	7	Spherical disproportion
	8	Sphericity
	9	Surface to volume ratio
	10	Eccentricity
Global intensity	11	Mean
	12	Median
	13	Maximum
	14	Minimum
	15	Root mean squre
	16	Energy
	17	Entropy
	18	Kurtosis
	19	Skewness
	20	Stand deviation
	21	Variance
GLCM texture	22	Correlation
	23	Autocorrelation
	24	Contrast
	25	Energy
	26	Entropy
	27	Cluster prominence
	28	Cluster shade
	29	Cluster tendency
	30	Dissimilarity
	31	Difference entropy
	32	Homogeneity 1
	33	Homogeneity 2
	34	Informational measure of correlation 1
	35	Informational measure of correlation 2
	36	Inverse difference moment normalized

Table 1. (*Continued*)

Group	Feature index	Feature name
GLCM texture	37	Inverse difference normalized
	38	Inverse variance
	39	Maximum probability
	40	Sum average
	41	Sum entropy
GLRLM texture	42	Short run emphasis
	43	Long run emphasis
	44	Gray level non-uniformity
	45	Run length non-uniformity
	46	Run percentage
	47	Low gray level run emphasis
	48	high gray level run emphasis
	49	Short run low gray level emphasis
	50	short run high gray level emphasis
	51	long run low gray level emphasis
	52	Long run high gray level emphasis
	53	Gray-level variance
	54	Run-length variance
GLSZM texture	55	Small zone emphasis
	56	Large zone emphasis
	57	Gray-level non-uniformity
	58	Zone-size non-uniformity
	59	Zone percentage
	60	Low gray-level zone emphasis
	61	High gray-level zone emphasis
	62	Small zone low gray-level emphasis
	63	Small zone high gray-level emphasis
	64	Large zone low gray-level emphasis
	65	Large zone high gray-level emphasis
	66	Gray-level variance
	67	Zone-size variance
NGTDM texture	68	Coarseness
	69	Contrast
	70	Busyness
	71	Complexity
	72	Strength

2.3   Features Clustering

Various cluster ensemble methods have emerged for analyzing gene expression microarray data. Among these methods, consensus clustering has been widely used in genomic studies, especially in discovering molecular subtypes for GBM [15]. It calculates how frequently two subsamples are clustered together in multiple runs, and uses the resulting pairwise "consensus rates" for visual evaluation, stability comparison, and optimal cluster number determination (K). The basic assumption is that if optimal cluster number K exists, the stability of different subsamples at K would achieve the best. The clustering consensus (range 0–1) is used to describe the stability. The consensus rate heatmap is used to visually validate the results. We employ hierarchical agglomerative ward linkage method with a Pearson correlation based dissimilarity measure and 2,000 resampling iterations. In order to determine the number of clusters, we first compute the cumulative distribution function (CDF) for different clustering numbers (range 1–15). The optimal clustering number is chosen as the converge number of the delta area under the CDF curve. The R package ConsensusClusterPlus was used for the clustering task [16].

3   Results and Discussions

An integrated evaluation of a radiomics model is out of the scope of this paper. Here we focus on demonstrating the performance of the proposed radiomics feature cluster, in terms of clinical relevance. We use the concordance index (C-index) to measure the prognostic performance of the radiomics features owing to its good discrimination ability [17]. C-index can be considered as a generalisation of the area under the receiver operating characteristic (ROC) curve (AUC). For each feature, univariate C-index can be calculated using R package Hmisc. To quantify the association of a cluster with the survival, the average C-index over all features included in that cluster is calculated.

We evaluate the proposed radiomics model using 83 GBM patient data in total from both The Cancer Genome Atlas (63 patients) and Sun Yat-Sen University Cancer Center (20 patients).

An automatic segmentation result for one patient is shown in Fig. 1. The average segmentation time for all four modalities of each patient is 502 s on a Lenovo X1 Carbon computer with Intel(R) Core i5-3317U 1.70 GHz CPU and 4 GB RAM, including the skull-stripping, registration, and classification.

The heatmaps in Fig. 2 respectively show the consensus map of the radiomics feature clustering, the expression level of the Z-score normalized radiomics feature clusters corresponding to the consensus map. From the delta area data, the cluster number was set to 10. There were seven clusters with high cluster consensus ≥ 0.75. Three clusters had a mean C-index ≥ 0.60. The cluster C-index are listed in Table 2. For each cluster we can obtain the medoid, i.e. the feature with highest average pairwise correlation. These medoids, representing their clusters, are candidates of promising radiomics signatures. The maximum and mean C-indices of the medoids are 0.75 and 0.68.

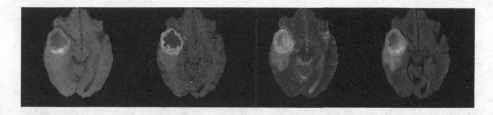

Fig. 1. Subregions in T1, T1C, T2 and FLAIR images are shown in red (necrosis), yellow (enhancing core), blue (non-enhancing core) and green (edema). All images are skull-stripped and registered using T1C as a template (Color figure online).

Table 2. Radiomics clustering results.

Cluster no	Cluster size	Cluster C-index	Cluster medoid
1	176	0.54	necrosis-GLCM-sumAverage
2	118	0.61	enhanced-energy
3	12	0.54	nonedema-maxValue
4	2	0.56	nonedema-disproportion
5	69	0.60	nonedema-GLCM-variance
6	55	0.57	necrosis-GLRLM-SRHGE
7	20	0.65	nonedema-GLRLM-HGRE
8	5	0.58	nonedema-GLCM-autocorrelation
9	3	0.56	necrosis-GLRLM-GLV
10	6	0.53	nonedema-NGTDM-complexity

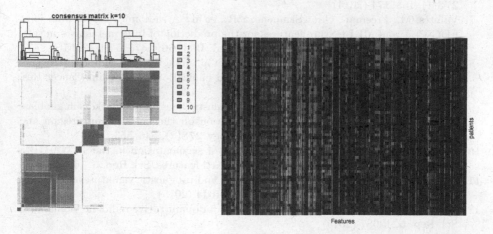

Fig. 2. Heatmaps for radiomics features ordered with respect to the clusters. Left: Cluster consensus map. Right: Radiomics feature expression with Z-score from −1 to 1.

4   Conclusions

Radiomics is a promising method for quantification of tumor phenotypes by extracting high-throughput imaging features. One challenge is to deal with the high dimensional radiomics features space. This study showed that the consensus clustering method reduced the feature redundancy and generated clinical-relevant radiomics clusters. In future, we will investigate the influence of different image processing parameters and feature selection methods with large population. The aim is to obtain a stable radiomics signature for MRI GBM.

References

1. Dolecek, T.A., Propp, J.M., Stroup, N.E., Kruchko, C.: CBTRUS statistical report: primary brain and central nervous system tumors diagnosed in united states in 2005–2009. Neuro-Oncol. **14**(Suppl. 5), v1–v49 (2012)
2. Reardon, D.A., Wen, P.Y.: Glioma in 2014: unravelling tumour heterogeneity-implications for therapy. Nat. Rev. Clin. Oncol. **12**, 69–70 (2015)
3. Kumar, V., Gu, Y., Basu, S., et al.: Radiomics: the process and the challenges. Magn. Reson. Imaging **30**, 1234–1248 (2012)
4. Gillies, R.J., Kinahan, P.E., Hricak, H.: Radiomics: images are more than pictures, they are data. Radiology **278**(2), 563–577 (2016)
5. Aerts, H.J.W.L., Velazquez, E.R., Leijenaar, R.T.H., et al.: Decoding tumour phenotype by noninvasive imaging using a quantitative radiomics approach. Nat. Commun. **5**, 4006 (2014)
6. Gevaert, O., Mitchell, L.A., Achrol, A.S., et al.: Glioblastoma multiforme: exploratory radiogenomic analysis by using quantitative image feature. Radiology **273**(1), 168–174 (2014)
7. Vallires, M., Freeman, C.R., Skamene, S.R., et al.: A radiomics model from joint FDG-PET and MRI texture features for the prediction of lung metastases in soft-tissue sarcomas of the extremities. Phys. Med. Biol. **60**, 5471–5496 (2015)
8. O'Connor, J.P., Rose, C.J., Waterton, J.C., et al.: Imaging intratumor heterogeneity: role in therapy response, resistance, and clinical outcome. Clin. Cancer Res. **21**(2), 249–257 (2015)
9. Cui, Y., Tha, K.K., Terasaka, S., et al.: Prognostic imaging biomarkers in glioblastoma: development and independent validation on the basis of multiregion and quantitative analysis of MR images. Radiology **278**(2), 546–553 (2016)
10. Velazquez, E.R., et al.: Fully automatic GBM segmentation in the TCGA-GBM dataset: prognosis and correlation with VASARI features. Sci. Rep. **5**, 16822 (2015)
11. Parmar, C., et al.: Radiomic feature clusters and prognostic signatures specific for lung and head & neck cancer. Sci. Rep. **5**, 11044 (2015)
12. Parmar, C., et al.: Machine learning methods for quantitative radiomic biomarkers. Sci. Rep. **5**, 13087 (2015)
13. Menze, B.H., Jakab, A., Bauer, S., et al.: The multimodal brain tumor image segmentation benchmark (BRATS). IEEE Trans. Med. Imaging **34**(10), 1993–2024 (2014)
14. Zhang, J., Barborial, D.P., Hobbs, H., et al.: A fully automatic extraction of magnetic resonance image features in glioblastoma patients. Med. Phys. **41**(4), 042301 (2014)

15. Monti, S., Tamayo, P., Mesirov, J., Golub, T.: Consensus clustering: a resampling-based method for class discovery and visualization of gene expression microarray data. Mach. Learn. **52**, 91–118 (2003)
16. Wilkerson, M.D., Hayes, D.N.: ConsensusClusterPlus: a class discovery tool with confidence assessments and item tracking. Bioinformatics **26**, 1572–1573 (2010)
17. Pencina, M.J., D'Agostino, R.B.: Overall C as a measure of discrimination in survival analysis: model specific population value and confidence interval estimation. Stat. Med. **23**, 2109–2123 (2004)

A Multi-resolution Multi-model Method for Coronary Centerline Extraction Based on Minimal Path

Dengqiang Jia[1], Wenzhe Shi[2], Daniel Rueckert[2], Liu Liu[1],
Sebastien Ourselin[3], and Xiahai Zhuang[1(✉)]

[1] School of Naval Architecture, Ocean and Civil Engineering,
Shanghai Jiao Tong University, Shanghai, China
zhuangxiahai@163.com
[2] Biomedical Image Analysis Group, Imperial College London, London, UK
[3] Centre for Medical Image Computing, University College London, London,
UK

Abstract. Extracting centerlines of coronary arteries is challenging but important in clinical applications of cardiac computed tomography angiography
(CTA). Since manual annotation of coronary arteries is time-consuming, labor-
intensive and subject to intra- and inter-variations, we propose a new method to
fully automatically extract the coronary centerlines. We first develop a new
image filter which generates pixels with salient vessel features within a given
window. This filter hence can capture sparsely distributed but important vessel
points, enabling the minimal path (MP) process to track the key centerline points
at different resolution of the images. Then, we reformulate the filter for
multi-resolution fast marching, which not only can speed up the coronary
tracking process, but also can help the front propagation to step over the indistinct
segments of the coronary artery such as at the locations of stenosis. We embed
this scheme into the MP framework to develop a multi-resolution multi-model
approach (MMP), where the extracted centerlines from low-resolution MP serve
as prior and constraints for the high-resolution process. We evaluated the performance of this method using the Rotterdam CTA training data and the coronary
artery algorithm evaluation framework. The average inside of our extraction was
0.51 mm and the overlap was 72.9 %. The mean runtime on the original resolution CTA images was 3.4 min using the MMP method.

1 Introduction

Extracting coronary centerlines from cardiac Computed Tomography Angiography
(CTA) is important in clinics, which facilitates the diagnosis and quantification of
coronary stenosis. A number of works have focused on extracting the complete coronary
artery tree [1]. However, it is difficult to automatically extract the main branches of the
coronary tree. The minimal path (MP) framework has been extended for this purpose,
either to extract a single branch [2–4] or multiple branches based on initialized seed
points [5]. However, the extraction could perform poorly at the indistinct segments, such
as due to the occlusion, calcifications, imaging artifacts, or insufficient contrast agent.

© Springer International Publishing Switzerland 2016
G. Zheng et al. (Eds.): MIAR 2016, LNCS 9805, pp. 320–328, 2016.
DOI: 10.1007/978-3-319-43775-0_29

The detection methods also tend to be challenged, when the seed points are off the coronary or the branch has discontinues segments due to bypass surgeries or image artifacts. Zheng et al. [6, 7] adopted a model-driven approach to automatically extract and recognize the main branches through a learning-based algorithm, which employed 108 CTA volumes, with manual annotations of the coronary centerlines, to train their learning algorithm. Liu et al. proposed a model-guided directional MP method for automatic extraction of coronary centerlines [8, 9]. The model used in this method helps tracking the coronary branch of interest correctly. However, the fast marching method (FMM) iteration is still computationally expensive and the front propagation can be blocked due to the indistinct segments of the coronary artery.

In this work, we develop a new method based on the multi-resolution and multi-model MP framework. First, we propose a new image filter which identifies points with salient vessel features within a given window. This filter can be used to generate feature maps at different resolutions, enabling the MP process to track the centerline key points at different resolutions of the images. This multi-resolution approach has two advantages:

(1) Finding one salient point within a big window, instead of all vessel points, can help stepping over the invisible sites of the coronary at some locations such as the severe stenosis, thus improve the performance of the MP method.
(2) It can speed up the FMM process and consequently the back tracking at a coarse resolution to provide a more efficient centerline extraction method.

Second, we develop a multi-model method, based on the multi-resolution MP framework, referred to as MMP, to extract multiple branches of the coronary arteries. The MMP method is capable of efficiently tracking the desired branches with great length.

The rest of the paper is organized as follows: Sect. 2 describes the proposed new filter. Section 3 introduces the MMP framework. We provide the experiments and results in Sect. 4 and finally conclude this work in Sect. 5.

2   A Filter Preserving Salient Vessel Features

In MP-based centerline extraction, one major issue is the indistinct segments in the vessel, which easily resulting a deviation of the FMM and consequently tracking into wrong path; and the other is the computation complexity of FMM iteration, which is $O(N\log N)$, where N denotes the number of pixel points [10, 18]. In this section, we introduce a new image filter which can provide CTA images with arbitrary low resolution while enhancing the vesselness of coronary arteries for MP process.

The original vesselness filter proposed by Frangi et al. enhances the tube structure of an image by computing the Hessian matrix and its eigenvalues [12]:

$$v(x) \triangleq \begin{cases} 0 & \text{if } \lambda_2 > 0 \text{ or } \lambda_3 > 0 \\ (1 - e^{-\frac{\mathcal{R}_A^2}{2\alpha^2}})e^{-\frac{\mathcal{R}_B^2}{2\beta^2}}(1 - e^{-\frac{S^2}{2c^2}}) & \text{otherwise} \end{cases} \tag{1}$$

where v is the vesselness at pixel x, λ_k denotes the ordered eigenvalues, $\mathcal{R}_A \triangleq \left|\frac{\lambda_2}{\lambda_3}\right|$, $\mathcal{R}_B \triangleq \frac{|\lambda_1|}{\sqrt{|\lambda_2\lambda_3|}}$, $S \triangleq \sqrt{\sum_j \lambda_j^2}$; α, β, and c tune the sensitivity of the filters.

To achieve the multi-resolution FMM, one needs to obtain the image intensity f and vesselness v with salient vessel features at different resolution. Since MP tracks the vessel centerlines based on the minimal cost of the potential function, we propose to compute the image intensity and vesselness within a given window as follows,

$$f_W(x) = f\left(\mathrm{argmin}_{x \in W_x} P(x)\right) \text{ and } v_W(x) = v\left(\mathrm{argmin}_{x \in W_x} P(x)\right), \tag{2}$$

where W_x denotes the volume defined by the given window, $P(x)$ is the potential function proposed in [13],

$$P(x) = \frac{1}{v(\mathrm{x})^{\alpha} * s(\mathrm{x})^{\beta} + \varepsilon} \tag{3}$$

Here, $s(x)$ is the intensity similarity term.

The proposed filter can down sample the intensity and vesselness images of a CTA volume into any resolutions, which is determined by the size of the given window W. The advantage of the proposed filter for down sampling the CTA images is that it can select the points with the most salient vessel features within the window to save the vessel information at the low-resolution images for MP tracking. This is unlike the

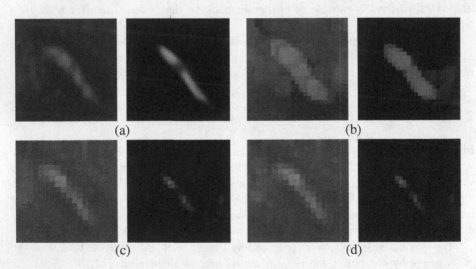

(a)   (b)

(c)   (d)

Fig. 1. Illustration of the vessel images: (a) the original resolution CTA image (left) and corresponding vesselness image (right); (b) the down-sampled images using the proposed filter; (c) the down-sampled images using the nearest interpolation; (d) the down-sampled images using the B-Spline interpolation.

conventional down-sampling methods which blur the original images and thus loose the important vessel characteristics after down-sampling. Figure 1 provides the examples of an original CTA and vesselness image pair and the down-sampled images by the proposed filter and the nearest and B-Spline interpolation methods. The occlusive vessel is then *connected* and enhanced by the proposed filter at low resolution images. By contrast, the other two methods blue weaken the vessel features in the resulting images.

3 Multi-resolution Multi-model Minimal Path for Centerline Extraction

3.1 The Minimal Path at Multi-resolution Images

In the MP framework [14], a decreasing potential function $P(x)$ is given to build an energy functional E: $\mathcal{C}_{a_1,a_2} \to \mathbb{R}^+$,

$$E(C) = \int_C \{P(C(s)) + w\}ds = \int_C \{\tilde{P}(C(s))\}ds, \tag{4}$$

where $\mathcal{C}_{a_1,a_2}$ is the set of all path joining a_1 to a_2, s is the arc-length parameter, w is a positive regularization factor. MP computes the minimal action map $U : \Omega \to \mathbb{R}^+$ associated to a_1 is used to solve the minimization problem. Conventional, U is updated on the neighbor pixels of the current propagation. In this work, we propose to update this map solely on one pixel within a given window W_x which controls the resolution of the action map, i.e. $U' : \Omega/|W| \to \mathbb{R}^+$. Since $\{W_x\}$ can be user-defined, the FMM and MP hence can *operate on a different resolution of the action map*, given the sizes of windows are set differently at different regions or iteration steps.

Furthermore, the potential function P is generally defined related to the intensity and vesselness such as in (3). In the model-guided MP, we further include the direction of the coronary model as follow,

$$P(x) = \frac{1}{v(x)^\alpha \cdot s(x)^\beta \cdot d(x) + \varepsilon} \tag{5}$$

where $d(x)$ is the direction information derived from the model [9].

3.2 Multi-resolution and Multi-model Minimal Path

To improve the performance of MP for coronary artery extraction, we propose to use multiple models for the model-guided MP, resembling the widely used multi-atlas segmentation strategy [16, 17], which operates on multi-resolution images using the proposed salient vesselness filter, i.e. MMP, which works as follows:

(1) MMP first performs the multi-model MP using the low-resolution intensity (LRI) images and low-resolution vesselness (LRV) images. This can efficiently generate a set of centerlines, each of which comes from one model-guided MP.
(2) Then an optimal centerline is identified based on the length of the centerline and closeness to the branch of interests. Based on the selected result, we identify the optimal model and generate a mask, as prior and a constraint for the next tracking using higher resolution images.
(3) The previous tracking-and-selecting step iterates until the original resolution intensity (ORI) and vesselness (ORV) images are reached. The final coronary centerline is generated from the original images. Figure 2 provides the illustration of the MMP method.

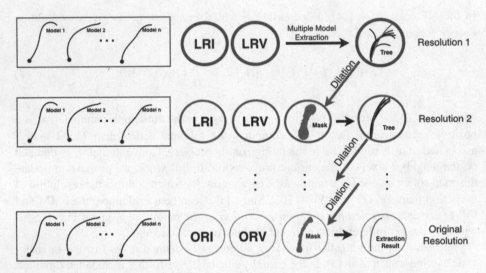

Fig. 2. Diagram illustrating the MMP method extracting the centerline of a main branch of the coronary artery tree.

3.3 Initialization of Coronary Model and Ostium Detection

The coronary model, a coronary centerline extracted from a training CTA, contains the shape of the artery and the line direction at any location. By mapping this coronary model to the target CTA using a hierarchical registration scheme [11], one can extract the direction information from the model for local direction-guided FMM [9]. We employ the learning-based ostium detection based on Haar-like features and the probability boosting tree framework [7, 8], and transform the coronary model to the target CTA by aligning the ostium of the coronary model to corresponding one in the target image. This ostium mapping is first initialized with a deformable registration between the segmented target image and the model CTA [11].

4   Results

To analyze the performance of the proposed method, we used the eight datasets with gold standard from the Rotterdam database [15]. Each of them has manually annotated right coronary artery (RCA), left anterior descending artery (LAD), left circumflex artery (LCX), and a randomly picked large side branch. Methods were evaluated with the overlap measurement and accuracy inside (AI) metrics [15]. The overlap metric includes overlap (OV), overlap until first error (OF), and overlap with the clinically relevant part of the vessel (OT). We used the leave-one-out strategy to perform our experiments, by considering one of them as the target image, and the others as models.

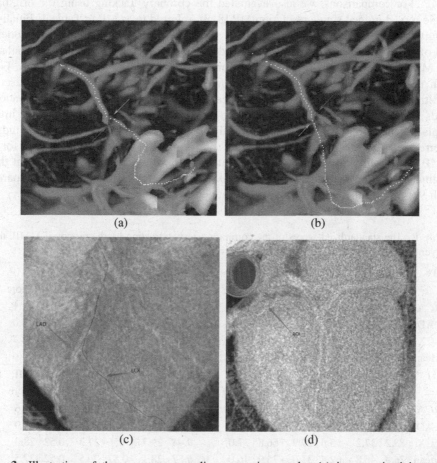

(a)   (b)

(c)   (d)

Fig. 3. Illustration of the coronary centerline extraction results: (a) is a maximal intensity projection (MIP) of the vesselness and the extracted centerline using the conventional method on the original vesselness images. The centerline goes into an undesired sub-branch due to the stenosis at a position of the main branch, which is pointed out by the red arrow. (b)is the MIP of the vesselness and the extracted centerline using the proposed method. The centerline is corrected and goes through the narrowed coronary artery thanks to the usage of the proposed filter and MMP method. (c) and (d) are the volume rendering results of a CTA image with extracted coronary centerlines. (Color figure online)

Figure 3 first provides an illustration of the coronary centerline extraction results. The CTA image has an indistinct segments of the coronary artery due to the stenosis. The conventional fast marching hence is prone to trace into the sub-branch which has no narrowed lumen, as the maximal intensity projection (MIP) image shows. By contrast, with the proposed filter, the indistinct vessel segment can be enhanced, helping the fast marching algorithm to pass the stenostic segment of the artery. Figure 3(b) provides the MIP of the vesselness and the extracted centerline result using the proposed filter and MMP method. Figure 3(c) and (d) visualize the volume rendering results of a CTA image with extracted coronary centerlines for demonstration.

Table 1 provides the results of the four measures and their scores by the proposed MMP. For comparisons, we also evaluated the coronary tracking using the original single model-guided single resolution MP [8, 9], referred to as MP in Table 1. Finally, to further investigate the robustness of the MMP, we deformed the coronary models and offset the detected ostia using random deformation and displacements, to simulate the MMP coronary tracking with less accurate registration and ostium detection. For each target centerline extraction, we simulated ten sets of deformations and offsets, resulting in eighty coronary extraction cases. Both the magnitudes of the deformation fields were set to less than the maximum errors we expected, for example the maximal displacement for offsetting the detected ostia was about 2 mm. The results of this study, referred to as SimuMMP, is presented in Table 1. Finally, the computation time for a MMP was about 1.6 min at the low resolution of $1 \times 1 \times 1$ mm and 3.4 min at the original resolution with the constraint mask from the previous result. This compares with 9.8 min by the conventional model-guided MP.

Table 1. The standardized scores of the coronary artery extraction by the proposed MMP, the conventional MP (MP), and the results of the simulated data by the MMP (SimuMMP).

OV	MMP		MP		SimuMMP		OF	MMP		MP		SimuMMP	
	%	Score	%	Score	%	Score		%	Score	%	Score	%	Score
RCA	**84.6**	48.4	73.3	38.7	87.6	49.2		**60.7**	42.6	57.3	38.4	60.0	41.1
LAD	**64.2**	33.0	39.2	20.3	67.8	34.9		**39.2**	26.9	24.2	14.1	34.6	24.0
LCX	**70.1**	41.5	45.6	25.2	63.0	37.3		**50.7**	35.7	46.2	34.0	51.8	38.7
Mean	**72.9**	41.0	52.7	28.0	72.7	40.5		**50.2**	35.1	42.6	28.8	48.8	34.6
OT	MMP		MP		SimuMMP		AI	MMP		MP		SimuMMP	
	%	Score	%	Score	%	Score		mm	Score	mm	Score	MM	Score
RCA	**88.8**	63.2	87.1	57.6	90.5	60.3		**0.54**	25.4	0.54	25.5	0.54	25.6
LAD	**67.3**	39.9	45.2	23.5	70.4	40.8		**0.51**	29.2	0.61	26.5	0.50	28.9
LCX	**73.2**	37.2	55.6	29.9	66.8	37.0		**0.48**	29.7	0.56	27.3	0.52	28.3
Mean	**76.4**	46.8	62.4	37.0	75.9	46.0		**0.51**	28.1	0.57	26.5	0.52	27.5

5   Conclusions

In this work, we have presented a new automatic method for extracting coronary centerlines, combining multi-model and multi-resolution within the MP framework, referred to as MMP. The multi-resolution is achieved using the new image filter which can generate low resolution coronary images while preserving the salient vessel features and enhancing the vesselness for fast and robust vessel tracking. MMP achieved 72.9 % overlap score and 0.51 mm AI accuracy, which are evidently better than 52.7 % and 0.57 mm by the conventional model-guided MP. In conclusion, the proposed MMP is efficient and effective in coronary centerline tracking and can be valuable in clinics for coronary disease analysis using cardiac CTA. For the future work, we will apply the method to more test cases from our hospital as well as the publically available data to validate the performance.

Acknowledgment. This work was partially supported by the Chinese NSFC research fund (81301283), the NSFC-RS fund (81511130090).

References

1. Schaap, M., Metz, C.T., van Walsum, T., van der Giessen, A.G., Weustink, A.C., Mollet, N. R., Dikici, E.: Standardized evaluation methodology and reference database for evaluating coronary artery centerline extraction algorithms. Med. Image Anal. **13**(5), 701–714 (2009)
2. Zhu, N., Chung, A.C.: Minimum average-cost path for real time 3D coronary artery segmentation of CT images. In: Fichtinger, G., Martel, A., Peters, T. (eds.) MICCAI 2011, Part III. LNCS, vol. 6893, pp. 436–444. Springer, Heidelberg (2011)
3. Deschamps, T., Cohen, L.D.: Minimal paths in 3D images and application to virtual endoscopy. In: Vernon, D. (ed.) ECCV 2000. LNCS, vol. 1843, pp. 543–557. Springer, Heidelberg (2000)
4. Wink, O., Frangi, A., Verdonck, B., Biergever, M., Niessen, W.: 3D MRA coronary axis determination using a minimum cost path approach. Magn. Reson. Med. **47**(6), 1169–1175 (2002)
5. Kaul, V., Yezzi, A., Tsai, Y.: Detecting curves with unknown endpoints and arbitrary topology using minimal paths. IEEE Trans. Pattern Anal. Mach. Intell. **34**(10), 1952–1965 (2012)
6. Zheng, Y., Tek, H., Funka-Lea, G.: Robust and accurate coronary artery centerline extraction in CTA by combining model-driven and data-driven approaches. In: Mori, K., Sakuma, I., Sato, Y., Barillot, C., Navab, N. (eds.) MICCAI 2013, Part III. LNCS, vol. 8151, pp. 74–81. Springer, Heidelberg (2013)
7. Zheng, Y., Tek, H., Funka-Lea, G., Zhou, S., Vega-Higuera, F., Comaniciu, D.: Efficient detection of native and bypass coronary ostia in cardiac CT volumes: anatomical vs. pathological structures. In: Fichtinger, G., Martel, A., Peters, T. (eds.) MICCAI 2011, Part III. LNCS, vol. 6893, pp. 403–410. Springer, Heidelberg (2011)
8. Liu, L., Shi, W., Rueckert, D., Hu, M., Ourselin, S., Zhuang, X.: Coronary centerline extraction based on ostium detection and model-guided directional minimal path. In: 2014 IEEE 11th International Symposium on Biomedical Imaging (ISBI), pp. 133–136. IEEE (2014)
9. Liu, L., Shi, W., Rueckert, D., Hu, M., Ourselin, S., Zhuang, X.: Model-guided directional minimal path for fully automatic extraction of coronary centerlines from cardiac CTA. In: Mori, K., Sakuma, I., Sato, Y., Barillot, C., Navab, N. (eds.) MICCAI 2013, Part I. LNCS, vol. 8149, pp. 542–549. Springer, Heidelberg (2013)
10. Kim, S.: An O(N) level set method for eikonal equations. SIAM J. Sci. Comput. **22**(6), 2178–2193 (2001)

11. Zhuang, X., Rhode, K., Razavi, R., Hawkes, D.J., Ourselin, S.: A registration-based propagation framework for automatic whole heart segmentation of cardiac MRI. IEEE Trans. Med. Imaging **29**(9), 1612–1625 (2010)

12. Frangi, A.F., Niessen, W.J., Hoogeveen, R.M., Van Walsum, T., Viergever, M.A.: Model-based quantitation of 3-D magnetic resonance angiographic images. IEEE Trans. Med. Imaging **18**(10), 946–956 (1999)

13. Tang, H., van Walsum, T., van Onkelen, R.S., Hameeteman, R., Klein, S., Schaap, M., van Vliet, L.J.: Semiautomatic carotid lumen segmentation for quantification of lumen geometry in multispectral MRI. Med. Image Anal. **16**(6), 1202–1215 (2012)

14. Cohen, L.D., Kimmel, R.: Global minimum for active contour models: a minimal path approach. Int. J. Comput. Vis. **24**(1), 57–78 (1997)

15. Metz, C., Schaap, M., van Walsum, T., van der Giessen, A., Weustink, A., Mollet, N., Niessen, W.: 3D segmentation in the clinic: a grand challenge II-coronary artery tracking. Insight J. **1**(5), 1–6 (2008)

16. Zhuang, X., Shen, J.: Multi-scale patch and multi-modality atlases for whole heart segmentation of MRI. Med. Image Anal. **31**, 77–87 (2016)

17. Zhuang, X., Bai, W., Song, J., Zhan, S., Qian, X., Shi, W., Rueckert, D.: Multiatlas whole heart segmentation of CT data using conditional entropy for atlas ranking and selection. Med. Phys. **42**(7), 3822–3833 (2015)

18. Yatziv, L., Bartesaghi, A., Sapiro, G.: O(N) implementation of the fast marching algorithm. J. Comput. Phys. **212**(2), 393–399 (2006)

Facial Behaviour Analysis in Parkinson's Disease

Riyadh Almutiry[1]([✉]), Samuel Couth[2], Ellen Poliakoff[2], Sonja Kotz[3],
Monty Silverdale[4], and Tim Cootes[1]

[1] Centre for Imaging Sciences, University of Manchester, Manchester M13 9PT, UK
r.almutiry@gmail.com
[2] Faculty of Life Sciences, University of Manchester, Manchester M13 9PT, UK
[3] School of Psychological Sciences, University of Manchester,
Manchester M13 9PT, UK
[4] Department of Neurology and Neurosurgery, Salford Royal Foundation Trust,
Greater Manchester, UK

Abstract. We describe a method for evaluating facial expressivity in
order to improve related clinical assessments of Parkinson's Disease (PD).
There is a controversial evidence in the literature that PD facial impairment can be detected on certain emotional expressions. This study aimed
to investigate the feasibility of discriminative and quantitive measures of
PD from the ability of a subject to express facial expressions. Video
clips of 8 subjects (4 healthy controls and 4 with patients with PD) were
recorded during daily sessions over several weeks. Observations covered
emotion variation over one week for control subjects and six weeks for
patients with PD. A statistical shape model was used to track facial
expressions and to measure the amount of expressivity exhibited by each
subject. The study suggests that measures of the amount of movement
during happiness, disgust and anger expressions are the most discriminative, with PD patients exhibiting less movement than controls. This work
demonstrates that it may be possible to measure day-to-day variations
in symptoms of PD automatically.

1 Introduction

Parkinson's disease (PD) is a neurodegenerative disease affecting around 10 million worldwide [31] and about 1 % of the population of people aged over 60 years
[18]. An important symptom is the loss of muscle control leading to movement
difficulties and effects on facial expressions.

Symptoms can vary significantly from one day to another. There are no quantitative measures of their severity, and so disease progression is usually evaluated
by observation and interview with a clinical expert. This usually happens infre-
quently, and the results are not reliable because of the day-to-day variation.
This makes it difficult to manage treatment - for instance to evaluate whether
the current drug regime is effective. An automatic method for measuring symptoms which could record them daily would enable much better management of
the disease. We explore whether it is possible to measure the severity of symptoms related to facial muscles based on tracking the facial expressions of people
with the disease.

© Springer International Publishing Switzerland 2016
G. Zheng et al. (Eds.): MIAR 2016, LNCS 9805, pp. 329–339, 2016.
DOI: 10.1007/978-3-319-43775-0_30

PD is associated with dopamine-deficiency due to the loss of dopaminergic neurons, brain cells responsible for producing the dopamine which plays a vital role in essential human daily functions such as movement, memory, cognition, behaviour and attention. The disease can be directly linked to the loss of motor-control neurons in substantia nigra. However it is still unclear whether this is because of the loss of nonmotor-control neurons in other parts of the brain or if it is just a side effect of the motor disorder [32].

Patients with PD can suffer from motor disorders such as tremors, rigidity, bradykinesia and postural instability. Other non-motor symptoms linked to PD are disorders in mode, cognition and emotional processing [4,28]. The Theory of Mind (ToM) [25] is a concept which many researchers use to evaluate non-motor disorder of PD patients such as emotion recognition. ToM illustrates the individual's ability to make inferences about their own mental state and that of others. Clearly awareness of such states can be advantageous in social communications. Whether or not PD can relate to low performance on ToM abilities is still heavily debated [21,34].

Currently there is no cure for PD [20]. Several treatments exist which aim to reduce the symptoms such as physiotherapy, which provides general muscle exercises, occupational therapy such as training to perform specific tasks and speech and language therapy to encounter speech and sallowness problems caused by PD [20].

There is no standard for diagnosing PD due to the lack of accurate measures [20,32]. Many PD patients seek a neurological examination even though it is difficult for neurologist to verify the existence of PD due to the similarity of symptoms with those of other neurological disorders [32]. The best examination of PD to date is done by studying the dopamine system and the metabolism through a specialised brain scan, which is an expensive process [32].

Currently many researchers are attempting to establish methods for assessing PD symptoms automatically using models which parameterise behavioural activities such as speech [5], emotional and non-emotional facial expressions [11] and emotional cognition processes [28,30]. Facial expressions, in terms of face anatomical structure, are produced by movements of the facial muscles [12]. Therefore, accurate automatic modelling of facial expressions raises the potential for capturing the adverse effects of PD on those muscles. Despite the vast literature on automatic modelling of facial expressions, it is still an active area of research as most of the state-of-the-art methods are still not robust or efficient enough for real-time applications [8].

The goal of this paper is to explore the potential of feasible discriminative and quantitive measures for PD through modelling several emotional facial expressions. We examine measures of facial movement in both healthy controls and patients with PD when making particular facial expressions. The study, though small, suggests that measures of the amount of movement during happiness, disgust and anger expressions are the most discriminative, with PD patients exhibiting less movement than healthy controls.

2 Previous Studies of Facial Movement in Parkinson's Disease

Prior to detecting PD impairment on any facial expression one has to model these expressions. Affect is regarded as expressed emotions or feelings [3]. The various movements of the human facial muscles convey emotional states of the observed subject [10]. This has led many studies to analyse the relationship between these movements and their corresponding affects using various scientific measures [10]. The number of emotional states that can be produced by facial muscle movements is vast. Thus, many attempts have been made to conceptualize these emotions [9,24]. Despite these efforts, researchers have not yet reached an agreement on what conceptualizes the idea of emotions [2]. In the context of facial behaviour analysis, the terms *affect* and *emotion* are not clearly distinguished and are interchangeably used in the literature [3,27].

Fontaine et al. [14] presented four dimensional model of emotions, resulted from a study of 24 universal English-based emotional terms, selected based on six components: appraisals of events, bodily sensations, action tendencies, subjective experiences, emotion regulation and motor expressions. For each term, 144 features were derived from participants' evaluations to emotional experience questions. A PCA analysis was then applied to the features. They found that four dimensions of the PCA results account for the majority (75 %) of the data variance. These dimensions describe measures for the degree of pleasantness, appraisal control, activation-arousal and unpredictability.

Automatic facial expression modelling can be classified to two categories: *geometrically-based* and appearance-based. Geometrically-based approaches rely on the geometrical properties of the face image, which are represented by a set of landmarks. One of the earliest attempts to quantify PD effects on a smile expression was conducted in 1988 by [16] using a geometrical approach [23]. They studied a group of 18 subjects (9 controls and 9 with PD) and recorded videos of subjects while viewing 11 video slides used as a stimuli of the expression. A manual filtering was applied to select the best animated smile produced in a still photograph. Each photograph was then scored based on 12 facial measures [23]. Depression scores were also evaluated using a questionnaire. Their findings suggested that smiling frequency was significantly higher in the control group.

Appearance-based approaches rely on image texture properties. A common morphological-based measure, which is widely used in automatic facial expression modelling, is to encode facial expressions using the Facial Action Coding System (FACS). FACS provides a general definition based on the movement of one or more facial muscles in terms of their contractions and relaxations to describe any facial expression. The FACS scheme has several drawbacks, which affect its adaptability. Firstly, FACS is error prone. The coding of action units (AUs) requires expert knowledge and skills [17]. An early version of FACS required approximately 100 hours of training. Furthermore the number of possible behaviour to encode by FACS can be very large. Alternatives guides for FACS have been proposed [13], which are more subjective- and time-oriented to a set of specific emotions.

An example of recent approach that adopted FACS scheme can be found in [33]. Their approach involves using geometrical-based and appearance-based features extracted by tracking 83 facial landmarks. The study involves a group of 15 subjects (8 controls and 7 with PD). The study suggests that people with PD showed less expressivity than healthy controls when experiencing disgust emotions.

The influence of PD on emotional facial expressions is still an active area of research [1,15,19,22,29]. Many researchers have claimed that impairments on certain facial expressions is often associated with PD. However this claim still not consistent [19,22,30]. Due to the high variability of the face and facial expressivity, automatic modelling and tracking of facial expressions is still challenging.

3   Method

3.1   Data Collection and Annotation

Eight subjects (4 healthy controls and 4 with PD) were involved in this study. The healthy controls group were aged between 67.3 and 69.7 years while PD group were aged between 56.3 and 72.1 years. All subjects were followed over several weeks. Once a day they sat before a computer and ran a program which prompted them to perform various facial expressions several times while a webcam recorded their face. They were encouraged to ensure that their face was in the middle of the recording area, but otherwise there were no constraints imposed. The recording was done in their own homes. The control subjects were recorded daily for one week while subjects with PD were followed for six weeks. Figure 1 shows a summary of data collection process.

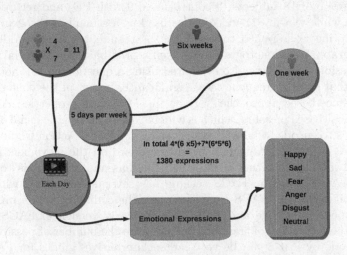

Fig. 1. Summary of data collection process

Each expression in every video clip was then reviewed and annotated with meta data indicating the beginning and the end of the expression development. All video frames containing expressions were then extracted for further processing to localise and track facial features.

3.2 Feature Extraction

Because of the unconstrained nature of the recording, facial feature detection and tracking on the data is challenging. To achieve accurate detection and tracking we adopted two facial feature tracking techniques: a generic Constrained Local Model (CLM) [6] and subject-specific Active Appearance Model (AAM), both were trained to localise 27 facial features. Subject-specific AAM models are used for extremely challenging conditions as they are easier to build and require fewer training examples than generic models.

A common approach for quantifying shape variations is to project the extracted landmarks to a statistical shape model (SSM) [7]. The SSM defines a linear model which define shape variations after filtering out all irrelevant shape information such as isotropic scaling, rotations and translations. Any shape then can be represented by

$$\mathbf{x} = \bar{\mathbf{x}} + \boldsymbol{\Phi}\mathbf{b} \tag{1}$$

Where $\mathbf{x}$ is the target shape, $\bar{\mathbf{x}}$ is the mean shape, $\boldsymbol{\Phi}$ is a set of eigenvectors which represents modes of variations and $\mathbf{b}$ is the shape parameter vector representing the weights on each mode.

Each extracted group of landmarks was converted to SSM representation, $\mathbf{b}$, by inverting (1). All computed shape parameters are then registered to in order to eliminate inter-subject shape variations by subtracting the identity shape of each subject as explained below.

Consider a set of subjects $\mathbf{S} \in \{s_1, ..., s_i, ..., s_p\}$ where $p =$ the number of subjects. And another set of expressions $\mathbf{E} = \{e_1, ...e_j, ...e_k\}$ where k is the index of different expressions in $\mathbf{E}$. $\forall s_i$ that has a set of vectors $\mathbf{B}_{ij} = \{\mathbf{b}_{ij1}, ..., \mathbf{b}_{ijm}, ..., \mathbf{b}_{ijn}\}$ where $\mathbf{b}_{ijm}$ is the shape model parameters for the ith subject, the jth expression for the mth sample.

We considered the mean of the shape parameter $\bar{\mathbf{b}}_{ir}$, where r is the index of the neutral expression, as the baseline for the shape variations of all expressions and $\forall \mathbf{b}_{ijm} \in \mathbf{B}_{ij}$ we compute the vector of residuals from the mean of the neutral shape per subject using (2).

$$\delta\mathbf{b}_{ijm} = \mathbf{b}_{ijm} - \bar{\mathbf{b}}_{ir} \tag{2}$$

3.3 Modelling Expresssion Variations

To model the expression variability we applied a Principal Component Analysis (PCA) on $\delta\mathbf{B}_j$ to identify the major modes of variations specific to each expression. Each can then be represented by a vector $\mathbf{c}$ which describes expression variations on a matrix of modes $\mathbf{Q}_j$ as shown in (3).

$$\mathbf{x}_{ijm} = \bar{\mathbf{x}} + \boldsymbol{\Phi}^T(\delta\bar{\mathbf{b}}_j + \mathbf{Q}_j^T\mathbf{c}_{ijm}) \tag{3}$$

Table 1. Effect of varying several modes between −4 to +4 standard deviations for happy, disgust and anger facial expressions.

Expressions	Mode No.	-4 to +4 Std.
happy	1	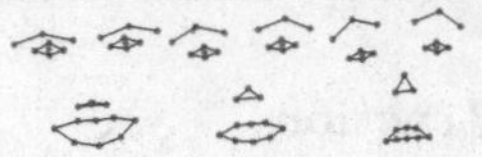
Disgust	3	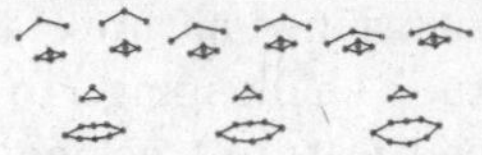
Anger	2	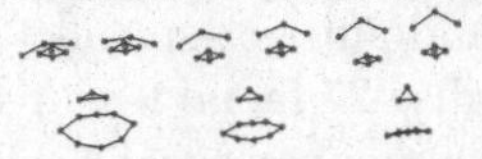
Anger	4	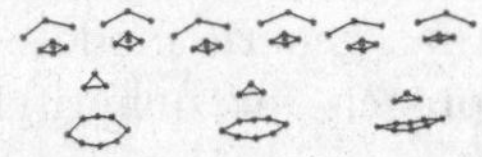

A sample of the resulting modes can be seen in Table 1 which shows the effects of varying each mode within ±4 standard deviations about the neutral point.

The table above shows how the facial expression model varies using a specific set of modes. Note that high facial expressivity can be in positive or negative direction for different modes. An example can be seen in mode 1 and 3 for expressions of happy and disgust respectively.

4   Observation and Evaluation

We examined to what extent measures of facial expressivity differ between the PD group and the controls. We computed the vector parameter $\mathbf{c}$ as in (4) for every frame in a sequence and plot every element of $\mathbf{c}$ against time. An example can be seen in Fig. 2. As every element of $\mathbf{c}$ describes the degree of facial expressivity using specific mode in $\mathbf{Q}$ as shown in Table 1, our aim is to evaluate how PD and controls scores on these modes in order to highlight PD-sensitive modes. An example can be seen in Fig. 2, which shows the variation of the first element of the vector $\mathbf{c}$ that describes the variation of the first mode in $\mathbf{Q}$. The figure shows parameter values per frame for PD (red) and controls (green) when performing a happy expression.

We compared all control data, (only available for one week), to the six weeks of data gathered from subjects with PD. We found that the PD group showed significantly less facial expressivity (a smaller range of parameter variation) on happy and disgust expressions specifically on mode 1 and 3 respectively.

$$\mathbf{c}_{ijm} = \mathbf{Q}_j^T (\delta\mathbf{b}_{ijm} - \delta\bar{\mathbf{b}}_j) \tag{4}$$

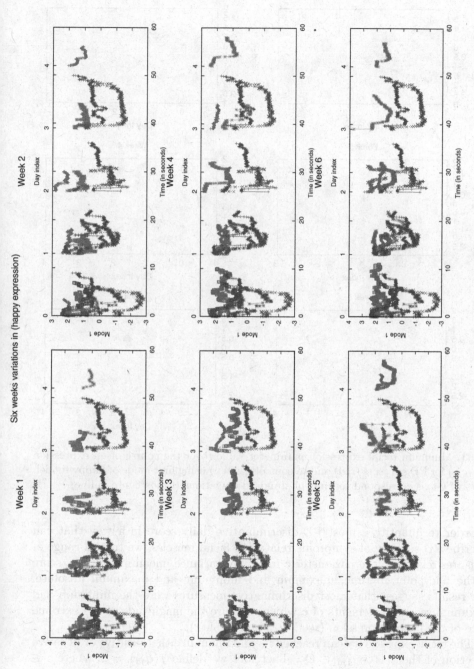

Fig. 2. Facial expression variation of PD subjects (red) compared to controls subjects (green) using first mode of happy model. Units of y-axis correspond to units of standard deviations (Color figure online).

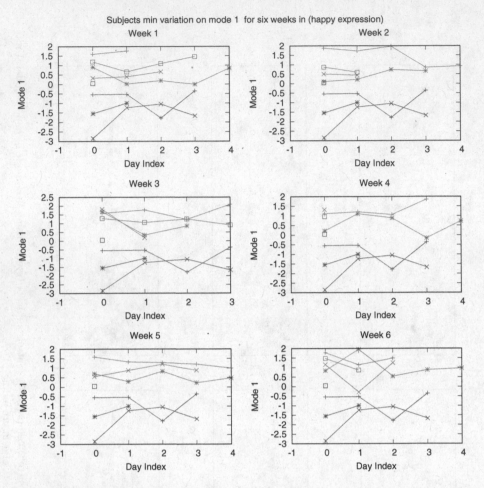

Fig. 3. Minimum facial expression parameter value (over the course of an expression $min_t c_{1t}$) for PD subjects (red) and to controls (green) using first mode of happy model. Units of y-axis correspond to units of standard deviations (Color figure online).

In order to quantify a most PD-discriminative daily score in a way that can describe PD severity of symptoms related to facial muscles, we tried a range of measures related to the parameter c including variance, mean magnitude, score at the mid-point in time, maximum and minimum, and maximum absolute. Our results suggest that most discriminative measures were the minimum and maximum scores of elements of c which measure the magnitude of the extreme state of the facial expression (see Fig. 3 and Table 1).

The facial expressivity can reached its maximum in either positive or negative direction of the vector $q_{jd} \in Q_j$. Therefore we define $f(q_{jd}) = z$, where $z \in \{-1, 1\}$ which indicate the direction sign to the maximum expressivity state of the mode q_{jd}. Daily score can then be defined as follows

$$d(\mathbf{c}_{ijm}) = \begin{cases} \min_m \ \mathbf{c}_{ijm,k}, & \text{if } f(\mathbf{q}_{jd}) = -1 \\ \max_m \ \mathbf{c}_{ijm,k}, & \text{if } f(\mathbf{q}_{jd}) = 1 \end{cases} \tag{5}$$

where k is the kth element of $\mathbf{c}_{ijm}$.

5 Discussion and Future Work

We have described analysis of data from a pilot experiment which suggests that (a) facial expressions exhibited by people with Parkinson's Disease involve less movement than those from healthy controls, and (b) that it is possible to track such expressions automatically.

The study suggests that happy, disgust and anger are the expressions most effected by the disease, and that by recording the range of a few model parameters associated with these expressions it may be possible to construct a measure related to the severity of the symptoms on that day.

Clearly this study is limited by the small sample size. We hope to gather a larger set in order to verify the approach.

References

1. Alonso-Recio, L., Serrano, J.M., Martín, P.: Selective attention and facial expression recognition in patients with Parkinson's disease. Arch. Clin. Neuropsychol.: Official J. Nat. Acad. Neuropsychologists **29**(4), 374–84 (2014). http://www.ncbi. nlm.nih.gov/pubmed/24760956
2. Baltrusaitis, T.: Automatic facial expression analysis. Technical report UCAM-CL-TR-861. University of Cambridge, Computer Laboratory, October 2014. http:// www.cl.cam.ac.uk/techreports/UCAM-CL-TR-861.pdf
3. Carlson, N.R., Heth, D., Miller, H., Donahoe, J., Martin, G.N.: Psychology: The Science of Behavior. Pearson, London (2009)
4. Chennamma, H., Yuan, X.: A survey on eye-gaze tracking techniques. arXiv preprint arXiv:1312.6410 4, 388–393 (2013)
5. Constantinescu, G., Theodoros, D., Russell, T., Ward, E., Wilson, S., Wootton, R.: Assessing disordered speech and voice in Parkinson's disease: a telerehabilitation application. Int. J. Lang. Commun. Disord./Roy. Coll. Speech Lang. Therapists **45**(6), 630–44 (2010). http://www.ncbi.nlm.nih.gov/pubmed/20102257
6. Cootes, T.F., Ionita, M.C., Lindner, C., Sauer, P.: Robust and accurate shape model fitting using random forest regression voting. In: Fitzgibbon, A., Lazebnik, S., Perona, P., Sato, Y., Schmid, C. (eds.) ECCV 2012, Part VII. LNCS, vol. 7578, pp. 278–291. Springer, Heidelberg (2012). http://link.springer.com/chapter/10.1007/978-3-642-33786-4_21
7. Cootes, T., Taylor, C., Cooper, D., Graham, J.: Active shape models-their training and application. Comput. Vis. Image Underst. **61**, 38–59 (1995). http://www. sciencedirect.com/science/article/pii/S1077314285710041
8. Danelakis, A., Theoharis, T., Pratikakis, I.: A survey on facial expression recognition in 3D video sequences. Multimedia Tools Appl. **74**(15), 5577–5615 (2015)
9. Ekman, P.: Basic emotions (1999). http://onlinelibrary.wiley.com//10.1002/0470013494.ch3/summary

10. Ekman, P., Friesen, W.V., Ellsworth, P.: Emotion in the Human Face, 2nd edn. Cambridge University Press, Cambridge (1982)

11. Ekman, P., Friesen, W.V.: The Facial Action Coding System. Consulting Psychologists Press, Stanford University, Palo Alto (1982)

12. Fehrenbach, M.J., Herring, S.W.: Illustrated Anatomy of the Head and Neck. Elsevier Health Sciences, London (2013)

13. Flores, V.C.: ARTNATOMY (anatomical basis of facial expression interactive learning tool). In: ACM SIGGRAPH 2006 Educators Program on - SIGGRAPH 2006, p. 22 (2006). http://www.scopus.com/inward/record.url?eid=2-s2.0-34548268121&partnerID=tZOtx3y1

14. Fontaine, J.R.J., Scherer, K.R., Roesch, E.B., Ellsworth, P.C.: The world of emotions is not two-dimensional. Psychol. Sci. 18(12), 1050–1057 (2007)

15. Kan, Y., Kawamura, M., Hasegawa, Y., Mochizuki, S., Nakamura, K.: Recognition of emotion from facial, prosodic and written verbal stimuli in Parkinson's disease. Cortex J. Devoted Study Nerv. Syst. Behav. 38(4), 623–630 (2002)

16. Katsikitis, M., Pilowsky, I.: A study of facial expression in Parkinson's disease using a novel microcomputer-based method. J. Neurol. Neurosurg. Psychiatry 51(3), 362–366 (1988). http://jnnp.bmj.com/cgi//10.1136/jnnp.51.3.362

17. Kring, A., Sloan, D.: The facial expression coding system (FACES): a users guide. Unpublished manuscript (1991). http://ist-socrates.berkeley.edu/~akring/FACESmanual.pdf

18. de Lau, L.M.L., Breteler, M.M.B.: Epidemiology of Parkinson's disease. Lancet Neurol. 5(6), 525–535 (2006). http://www.sciencedirect.com/science/article/pii/S1474442206704719

19. Marsili, L., Agostino, R., Bologna, M., Belvisi, D., Palma, A., Fabbrini, G., Berardelli, A.: Bradykinesia of posed smiling and voluntary movement of the lower face in Parkinson's disease. Parkinsonism Relat. Disord. 20(4), 370–375 (2014)

20. NHS: Parkinson's disease - Treatment (2014). http://www.nhs.uk/Conditions/Parkinsons-disease/Pages/Treatment.aspx

21. Parrish, A., Brosnan, S.: Primate cognition. In: Encyclopedia of Human Behavior, pp. 174–180. Elsevier (2012). http://www.sciencedirect.com/science/article/pii/B9780123750006002895

22. Pell, M.D., Leonard, C.L.: Facial expression decoding in early Parkinson's disease. Brain Res. Cogn. Brain Res. 23(2–3), 327–340 (2005)

23. Pilowsky, I., Thornton, M., Stokes, B.: A microcomputer based approach to the quantification of facial expressions. Australas. Phys. Eng. Sci. Med./Support. Australas. Coll. Phys. Scientists Med. Australas. Assoc. Phys. Sci. Med. 8(2), 70 (1985)

24. Plutchik, R.: The nature of emotions: human emotions have deep evolutionary roots. Am. Sci. 89(4), 344–350 (2001)

25. Premack, D., Woodruff, G.: Does the chimpanzee have a theory of mind? Behav. Brain Sci. 4, 515–526 (1978)

26. Smith, M., Smith, M., Ellgring, H.: Spontaneous and posed facial expression in Parkinson's disease. J. Int. Neuropsychol. Soc. 2, 383–391 (1996)

27. de Spinoza, B.: Ethics. Classics of World Literature Series, Wordsworth Editions (2001). https://books.google.co.uk/books?id=FJrOf7k44NMC

28. Sprengelmeyer, R., Young, A.W., Mahn, K., Schroeder, U., Woitalla, D., Büttner, T., Kuhn, W., Przuntek, H.: Facial expression recognition in people with medicated and unmedicated Parkinson's disease. Neuropsychologia 41(8), 1047–1057 (2003)

29. Sprengelmeyer, R., Young, A.W., Pundt, I., Sprengelmeyer, A., Calder, A.J., Berrios, G., Winkel, R., Vollmöeller, W., Kuhn, W., Sartory, G., Przuntek, H.: Disgust implicated in obsessive-compulsive disorder. Proc. Biol. Sci./Roy. Soc. **264**(1389), 1767–1773 (1997)
30. Suzuki, A., Hoshino, T., Shigemasu, K., Kawamura, M.: Disgust-specific impairment of facial expression recognition in Parkinson's disease. Brain **129**(3), 707–717 (2006)
31. The Parkinson's Disease Foundation: Statistics on Parkinson's (2015). http://www.pdf.org/en/parkinson_statistics
32. The Parkinson's Disease Foundation: Diagnosis (2016). http://www.pdf.org/en/diagnosis
33. Wu, P., Gonzalez, I., Patsis, G., Jiang, D., Sahli, H., Kerckhofs, E., Vandekerckhove, M.: Objectifying facial expressivity assessment of parkinson's patients: preliminary study. Comput. Math. Methods Med. **2014**, Article ID 427826 (2014)
34. Yu, R.L., Wu, R.M.: Social brain dysfunctions in patients with Parkinson's disease: a review of theory of mind studies. Transl. Neurodegeneration **2**(1), 2–7 (2013). http://www.pubmedcentral.nih.gov/articlerender.fcgi?artid=3621839&tool=pmcentrez&rendertype=abstract

Medical Image Computing

Weighted Robust PCA for Statistical Shape Modeling

Jingting Ma[1,2], Feng Lin[1], Jonas Honsdorf[2], Katharina Lentzen[2],
Stefan Wesarg[3], and Marius Erdt[2(✉)]

[1] School of Computer Science and Engineering, Nanyang Technological University,
50 Nanyang Avenue, 639798 Singapore, Singapore
[2] Fraunhofer IDM@NTU Nanyang Technological University, 50 Nanyang Avenue,
639798 Singapore, Singapore
marius.erdt@fraunhofer.sg
[3] Visual Healthcare Technologies, Fraunhofer IGD, Darmstadt, Germany

Abstract. Statistical shape models (SSMs) play an important role
in medical image analysis. A sufficiently large number of high quality datasets is needed in order to create a SSM containing all possible shape variations. However, the available datasets may contain corrupted or missing data due to the fact that clinical images are often
captured incompletely or contain artifacts. In this work, we propose a
weighted Robust Principal Component Analysis (WRPCA) method to
create SSMs from incomplete or corrupted datasets. In particular, we
introduce a weighting scheme into the conventional Robust Principal
Component Analysis (RPCA) algorithm in order to discriminate unus-
able data from meaningful ones in the decomposition of the training data
matrix more accurately. For evaluation, the proposed WRPCA is compared with conventional RPCA on both corrupted (63 CT datasets of
the liver) and incomplete datasets (15 MRI datasets of the human foot).
The results show a significant improvement in terms of reconstruction
accuracy on both datasets.

Keywords: Statistical shape models · Corrupted data · Missing data ·
Weighted robust principal component analysis

1 Introduction

Statistical shape models (SSMs) are frequently used in medical image analysis
tasks (e.g. segmentation). A good quality SSM aims to represent the variability of
a specific object over a training population. To create such a model, a sufficiently
large subset of training data needs to be collected. However, often the number
of datasets that can be used for creating SSMs is limited, because often clinical
images contain artifacts or do not cover the anatomical structures of interest
completely. Discarding these datasets results in a great loss of useful statistics
inherent in the incomplete shapes. The goal of this work is to create a SSM of
good quality based on training datasets that contain corrupted and/or missing
data.

© Springer International Publishing Switzerland 2016
G. Zheng et al. (Eds.): MIAR 2016, LNCS 9805, pp. 343–353, 2016.
DOI: 10.1007/978-3-319-43775-0_31

There are already a number of approaches addressing the handling of missing data in Principal Component Analysis [1–3]. In the work of Luthi et al. [4], the training surfaces are divided into several patches and each patch is assigned a probability of being an outlier via PCO_{ut} using the approach of Filzmoser et al. [5]. Only the non-outlier patches remain for the creation of the SSM. However, a part of the corrupted data may cause a complete patch to be identified as an outlier leading to a loss of correct information. Instead of discarding all the outliers, imputation methods [1,6] aim at replacing the missing data with data estimated from the remaining valid population at that position. In the work of Ma et al. [7], each landmark is assigned a probability of being an outlier. Each landmark is replaced by a weighted overall mean afterwards. Landmarks with higher probability have more influence on the weighted overall mean. Such imputation methods provide reasonable results. However, they assume the outliers to have a normal distribution. Robust Principal Component Analysis (RPCA) [8] handles outliers and missing data by decomposing the training data matrix into a low-rank subspace containing the correct data and a high-rank subspace containing the corrupted observations by convex optimization [9–11]. In the work of Gutierrez [12], RPCA is applied to 43 corrupted CT scans to create a SSM and outperforms other approaches. However, often some correct high frequency information may be considered an outlier and therefore may get lost in RPCA in case this information is not sufficiently present in other datasets of the training set. As a result, the SSM built from the constructed low-rank subspace will lose some modes of variation.

To address these drawbacks of RPCA, we propose a weighted Robust Principal Component Analysis (WRPCA) method where a probability of being an outlier is assigned to each landmark. The weighting is then used to favor the landmarks with high probability in the construction of the low-rank subspace. Landmarks of missing parts can be set to zero. They will therefore be considered outliers. Using this WRPCA, more relevant information of the training data can be preserved and therefore, SSMs of higher accuracy can be built.

2   Method

In this section, we will recall the idea of the RPCA approach and formulate our new WRPCA to create shape models. First, a point-to-point groupwise correspondence method [13] is applied to a set of training shapes $S^{(n_S)} \in \{x_1, ..., x_{n_S}\}$ in order to generate n_p corresponding landmarks among all the instances. A shape is represented as a column vector $x_i = (x^{(1)}, y^{(1)}, z^{(1)}, ..., x^{(n_p)}, y^{(n_p)}, z^{(n_p)})^T$ in Point Distribution Model (PDM), where $(x^{(j)}, y^{(j)}, z^{(j)})$ are the Cartesian coordinates of the jth landmark. Next, all shape vectors are stacked into a training observation matrix $M = [m_1, ..., m_{n_S}]$, with m_j denoting the jth training shape vector and m_{ij} denoting the ith landmark of the jth training shape.

RPCA decomposes the training observation matrix M into a low-rank matrix L containing correct data and a sparse matrix S corresponding to the entries of corrupted data, where L and S are unknown. The RPCA problem can be solved via convex optimization and be formulated as

$$\begin{aligned}
\text{minimize} \quad & \|L\|_* + \lambda \|S\|_1 \\
\text{subject to} \quad & L + S = M.
\end{aligned} \tag{1}$$

A positive factor λ is used to balance the nuclear norm of L and l^1-norm of S. Often the value of $\lambda = 1/\sqrt{n}$, where n is the largest dimension of matrix M inspired in [8]. The output low-rank matrix L is assumed to be outlier-free and used to compute the variation modes of the shape via Principal Component Analysis (PCA) [14].

2.1 WRPCA for Statistical Shape Modeling

In conventional RPCA, the low-rank matrix L is recovered automatically which leads to a loss of information that are non-outlier but not statistically significant in the datasets. Our assumption is that prior knowledge can be obtained from the original clinical images to determine the possibility of being an outlier for each landmark. In a simple case, the probability of being an outlier for the parts that are not visible in the image is naturally 100 %. However, our formulation allows all probabilities between 0 and 100 %, e.g. to describe areas with noisy or fuzzy boundaries. In order to account for these different probabilities and therefore to raise the accuracy of the low-rank matrix L, we propose a WRPCA method by introducing a weighting scheme in the solution of RPCA. Let $W = [w_1, ..., w_{n_S}]$ be the weighting matrix with the same dimensions as M; each column vector w_j is associated with the jth training shape and matrix element w_{ij} denotes the weighting of the ith landmark on the jth shape, where w_{ij} is in the interval of $[0, 1]$. Figure 1 shows the improvement of WRPCA in the construction of low-rank subspace by preserving landmarks with high probability.

We now describe how Eq. 1 can be solved and then describe how the weighting matrix W can be incorporated. We apply the inexact augmented Lagrange multiplier (IALM) [15] to solve Eq. 1, leading to the Lagrange function:

$$\mathcal{L}(L, S, Y, \mu) = \|L\|_* + \lambda \|S\|_1 + \langle Y, M - L - S \rangle + \frac{\mu}{2} \|M - L - S\|_F^2, \tag{2}$$

where M is the training observation matrix, Y is the Lagrange multiplier, μ is a positive scalar that penalizes the violation of the linear constraint, the notation $\langle \cdot, \cdot \rangle$ denotes the standard trace inner product between two matrices of the same size and $\|\cdot\|_F$ is the induced Frobenius norm of a matrix. An iteration strategy is adopted to minimize the Lagrange function in Eq. 2; given a sequence $\{(L_k, S_k, Y_k, \mu_k)\}$ of the kth iteration, the Lagrange function is solved by the following subproblems to get the $(k + 1)^{th}$ iteration:

$$L_{k+1} = \underset{L}{\operatorname{argmin}} \, \mathcal{L}(L, S_k, Y_k, \mu_k) \tag{3a}$$

$$S_{k+1} = \underset{S}{\operatorname{argmin}} \, \mathcal{L}(L_{k+1}, S, Y_k, \mu_k). \tag{3b}$$

L_{k+1} in Eq. 3a can be efficiently solved via a singular value shrinkage operator $\mathcal{D}_\tau[X]$ proposed in [16], which limits the number of retained singular values in

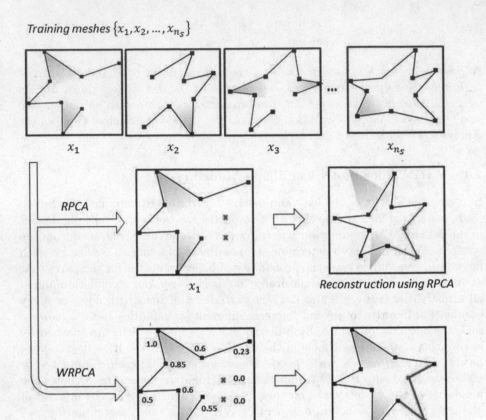

Training meshes $\{x_1, x_2, ..., x_{n_s}\}$

Fig. 1. Difference between reconstructions using WRPCA and RPCA. Note that the shading indicates the areas of mesh that are approximately ground truth and the red bits are the reconstruction of missing parts. (Color figure online)

the matrix X with τ being a positive thresholding parameter. Let us consider the singular value decomposition of a matrix X with rank r as $X = U\Sigma V^T$, of which $\Sigma = diag(\sigma_1, ..., \sigma_r)$ is a rectangle diagonal matrix containing positive singular values $\{\sigma_i\}$. This singular value shrinkage operator is then defined as:

$$\mathcal{D}_\tau[X] = U\mathcal{S}_\tau[\Sigma]V^T, \tag{4}$$

where $\mathcal{S}_\tau[X]$ is a soft-thresholding operator inspired by [15]:

$$\mathcal{S}_\tau[X] = \max(X - \tau, 0) + \min(X + \tau, 0) = \begin{cases} X - \tau, & \text{if } X > \tau, \\ X + \tau, & \text{if } X < -\tau, \\ 0, & \text{otherwise.} \end{cases} \tag{5}$$

Thus, L_{k+1} is estimated by computing:

$$L_{k+1} = \mathcal{D}_{\mu_k^{-1}}[M - S_k + \mu_k^{-1}Y_k]. \tag{6}$$

Now, the weighting matrix W is introduced to turn the RPCA into a WRPCA formulation. S_{k+1} in Eq. 3b is now computed as:

$$S_{k+1} = \mathcal{S}_{\lambda\mu_k^{-1}}[(1 - W) \circ (M - L_{k+1} + \mu_k^{-1}Y_k)], \tag{7}$$

where $\circ$ is the Hadamard product. The purpose of introducing the weighting matrix W is to influence the likelihood of being identified as an outlier for each landmark. Therefore, each entry S_{k+1}^{ij} of S_{k+1} in Eq. 7 is computed as:

$$S_{k+1}^{ij} = \max((1 - w_{ij}) \cdot x'_{ij} - \lambda\mu_k^{-1}, 0) + \min((1 - w_{ij}) \cdot x'_{ij} + \lambda\mu_k^{-1}, 0), \tag{8}$$

where x'_{ij} is the matrix element in $X' = M - L_{k+1} + \mu_k^{-1}Y_k$. That is if a weighting value w_{ij} of the landmark x_{ij} is closer to 1, $(1 - w_{ij})$ is closer to 0, i.e. the corresponding element in the sparse matrix S_{k+1}^{ij} is more likely to be set to 0. A higher weighting value decreases the possibility to be identified as an outlier. Conversely, smaller weighting leads to a larger result of S_{k+1}^{ij}, indicating that the landmark x_{ij} is more likely to be an outlier. After separating the outliers and non-outliers in the kth iteration, the multiplier Y_k is updated by:

$$Y_{k+1} = Y_k + \mu_k(M - L_{k+1} - S_{k+1}). \tag{9}$$

By updating the sequence $\{(L_k, S_k, Y_k, \mu_k)\}$ with $\{(L_{k+1}, S_{k+1}, Y_{k+1}, \mu_{k+1})\}$, the process is repeated until convergence is reached. Subsequently, in order to build the SSM, PCA is applied to the output low-rank matrix L to capture the significant modes of variance of the input shapes.

3   Evaluation

The proposed WRPCA method is evaluated by two experiments. One uses complete training shapes whereas parts of the shapes are considered unreliable due to fuzzy boundaries, and the other experiment uses incomplete shapes where data is missing because the object of interest is not fully contained in the image. Measures of *Specificity S*, *Generalization ability G* [17] and *Reconstruction Error RE* are used for evaluation. *Specificity* and *Generalization* evaluate the quality of a SSM and are defined as

$$S = \frac{1}{M}\sum_{A=1}^{M}\min_i(\Psi(y_A, x_i)) \quad \text{and} \quad G = \frac{1}{n_S}\sum_{i=1}^{n_S}\min_A(\Psi(y_A, x_i)). \tag{10}$$

$Y = \{y_A : A = 1, ...M\}$ is a set of shapes sampled from the model's probability density function (pdf), where 1000 samples each are randomly generated in the tests. $X = \{x_i : i = 1, ...n_S\}$ is the set of ground truth training shapes. $\Psi(y_A, x_i)$ denotes the Euclidean distance between the shape y_A and x_i.

Furthermore, the reconstruction error is a measure to check whether the training datasets can be adequately reconstructed by the built model. The reconstruction error is calculated by measuring the similarity of a training shape with its reconstruction from the model's pdf.

Ground truth data $X = \{x_i : i = 1, ...n_S\}$ is used and projected back on to the built model by $N^T(x_i - \bar{x}) \doteq b_i$, where the covariance matrix N determines the mapping between physical shapes $\{x_i\}$ and parameter vectors $\{b_i\}$ in shape space. Afterwards, the reconstruction $\{\tilde{x}_i\}$ is computed by $\bar{x} + Nb_i \doteq \tilde{x}_i$. Hence the reconstruction error of the ith ground truth shape is defined as:

$$ME_i = \frac{1}{n_p} \sum_{j=1}^{n_p} \|x_{ij} - \tilde{x}_{ij}\|_2 . \tag{11}$$

Here the mean squared Euclidean distance $\|\cdot\|_2$ among all n_p corresponding landmarks is calculated. A smaller reconstruction error indicates higher quality of representations and therefore indicates higher quality of the built model.

3.1 Evaluation on Corrupted Shapes

To evaluate WRPCA with corrupted data, 63 clinical CT scans are used. 17 datasets were taken from the MICCAI07 liver challenge [18], 19 datasets were taken from the public 3D-IRCAD data base (www.ircad.fr), and 27 non public datasets were used. First, an existing automatic liver segmentation [19] is chosen to create 63 initial liver shapes. Depending on the algorithm, the shapes contain erroneous points to a lower or higher degree. The boundary assessment method proposed in [7] is used to compute a probability for each landmark to be an outlier based on the boundary fuzzyness. The probabilities are used to fill the weighting matrix. We create statistical shape models SSM_{RPCA} and SSM_{WRPCA} with the conventional RPCA and the new WRPCA, respectively. Figure 2 shows the generalization ability and specificity results for the built models for the first 10 modes.

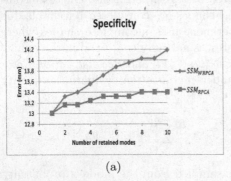
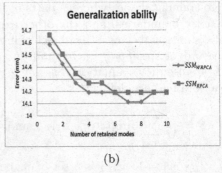

(a)   (b)

Fig. 2. (a) Shows the specificity errors for the built models of the liver. Smaller values indicate that the model is more specific; (b) shows the generalization ability of the built models of the liver. Smaller values indicate that the model is more general.

Furthermore, Fig. 3 shows the amount of variance captured by the single modes for each model. The SSM_{WRPCA} model can capture around 2 times more variation than SSM_{RPCA}. Because the variance covered by the modes of SSM_{RPCA} is so small, the specificity of SSM_{RPCA} is better than SSM_{WRPCA}. This is because the samples generated from SSM_{RPCA} are distributed in a small range around the mean, i.e. each sample is more likely to find a similar ground truth shape. On the other hand, $WRPCA$ preserves larger variance and this explains why SSM_{WRPCA} has a larger specificity error. In terms of generalization, SSM_{WRPCA} shows the smaller error of all models.

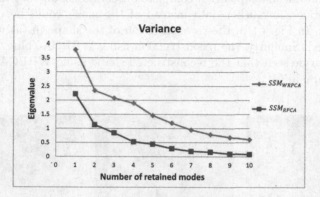

Fig. 3. The eigenvalues of each mode for the built modes, i.e. the retained variance of the built models.

In order to evaluate the ability of the models to reconstruct the original non corrupted shapes, the ground truth shapes for all livers are taken into account. These ground truth shapes are reprojected by the models. The mean reconstruction error is calculated by:

$$ME = \frac{1}{n_S} \sum_{i=1}^{n_S} ME_i. \tag{12}$$

Table 1 shows the average reconstruction errors of the 63 ground truth CT livers for the built models. SSM_{WRPCA} shows the smaller and SSM_{RPCA} the larger average reconstruction error. Since WRPCA uses weights to denote the probability of outliers, it is dependent on the quality of the probabilities. SSM_{WRPCA} performs better than SSM_{RPCA} in this test which indicates that the probability assignment used [7] is sufficient.

Table 1. The average reconstruction error of the 63 liver ground truth data for the built models with the standard deviation. Lower value indicates better performance.

Average reconstruction errors for built models (mm)	
SSM_{WRPCA}	SSM_{RPCA}
5.19 ± 2.08	6.49 ± 2.33

3.2   Evaluation on Incomplete Shapes

To test the performance of WRPCA with incomplete shapes, we take 15 non public labeled human foot MRI scans. In 10 of the 15 scans, one or multiple parts of the foot are missing. For the existing ground truth data, the weighting is set to 1; otherwise, for the missing data, the weighting is set to 0. In Fig. 4-(a) we show an incomplete ground truth human foot shape (green) with some parts missing (yellow). For the convenience of the visual appearance when constructing the observation matrix M, we fill the missing parts with the corresponding data from the overall mean shape of all complete observations, and set the weighting to 0. In practices, any other data instead of the mean could be used for the missing parts. In Fig. 4-(b), the reconstruction of the shape in (a) using RPCA is shown in red. Similarly, the reconstruction using WRPCA (blue) is shown In Fig. 4-c. It can be seen that the reconstructed shape using WRPCA is closer to the green shape in (a).

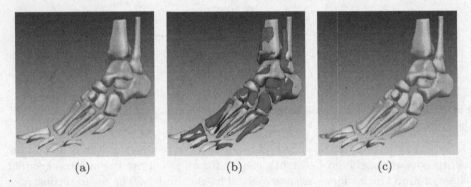

(a)   (b)   (c)

Fig. 4. (a) shows an incomplete human foot shape, where the green parts are the existing ground truth data and the yellow parts represent missing data (for visual convenience shown as the mean of all complete datasets); the red shape in (b) represents its reconstruction using RPCA; the blue shape in (c) represents its reconstruction using WRPCA. (Color figure online)

Furthermore, we create SSM_{RPCA} and SSM_{WRPCA} using standard RPCA and WRPCA, respectively. Figure 5 shows the generalization ability and specificity for the models SSM_{RPCA} and SSM_{WRPCA} and Fig. 6 shows the reconstruction errors of each data set from pdf of SSM_{RPCA} and SSM_{WRPCA}. Note that only the existing ground truth data is considered in the computation of specificity, generalization ability and the reconstruction error. This is because there is no ground truth for the non visible areas. Therefore, $\Psi(y_A, x_i)$ in Eq. 10 and the reconstruction error in Eq. 11 are all performed on the existing ground truth data, of which the weighting is set to 1.

In Fig. 5, SSM_{WRPCA} shows a smaller generalization error but a larger specificity error compared with the standard RPCA. SSM_{WRPCA} contains 12 variation modes but SSM_{RPCA} only captures 3 variation modes on the same training

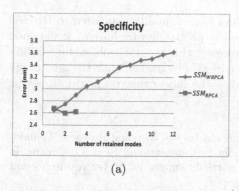
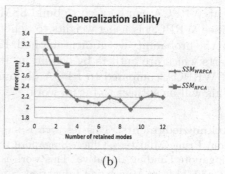

(a) (b)

Fig. 5. (a) Shows the specificity errors for the built models of human foot. Smaller values indicate the model is more specific; (b) shows the generalization ability results for the built models of human foot. Smaller values indicate the model is more general.

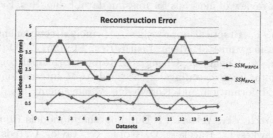

Fig. 6. Reconstruction error of human foot for the built models. Lower values indicate better performance.

data. Thus, SSM_{WRPCA} has more ability to cover significant shape variations and this explains for the larger specificity error as discussed above. As Fig. 6 shows, SSM_{WRPCA} has a significant smaller mean reconstruction error compared to SSM_{RPCA}.

To conclude the results, SSM_{WRPCA} performs better than SSM_{RPCA} in terms of generalization. Moreover, WRPCA captures more variation which leads to significantly smaller reconstruction errors. This can also be seen visually in Fig. 4, where the reconstruction using WRPCA almost provides a perfect overlap with the ground truth data in comparison to the result using RPCA. The specificity errors are higher for SSM_{WRPCA} than for SSM_{RPCA}. This can be explained with the smaller sample space of SSM_{RPCA} due to the lower variance captured.

4   Discussion

In this work, we proposed a new method weighted Robust PCA (WRPCA) as an extension of Robust PCA (RPCA) to handle both corrupted and missing data in medical images for statistical shape modeling. Evaluation results demonstrate that WRPCA can be used to build SSMs of higher quality compared to RPCA. Since WRPCA is using weights to denote the probability of outliers, it depends on the probability assignment method. However, this is not a problem for missing parts which are outliers by definition. It can also be argued that the advantage of WRPCA compared to RPCA diminishes the larger the training data set is. This will be subject to future work.

Acknowledgments. This research is supported by the National Research Foundation, Prime Minister's Office, Singapore under its International Research Centres in Singapore Funding Initiative. This work is partially supported by the research grant RG139/14 from Ministry of Education, Singapore.

References

1. Pigott, T.D.: A review of methods for missing data. Educ. Res. Eval. **7**(4), 353–383 (2001)
2. Ilin, A., Raiko, T.: Practical approaches to principal component analysis in the presence of missing values. J. Mach. Learn. Res. **11**, 1957–2000 (2010)
3. Shang, F., Liu, Y., Cheng, J., Cheng, H.: Robust principal component analysis with missing data. In: Proceedings of the 23rd ACM International Conference on Conference on Information and Knowledge Management, pp. 1149–1158. ACM (2014)
4. Lüthi, M., Albrecht, T., Vetter, T.: Building shape models from lousy data. In: Yang, G.-Z., Hawkes, D., Rueckert, D., Noble, A., Taylor, C. (eds.) MICCAI 2009, Part II. LNCS, vol. 5762, pp. 1–8. Springer, Heidelberg (2009)
5. Filzmoser, P., Maronna, R., Werner, M.: Outlier identification in high dimensions. Comput. Stat. Data Anal. **52**(3), 1694–1711 (2008)
6. Donders, A.R.T., van der Heijden, G.J.M.G., Stijnen, T., Moons, K.G.: Review: a gentle introduction to imputation of missing values. J. Clin. Epidemiol. **59**(10), 1087–1091 (2006)
7. Jingting, M., Lentzen, K., Honsdorf, J., Feng, L., Erdt, M.: Statistical shape modeling from gaussian distributed incomplete data for image segmentation. In: Oyarzun Laura, C., et al. (eds.) CLIP 2015. LNCS, vol. 9401, pp. 113–121. Springer, Heidelberg (2016). doi:10.1007/978-3-319-31808-0_14
8. Candès, E.J., Li, X., Ma, Y., Wright, J.: Robust principal component analysis? J. ACM (JACM) **58**(3), 11 (2011)
9. Wright, J., Peng, Y., Ma, Y.: Robust principal component analysis: exact recovery of corrupted low-rank matrices via convex optimization (2009)
10. Bouwmans, T., Zahzah, E.H.: Robust PCA via principal component pursuit: a review for a comparative evaluation in video surveillance. Comput. Vis. Image Underst. **122**, 22–34 (2014)
11. Lin, Z., Liu, R., Zhixun, S.: Linearized alternating direction method with adaptive penalty for low-rank representation (2011)
12. Gutierrez, B., Mateus, D., Shiban, E., Meyer, B., Lehmberg, J., Navab, N.: A sparse approach to build shape models with routine clinical data. In: IEEE 11th International Symposium on Biomedical Imaging (ISBI), pp. 258–261. IEEE (2014)
13. Kirschner, M., Wesarg, S.: Construction of groupwise consistent shape parameterizations by propagation. In: Proceedings of the SPIE Medical Imaging 2010: Image Processing (2010)

14. Cootes, T.F., Taylor, C.J., Cooper, D.H., Graham, J.: Active shape models - their training and application. Comput. Vis. Image Underst. **61**(1), 38–59 (1995)
15. Lin, Z., Chen, M., Ma, Y.: The augmented lagrange multiplier method for exact recovery of corrupted low-rank matrices (2010). arXiv preprint arXiv:1009.5055
16. Cai, J.-F., Candès, E.J., Shen, Z.: A singular value thresholding algorithm for matrix completion. SIAM J. Optim. **20**(4), 1956–1982 (2010)
17. Davies, R.H., Twining, C.J., Taylor, C.J.: Statistical Models of Shape - Optimization and Evaluation. Springer, Heidelberg (2008)
18. Heimann, T., Meinzer, H.-P.: Statistical shape models for 3D medical image segmentation: a review. Med. Image Anal. **13**(4), 543–563 (2009)
19. Erdt, M., Kirschner, M., Steger, S., Wesarg, S.: Fast automatic liver segmentation combining learned shape priors with observed shape deviation. In: IEEE CBMS, pp. 249–254 (2010)

Intra-Operative Modeling of the Left Atrium: A Simulation Approach Using Poisson Surface Reconstruction

Rafael Palomar[1,2(✉)], Faouzi A. Cheikh[1], Azeddine Beghdadi[3], and Ole J. Elle[2,4]

[1] Norwegian Media Technology Lab,
Faculty of Computer Science and Media Technology, NTNU,
Teknologivegen 22, 2815 Gjøvik, Norway
{rafael.palomar,faouzi.cheikh}@ntnu.no
[2] The Intervention Centre, Oslo University Hospital,
Rikshospitalet, Postboks 4950, Nydalen, 0424 Oslo, Norway
oelle@ous-hf.no
[3] L2TI, Institut Galilée, Université Paris 13,
9, Avenue J.B. Clément, 93430 Villetaneuse, France
beghdadi@univ-paris13.fr
[4] Department of Informatics, University of Oslo,
Postboks 1080, Blindern, 0316 Oslo, Norway

Abstract. Electroanatomic Mapping (EAM) is an important process in Radio-frequency Catheter Ablations. In EAM, sample points are collected from the patient's atrium during intervention. This process is subject to inaccuracies contributed by different sources (e.g. tissue deformations and tracking errors). Poisson Surface Reconstruction (PSR) has recently been applied for intra-operative modeling of the left atrium through highly-dense clouds of points extracted from intra-operative and pre-operative imaging. In this work, we study the application of PSR under low-density sampling conditions which occur in some clinical work-flows. For this study we propose a simulation framework that is employed to characterize PSR in terms of accuracy of reconstruction. Our results show that a median error as low as 2.28 mm can be obtained for a maximum of 600 sampled points. These results indicate the feasibility of applying PSR for low-dense clouds of points.

1 Introduction

Atrial Fibrillation (**AF**) is the most common heart rhythm disorder of clinical significance. Fibrillation of the aria is not only associated with a higher risk of stroke, but also contributes to heart failure and death. Around 8 million individuals in United States and Europe are affected by this condition—a higher life expectancy will increase this incidence up to more than 15 million individuals by 2050 [1]. Radio-frequency catheter ablation (**RFCA**), together with medication and cardioversion are the treatments of choice for AF.

© Springer International Publishing Switzerland 2016
G. Zheng et al. (Eds.): MIAR 2016, LNCS 9805, pp. 354–365, 2016.
DOI: 10.1007/978-3-319-43775-0_32

RFCA (Fig. 1) is a minimally invasive surgical procedure generally occurring under local anesthesia. Ablation catheters are inserted into a femoral vessel and advanced to the left atrium under fluoroscopy guidance. Once in the atrium, sample points and electrophysiological data are acquired when the mapping catheter is in contact with the endocardium in a process known as electroanatomic mapping (**EAM**). The electrophysiological data associated with the geometry of the atrium is then reconstructed in a 3D model that will guide the ablation process. The aim of this process is the isolation of areas triggering atrial fibrillation, typically located around the pulmonary veins (**PVs**) ostia, by delivering energy through radio-frequency, thus causing ablation lesions.

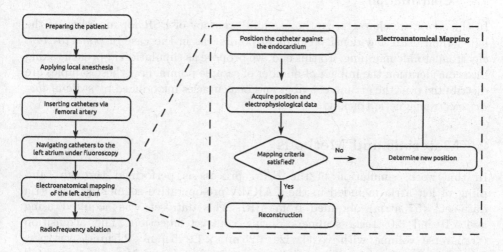

Fig. 1. RFCA procedure: clinical work-flow (left) and electroanatomic mapping of the left atrium (right).

EAM is an essential process during RFCA interventions. Several studies show the advantages of EAM compared to non-EAM guided approaches (e.g. [2]). 3D reconstructions from EAM are often merged with pre-operative models obtained from magnetic resonance imaging (**MRI**) or computed tomography (**CT**). This provides electrophysiologists with visualization of great anatomical detail. However, factors like added cost, patient's discomfort and possible additional exposure to radiation, have to be considered in order to decide on the use of pre-operative images [3].

It is known that the EAM process is subject to errors contributed by different sources. Several works in the literature have assessed the accuracy of EAM [4,5]. One source of errors is the underlying catheter tracking technology employed (usually based on electromagnetic tracking). Another source of errors is physiological factors like the heart motion caused by cardiac contractions and breathing [6].

Anatomical mapping of the left atrium is currently performed under two different strategies: *point-to-point* acquisition with triangulation-based reconstructions, and *progressive* reconstructions [7,8]. Recently, *Poisson surface reconstruction* (**PSR**) [9] has been used as an alternative to obtain intra-operative patient-specific models of the left atrium from clouds of points [10,11]. As opposed to the *point-to-point* acquisition approach, where a low density cloud of points is acquired, approaches based on PSR are supported on high-density clouds of points obtained either by intra-operative ultrasound or pre-operative models, which may not be available in some clinical work-flows.

1.1 Contribution

In this work, we characterize the use and accuracy of PSR for modeling of the left atrium using low-density clouds of points—as in the case of *point-to-point* electroanatomic mapping. To this end, we propose as simulation approach taking into consideration the impact of number of sample points, how these samples are distributed over the atrium chamber and inaccuracies introduced by *state-of-the-art* electromagnetic tracking.

2 Materials and Methods

In this work, simulation of the EAM process is performed through sampling of left atria included in the CARMA pre-operative segmented left atria data-set[1] (57 atria) obtained from MRI. This data-set was acquired using a 1.5 T and 3.0 Tesla scanners during contrast injection. The acquisition (transverse volume with voxel size $1.25\,mm \times 1.2\ 5\,mm \times 2.5\,mm$) was performed under free-breathing using navigator gating and then reconstructed to $0.625\,mm \times 0.625\,mm \times 1.25\,mm$ (3D inverse recovery GRE, $TR/TE = 5.4/2.3\,ms$).

An evaluation framework (Fig. 2) consisting of several processing stages is applied. In this process:

1. A 3D reference set is generated from the original segmented data-set.
2. The reference set is sampled under different conditions.
3. The sampled set is reconstructed using PSR under different parameters.
4. The reconstructed set is compared to the reference. Reconstruction error measurements are derived from this comparison.

2.1 Reference Set Generation

Given the set $\mathbf{A} = \{A_1, A_2, ..., A_{57}\}$ of segmented atria, a set of reference tetrahedral meshes $\mathbf{R} = \{\mathcal{R}_1, \mathcal{R}_2, ..., \mathcal{R}_{57}\}$ is obtained from the application of *Marching Cubes*.

---

[1] CARMA Left Atria MRI data-set available on (http://www.insight-journal.org/midas/collection/view/197).

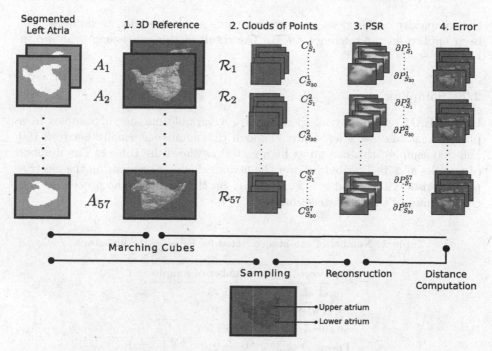

Fig. 2. Proposed simulation process. First, a reference mesh models $\mathcal{R}_i$, and clouds of points $C^i_{S_j}$ are generated from the original segmented atria A_i. PSR models $\partial P^i_{S_j}$ are then generated from the clouds of points. Finally PSR errors are computed.

MRI acquisition presents anisotropic resolution, this is, different resolution over different axis. The effect of anisotropic resolution on the reconstruction leads to staircase artifacts (Fig. 3a). In order to palliate this effect and to reduce

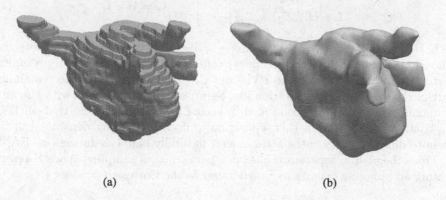

(a)   (b)

Fig. 3. Generation of the reference set: (a) Marching cubes, where staircase artifacts are visible and (b) Marching cubes with smoothing and decimation post-processing (staircase artifacts removed).

the complexity of the mesh, surface smoothing and decimation techniques have been applied on the reference set **R**. The result of this processing is shown in Fig. 3b.

2.2 Sampling

During EAM, electrophysiologists acquire a variable number of samples in a process that can last a few hours. Though this number is usually between 100 and 200 samples, this can go as high as 600 as shown in Table 1. The number of samples and its distribution over the atrium chamber depends on the electro-physiologists criteria and it has an impact on the length of the procedure and the accuracy of the reconstructions.

Table 1. Number of samples collected for EAM in the literature.

Reference	Number of samples
Sra *et al.* [12]	126 ± 13
Sy *et al.* [5]	90 ± 10
Smeets *et al.* [4]	110 ± 60
Porras *et al.* [13]	380 ± 219

In order to evaluate the impact of the sampling process in the atrium recon-struction, first, all the atria from the segmented set **A** are converted to oriented clouds of points $\mathbf{C} = \{C_1, C_2, ... C_{57}\}$ using gradient operators. Each of these clouds of points are then split into two separate clouds of points (upper and lower part of the atrium):

$$\mathbf{U} = \{\mathcal{U}_1, \mathcal{U}_2, ..., \mathcal{U}_{57}\} \qquad \mathbf{C} = \mathbf{U} \uplus \mathbf{L} \qquad (1)$$
$$\mathbf{L} = \{\mathcal{L}_1, \mathcal{L}_2, ..., \mathcal{L}_{57}\}$$

with $\mathbf{U} \uplus \mathbf{L} = \{\mathcal{U}_1 \cup \mathcal{L}_1, \mathcal{U}_2 \cup \mathcal{L}_2, ..., \mathcal{U}_{57} \cup \mathcal{L}_{57}\}$, where $\mathcal{U}_i \cup \mathcal{L}_i$ represents the union of the cloud of points $\mathcal{U}_i$ (upper) containing most geometrically complex part of the atrium, this is, the PVs; and $\mathcal{L}_i$ (lower) containing the remaining part of the atrium. The separation has been performed manually, with the aim of maximizing the volume contained in each $\mathcal{L}_i$, but making sure that all PVs are contained in $\mathcal{U}_i$. With this separation, different sampling densities can be given to different parts of the atrium, as it naturally happens during real EAM.

Once the atrium separation has been performed, a sampling space **S** repre-senting all sampling conditions is generated as the Cartesian product ($\times$):

$$\mathbf{S} = \mathbf{P} \times \mathbf{D} = \{S_0, ..., S_{30}\} \qquad (2)$$

with $\mathbf{P} = \{100, 200, ..., 600\}$ the set of number of samples approximating the space of samples in Table 1, and $\mathbf{D} = \{0.5, 0.6, ..., 0.9\}$ the distribution set in which $u \in \mathbf{D}$ is the proportion of samples taken from the upper part of the atrium ($\mathcal{U}_i$) and $l = 1 - u$ represents the proportion of samples taken from the lower part of the atrium ($\mathcal{L}_i$). This sampling space therefore, considers both, variability of samples and variability of distribution of samples.

For each atrium i in the data-set, a set of clouds of points $\mathbf{C}^i$ is generated by sampling according to the sampling conditions in $\mathbf{S}$:

$$\mathbf{C}^i = \{C^i_{S_0}, C^i_{S_1}, ..., C^i_{S_{30}}\} \tag{3}$$

2.3 Poisson Surface Reconstruction

Figure 4 shows the general idea behind PSR. To obtain the surface, PSR uses the oriented cloud of points $C^i_{S_j}$ to reconstruct an indicator function $\mathcal{X}_M : \mathbb{R}^3 \rightarrow \mathbb{R}$ of an atrium model M. This indicator function resembles the segmented image A_i, this is, a function in which the values inside the atrium are $a_i = 0$ and the values outside the atrium are $a_o = 1$. The oriented cloud of points $C^i_{S_j}$ can be thought of as a set of samples taken from the gradient of the indicator function $\nabla \mathcal{X}_M$. Then the problem can be stated as finding the scalar function $\mathcal{X}_M$ whose gradient best matches the cloud of points $C^i_{S_j}$:

$$\tilde{\mathcal{X}}_M = \arg \min_{\mathcal{X}_M} \|\nabla \mathcal{X}_M - C^i_{S_j}\| \tag{4}$$

with $\|.\|$ the Euclidean norm.

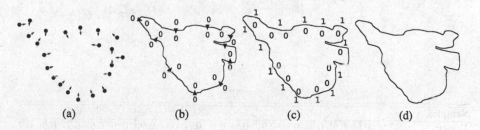

(a)   (b)   (c)   (d)

Fig. 4. Overview of Poisson surface reconstruction in 2D contour of a left atrium: (a) oriented set of points $C^i_{S_j}$; (b) gradient of the indicator function $\nabla \mathcal{X}_M$; (c) indicator function $\mathcal{X}_M$; (d) Poisson surface reconstruction ∂P.

The solution is represented through an adaptive and multi-resolution basis. More precisely, PSR constructs the minimal octree $\mathcal{O}$ with the property that every point sample falls into a leaf node at depth d. Intuitively, one can think of the depth as a parameter controlling the granularity of the mesh. Higher depth values thus lead to more complex models able to represent smaller features (and vice versa).

2.4   Error Estimation

In this work, the error between two meshes is approximated as the *surface-to-surface* distance:

$$D_s(\mathcal{S}, \mathcal{S}') = \max_{p \in \mathcal{S}} D_p(p, \mathcal{S}') \tag{5}$$

where p is a point contained in the surface described by $\mathcal{S}$. D_p is the *point-to-surface* distance defined as:

$$D_p(p, \mathcal{S}') = \min_{p' \in \mathcal{S}'} \| p - p' \| \tag{6}$$

with $\| . \|$ denoting the Euclidean norm. Since generally $D_s(\mathcal{S}, \mathcal{S}') \neq D_s(\mathcal{S}', \mathcal{S})$, we always calculate the distance from the reference mesh to the reconstructed meshes.

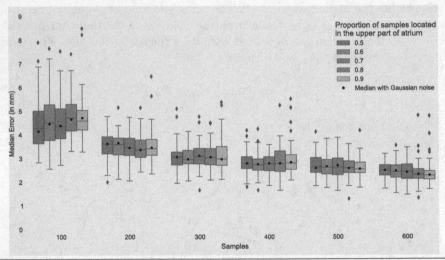

Samples	100					200					300				
Upper	0.5	0.6	0.7	0.8	0.9	0.5	0.6	0.7	0.8	0.9	0.5	0.6	0.7	0.8	0.9
Median (no noise)	4.30	4.54	**4.37**	4.74	4.61	3.63	3.61	3.48	**3.39**	3.43	3.08	**2.98**	3.11	3.05	3.00
Median (noise)	**4.17**	4.48	4.40	4.67	4.73	3.63	3.66	3.46	**3.37**	3.47	3.08	2.98	3.13	3.07	**2.98**
Samples	400					500					600				
Upper	0.5	0.6	0.7	0.8	0.9	0.5	0.6	0.7	0.8	0.9	0.5	0.6	0.7	0.8	0.9
Median (no noise)	2.80	**2.75**	2.79	2.80	2.82	2.67	2.64	2.64	2.62	**2.56**	2.51	2.44	2.46	2.33	**2.28**
Median (noise)	2.80	**2.76**	2.80	2.80	2.85	2.60	2.67	2.72	2.60	**2.57**	2.51	2.48	2.42	2.33	**2.30**

Minimum values per number of samples are highlighted in bold typeface.

Fig. 5. Median reconstruction error using PSR ($d = 5$) under different sampling conditions (number of samples and distribution of samples over the atrium). The results in the table correspond to median values relative to the population of atria reconstructed.

3   Results

The results presented in this section were obtained from the simulation process detailed in Sect. 2 to the *CARMA MRI Left Atria* data-set. The simulation sampling process, lead to the generation and reconstruction of 1710 atrium models. Additionally, the experiment was repeated for different PSR depth parameters ($d = \{4, 5, 6, 7, 8\}$) with the aim to find the best parameter in terms of accuracy. For $d > 4$ difference in results were negligible and therefore our results are based in PSR with $d = 5$. From the *point-to-surface* distance (Sect. 2.4), we derived the median error for every atrium reconstruction, which is employed to serve as a basis for our results (Fig. 4).

In order to provide results for more realistic sampling conditions, we introduce Gaussian noise ($\mu = 0.76, \sigma = 0.67$) to every point in the cloud. This noise matches the characterization of the inaccuracies introduced by electromagnetic tracking in interventional radiology environments [14].

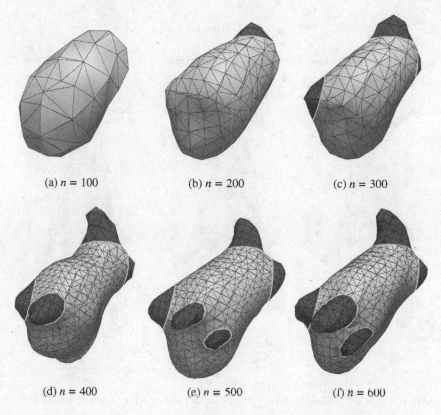

(a) $n = 100$ (b) $n = 200$ (c) $n = 300$

(d) $n = 400$ (e) $n = 500$ (f) $n = 600$

Fig. 6. PSR ($d = 5, upper = 0.8$) of CARMA0046 atrium for different number of samples. Red areas indicate clear visibility of PVs and yellow contour indicate clear visibility of PVs ostia. (Color figure online)

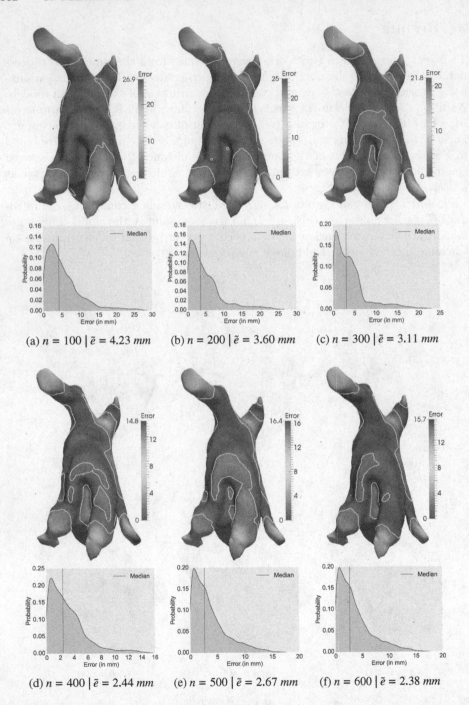

Fig. 7. Error distribution PSR for CARMA0046 ($d = 5, upper = 0.8$), projected in the reference mesh. The contour (yellow) corresponds to the median error ($\tilde{e}$) without noise. (Color figure online)

There is a clear trend of error reduction as the number of samples is increased. As shown in Fig. 5, the mean error (considering different sampling proportions) ranges from: 4.52 ± 0.22 mm for 100 samples, 3.51 ± 0.12 mm for 200 samples, 3.04 ± 0.06 mm for 300 samples, 2.78 ± 0.03 mm for 400 samples, 2.61 ± 0.05 mm for 500 samples and 2.39 ± 0.11 mm for 600 samples. The proportions of upper atrium leading to the best reconstructions in terms of median error were: 0.7 for 100 samples, 0.8 for 200 samples, 0.6 for 300 samples, 0.6 for 400 samples, 0.9 for 500 samples and 0.9 for 600 samples. Including Gaussian noise does not change significantly the median errors (Fig. 5).

The geometry of important features of the atrium, like the PVs ostia, where the ablation takes place, are not geometrically described for low number of samples. In this line, Fig. 6 illustrates the reconstruction of CARMA0046 where the PVs are only visible for high number of samples (e.g. $n \geq 400$), while the PVs ostia can be visible for a relatively low number of samples (e.g. $n \geq 200$). For low number of samples (e.g. $n < 200$), PVs and PVs ostia are not visible.

As shown in Fig. 7, reconstruction errors over the atrium are not uniformly distributed. A low number of prominent errors are located deep in the PVs. Moderate errors were located in areas of relatively high curvature, like the PVs and small features of the atrium. As shown in the figure, these areas are close to the median error ($\tilde{e}$) contours. Finally, an elevated number of small errors were located in low-curvature areas of the atrium chamber.

Computing time for PSR, including input/output data transfers was within the range $[0.31, 2.5]$ s (median time $t_m = 0.60$ s).

4   Discussion and Conclusion

In this work, the use of PSR for intra-operative modeling of left atria with application to RFCA is studied. The study is performed through a simulation approach, which is employed to isolate and analyze the errors introduced by solely the reconstruction method (PSR) and the sampling process. This, which is achieved by sampling static segmented MRI volumes (process that is not subject to motion and tracking errors), avoids errors contributed by other sources like breathing, cardiac motion or tracking technologies, thus leading to a better characterization of the error solely introduced by the method and the sampling process. This framework is applied for the evaluation of PSR from oriented clouds of points generated by sampling left atria under different sampling conditions. Clinically, as acquisition of points might not include normals, these can be estimated using techniques like in [15]. PSR has been previously used for the reconstruction of left atria under conditions of high density of samples [10,11], which requires the use of pre-operative models or intra-operative imaging technologies. In our work, we analyze the PSR reconstruction under low-density sampling to obtain intra-operative models not requiring intra-operative imaging or pre-operative models. This approach, can be combined with different *state-of-the-art* techniques like image registration and image fusion, thus providing with more flexibility to reach a wider scope of clinical work-flows.

Our results show that, under low number of samples a median error in the range of 4.52 ± 0.22 mm is expected. This error can decrease down to 2.61 ± 0.05 mm provided that a high number of samples is acquired ($n = 600$). Though our results do not show any specific sampling proportion that should be employed in all cases, approaches where more samples are taken from the upper part of the atrium ($upper > 0.5$) generally present better behavior than just uniform sampling ($upper = 0.5$). This behavior is expected since the more complex geometry of the upper part of the atrium (local features and high curvature) would be better described by a higher number of sample points, in contrast to the relatively smooth and low-curvature shape of the lower part of the atrium. The number of samples considered in this study ($n = \{100, 200, ..., 600\}$) matches the range of those reported in the literature [4,5,12,13]. When using PSR, our results shows the convenience of using a *moderate-to-high* number of samples to capture the geometry of the PVs ostia, which are the most important anatomic structures for EAM. Including Gaussian noise ($\mu = 0.76, \sigma = 0.67$) as expected in real acquisitions using electromagnetic tracking technologies does not increase the median errors significantly. This supports the adequacy of PSR for EAM.

The median accuracy reported in this work, is similar to the accuracy levels of other methods reported in the literature (Table 2). While this comparison can be used as indicator of adequacy of PSR for EAM, a careful comparison where all methods are evaluated in the same conditions would be needed to perform a more accurate assessment of the method. Furthermore, for anatomies where median errors are high (e.g. outliers in Fig. 5) elevating the number of samples is indicated. Detection of these complex anatomies, as well as the separation in upper/lower atrium, could potentially be detected automatically by prior shape analysis (e.g. curvature and local features). Such analysis could also help performing non-uniform sampling based on curvature/complexity criteria.

Table 2. Instances of errors (accuracy) reported in related works in the literature.

Reference	Errors reported	Type of error
[11]	1.68 mm RMS	Reconstruction from highly-dense cloud of points
[10]	0.88 ± 0.03 mm RMS	Reconstruction from highly-dense clouds of points
[5]	[2 − 6 mm]	Registration error
[6][a]	5.4 ± 2.5 mm	Reconstruction in PVs (long axis) with motion compensation
	3.3 ± 2.7 mm	Reconstruction in PVs (short axis) with no motion compensation

[a] Authors made a much richer report of error values in this work. Here, for simplicity, only a sample of these was included.

New technologies like catheters with force-sensing capabilities [16], together with motion compensation techniques have the potential to enable the acquisition of more sample points and therefore, the possibility of reducing the reconstruction error beyond the results presented in this work. The framework presented in this work can be employed to characterize these reconstructions which can fill the gap between our approach and that of reconstructions using high-density clouds of points.

Acknowledgments. The authors would like to thank the Comprehensive Arrhythmia Research and Management (CARMA) Center, the Center for Integrative Biomedical Computing (CIBC) and the National Institute of Health (NIH), for providing the *CARMA Left Atria MRI* data-set employed in this research.

References

1. Miyasaka, Y., Barnes, M.E., Gersh, B.J., Cha, S.S., Bailey, K.R., Abhayaratna, W.P., Seward, J.B., Tsang, T.S.M.: Secular trends in incidence of atrial fibrillation in Olmsted County, Minnesota, 1980 to 2000, and implications on the projections for future prevalence. Circulation **114**(2), 119–125 (2006)
2. Miller, M.: Principles of electroanatomic mapping. Indian Pacing Electrophysiol. J. **8**(1), 32–50 (2008)
3. Gregory, F.M., John, R.: Percutaneous pulmonary vein isolation for atrial fibrillation ablation. Circulation **123**(20), e596–e601 (2011)
4. Smeets, J.L.R.M., Ben-Haim, S.A., Rodriguez, L.-M., Timmermans, C., Wellens, H.J.J.: New method for nonfluoroscopic endocardial mapping in humans: accuracy assessment and first clinical results. Circulation **97**(24), 2426–2432 (1998)
5. Raymond, W., Sy, A.T., Stiles, M.K.: Modern electrophysiology mapping techniques. Heart, Lung Circ. **21**(6–7), 364–375 (2012)
6. Beinart, R., Kabra, R., Heist, K.E., Blendea, D., Barrett, C.D., Danik, S.B., Collins, R., Ruskin, J.N., Mansour, M.: Respiratory compensation improves the accuracy of electroanatomic mapping of the left atrium, pulmonary veins during atrial fibrillation ablation. J. Interv. Card. Electrophysiol. Int. J. Arrhythm. Pacing **32**, 105–110 (2011)
7. Reisfeld, D.: Three-Dimensional Reconstruction of Intra-Body Organs (2001)
8. Chiang, P., Zheng, J., Mak, K.H., Thalmann, N.M., Cai, Y.: Progressive surface reconstruction for heart mapping procedure. Comput. Aided Des. **44**(4), 289–299 (2012)
9. Kazhdan, M., Bolitho, M., Hoppe, H.: Poisson surface reconstruction. In: Eurographics Symposium on Geometry Processing 2006, pp. 61–70 (2006)
10. Sun, D., Rettmann, M.F., Holmes III, D.R., Linte, C., Cameron, B., Liu, J., Packer, D., Robb, R.A.: Anatomic surface reconstruction from sampled point cloud data and prior models. Stud. Health Technol. Inform. **196**, 387–393 (2014)
11. Sun, D., Rettmann, M.E., Packer, D., Robb, R.A., Holmes, D.R.: Simulated evaluation of an intraoperative surface modeling method for catheter ablation by a real phantom simulation experiment. In: SPIE Medical Imaging, p. 94152N. International Society for Optics and Photonics (2015)
12. Sra, J., Akhtar, M.: Mapping techniques for atrial fibrillation ablation. Curr. Probl. Cardiol. **32**(12), 669–767 (2007)
13. Porras, A.R., Piella, G., Cámara, O., Silva, E., Andreu, D., Berruezo, A., Frangi, A.F.: Cardiac deformation from electro-anatomical mapping data: application to scar characterization. In: Metaxas, D.N., Axel, L. (eds.) FIMH 2011. LNCS, vol. 6666, pp. 47–54. Springer, Heidelberg (2011)
14. Yaniv, Z., Wilson, E., Lindisch, D., Cleary, K.: Electromagnetic tracking in the clinical environment. Med. Phys. **36**(3), 876 (2009)
15. Mitra, N.J., Nguyen, A., Guibas, L.: Estimating surface normals in noisy point cloud data. Int. J. Comput. Geom. Appl. **14**(4–5), 261–276 (2004)
16. Hoffmayer, K.S., Gerstenfeld, E.P.: Contact force-sensing catheters. Curr. Opin. Cardiol. **30**(1), 74–80 (2015)

Atlas-Based Reconstruction of 3D Volumes of a Lower Extremity from 2D Calibrated X-ray Images

Weimin Yu and Guoyan Zheng[✉]

Institute for Surgical Technology and Biomechanics,
University of Bern, 3014 Bern, Switzerland
{weimin.yu,guoyan.zheng}@istb.unibe.ch

Abstract. In this paper, reconstruction of 3D volumes of a complete lower extremity (including both femur and tibia) from a limited number of calibrated X-ray images is addressed. We present a novel atlas-based method combining 2D-2D image registration-based 3D landmark reconstruction with a B-spline interpolation. In our method, an atlas consisting of intensity volumes and a set of predefined, sparse 3D landmarks, which are derived from the outer surface as well as the intramedullary canal surface of the associated anatomical structures, are used together with the input X-ray images to reconstruct 3D volumes of the complete lower extremity. Robust 2D-2D image registrations are first used to match digitally reconstructed radiographs, which are generated by simulating X-ray projections of an intensity volumes, with the input X-ray images. The obtained 2D-2D non-rigid transformations are used to update the locations of the 2D projections of the 3D landmarks in the associated image views. Combining updated positions for all sparse landmarks and given a grid of B-spline control points, we can estimate displacement vectors on all control points, and further to estimate the spline coefficients to yield a smooth volumetric deformation field. To this end, we develop a method combining the robustness of 2D-3D landmark reconstruction with the global smoothness properties inherent to B-spline parametrization.

1 Introduction

Good clinical outcomes of hip and knee arthroplasties demand the ability to plan a surgery precisely and measure the outcome accurately. In comparison with plain radiograph, CT-based three-dimensional (3D) planning offers several advantages. More specifically, CT has the benefits of avoiding errors resulting from magnification and inaccurate patient positioning. Additional benefits include the assessment in the axial plane, replacement of two-dimensional (2D) projections with 3D data, and the availability of information on bone quality including accurate differentiation between cortical and cancellous bone. The concern on 3D CT-based planning, however, lies in the increase of radiation dosage to the patients [1]. An alternative is to reconstruct a patient-specific 3D volume data from 2D X-rays (Fig. 1).

© Springer International Publishing Switzerland 2016
G. Zheng et al. (Eds.): MIAR 2016, LNCS 9805, pp. 366–374, 2016.
DOI: 10.1007/978-3-319-43775-0_33

Depending on the output, 2D-3D reconstruction methods can be largely classified into two categories [2]: 3D surface model reconstruction methods [3,4] and 3D volume reconstruction methods [5–9]. The methods in the former category compute 3D patient-specific surface models from one or multiple 2D X-ray images. No intensity information or information about cortical bone is available. The methods in the second category generate 3D patient-specific volumes from a limited number of X-ray images. When two or more C-arm/X-ray images are available, Yao and Tayor [5] and Sadowsky et al. [6] proposed an iterative registration process to estimate the pose, scale and modes of variation of a tetrahedral meshes-based Statistical Shape and Intensity Model (SSIM) by minimizing the difference between the simulated Digitally Reconstructed Radiographs (DRRs) and the real X-ray images. Mutual information was used as the similarity measure. With leave-one-out tests, an average registration error of 2.0 mm was reported in [6]. Zhéng [8] proposed to reconstruct a patient-specific 3D volume by matching independent shape and appearance models that are learned from a set of training data to a limited number of C-arm/X-ray images. An intensity-based nonrigid 2D-3D registration algorithm was proposed to deformably fit the learned models to the input images. When two C-arm images were used, a mean reconstruction accuracy of 1.5 mm was reported in [8]. To the best knowledge of the authors, none of the above mentioned methods have been applied to reconstruct volumes of a complete lower extremity.

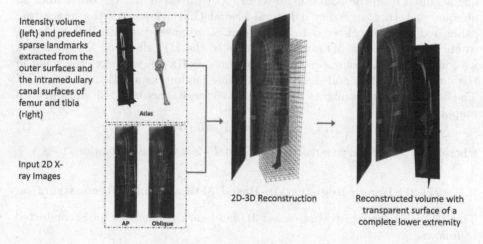

Intensity volume (left) and predefined sparse landmarks extracted from the outer surfaces and the intramedullary canal surfaces of femur and tibia (right)

Atlas

Input 2D X-ray Images

AP   Oblique

2D-3D Reconstruction

Reconstructed volume with transparent surface of a complete lower extremity

Fig. 1. A schematic view of the present 2D-3D reconstruction pipeline.

The contribution of this paper is an atlas-based approach for reconstructing 3D volumes of a complete lower extremity (including both femur and tibia) from a limited number of calibrated X-ray images. Figure 2 shows a schematic view of the present 2D-3D reconstruction method. Our method combines 2D-2D image registration-based 3D landmark reconstruction with a B-spline interpolation.

In our method, an atlas consisting of intensity volumes and a set of pre-defined, sparse 3D landmarks, which are derived from the outer surface as well as the intramedullary canal surface of the associated anatomical structures, are used together with the input X-ray images to reconstruct 3D volumes of the complete lower extremity. Robust 2D-2D image registrations are first used to match digitally reconstructed radiographs (DRRs), which are generated by simulating X-ray projections of the intensity volumes, with the input X-ray images. The obtained 2D-2D non-rigid transformations are used to update the locations of the 2D projections of the 3D landmarks in the associated image views. Combining updated positions for all sparse landmarks and given a grid of B-spline control points, we can estimate displacement vectors on all control points, and further to estimate the spline coefficients to yield a smooth volumetric deformation field.

The paper is organized as follows. Section 2 presents the 2D-3D reconstruction techniques. Section 3 describes the 2D-3D reconstruction algorithm. Section 4 presents the experimental results, followed by the conclusions in Sect. 5.

2   2D-3D Reconstruction Techniques

Below we first present two 2D-3D reconstruction techniques that are used in our method. We assume that we are given a pair of calibrated X-ray images, one acquired from the Anterior-Posterior (AP) direction and the other from an oblique view (not necessary a Lateral-Medial (LM) view). All the images are calibrated and co-registered to a common coordinate system called $\mathbf{c}$. As we would like to match a 3D intensity volume to the 2D calibrated X-ray images, we consider the 3D volume as the floating image $\{\mathbf{I}(\mathbf{x}_f)\}$, where $\mathbf{x}_f$ is a point in the intensity volume, and the set of predefine landmarks as $\{\mathbf{l}_f^i\}, i = 1, 2, ..., L$. The floating volume is aligned to the X-ray reference space $\mathbf{c}$ by following forward mapping:

$$\mathbf{I}(\mathbf{x_c}\,(T_g, T_d)) = \mathbf{I}(T_g \circ T_d \circ \mathbf{x_f}) \tag{1}$$

where T_g is a similarity transformation and T_d is a local deformation.

2.1   2D-2D Image Registration-Based 3D Landmark Reconstruction

The 2D-2D image registration-based 3D landmark reconstruction is conducted as follows.

– Step 1: DRR generation and landmark projection. Based on the current estimation of the registration transformation, we generate DRRs using Nvidias CUDA environment. At the same time, we transform all landmarks from the floating volume space to the X-ray reference space. We denote an arbitrary landmark with index i as $\mathbf{l}_\mathbf{c}^{i,t}$. After that, we do a forward projection of all transformed landmarks to the X-ray image reference space.

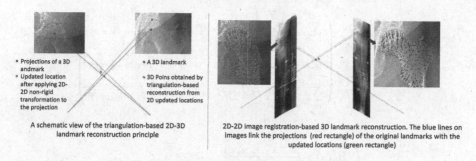

Fig. 2. A schematic view of the 2D-2D image registration-based 3D landmark reconstruction. Left: triangulation-based 2D-3D reconstruction of a single landmark; right: reconstruction of all landmarks.

- Step 2: 2D-2D Intensity-based Image Registration. At this step, we conduct an intensity-based affine 2D-2D registration first, followed by a deformable B-spline 2D-2D registration of each DRR with the associated X-ray image. In both stages, we choose to use Mattes mutual information [10] as the similarity metric and the adaptive stochastic gradient descent optimization [11] as the optimization method. The estimated 2D-2D transformations are used to update the localizations of the 2D projections of all landmarks.
- Step 3: Triangulation-based Point Reconstruction. Given the updated 2D locations of the projections of a 3D landmark $l_c^{i,t}$, an updated 3D position $l_c^{i,t+1}$ can be reconstructed from those updated 2D locations via a triangulation strategy as shown in Fig. 2.

2.2   B-Spline Interpolation

Before we present the details of our 3D B-spline interpolation algorithm, we introduce here the notations first.

- $\{c_{l,m,n}, \ l = -1 \sim L + 1, \ m = -1 \sim M + 1, \ n = -1 \sim N + 1\}$: To be computed B-spline coefficients.
- $\{d_{l,m,n}\}$: displacements at the positions of the B-spline control points are obtained with thin-plate spline interpolation from the sparse landmarks using the positions before and after triangulation-based landmark reconstruction.
- (S_x, S_y, S_z): spacing of the B-spline lattice.
- (O_x, O_y, O_z): origin of a volume data.

Given a volume space with a compact support $\Omega = [O_x, X_{Upper}] \times [O_y, Y_{Upper}] \times [O_z, Z_{Upper}] \subset \mathbb{R}^3$, for any point $(x, y, z) \in \Omega$ and its deformed position $(x', y', z') \in \Omega$, we can calculate the displacement $(x' - x, y' - y, z' - z)$ via a B-spline tensor product as follows:

$$
\begin{pmatrix} x' - x \\ y' - y \\ z' - z \end{pmatrix} = \begin{pmatrix} \sum_{r=0}^{3}\sum_{s=0}^{3}\sum_{t=0}^{3} B_r(u)B_s(v)B_t(w)c^x_{l+r,m+s,n+t} \\ \sum_{r=0}^{3}\sum_{s=0}^{3}\sum_{t=0}^{3} B_r(u)B_s(v)B_t(w)c^y_{l+r,m+s,n+t} \\ \sum_{r=0}^{3}\sum_{s=0}^{3}\sum_{t=0}^{3} B_r(u)B_s(v)B_t(w)c^z_{l+r,m+s,n+t} \end{pmatrix}
\tag{2}
$$

where

$$
\begin{cases}
B_0(s) = \frac{-s^3+3s^2-3s+1}{6} \\
B_1(s) = \frac{3s^3-6s^2+4}{6} \\
B_2(s) = \frac{-3s^3+3s^2+3s+1}{6} \\
B_3(s) = \frac{s^3}{6}
\end{cases}
\qquad (0 \le s < 1)
\tag{3}
$$

are the B-spline basis functions.

At the positions of the B-spline control points, it can be derived that $u = v = w = 0$. Then, we have $B_3(u) = B_3(v) = B_3(w) = 0$, and the tensor product at the positions of these B-spline control points can be written as

$$
\mathbf{d}_{l,m,n} = \begin{pmatrix} d_{l,m,n} \\ d_{l,m,n} \\ d_{l,m,n} \end{pmatrix} = \begin{pmatrix} \sum_{r=0}^{2}\sum_{s=0}^{2}\sum_{t=0}^{2} a_r a_s a_t c^x_{l+r,m+s,n+t} \\ \sum_{r=0}^{2}\sum_{s=0}^{2}\sum_{t=0}^{2} a_r a_s a_t c^y_{l+r,m+s,n+t} \\ \sum_{r=0}^{2}\sum_{s=0}^{2}\sum_{t=0}^{2} a_r a_s a_t c^z_{l+r,m+s,n+t} \end{pmatrix}
\tag{4}
$$

where $a_0 = B_0(0) = \frac{1}{6}$, $a_1 = B_1(0) = \frac{2}{3}$ and $a_2 = B_2(0) = \frac{1}{6}$.

Equation 4 defines 3 sets of $(L + 3) \times (M + 3) \times (N + 3)$ equations with $3 \times (L + 3) \times (M + 3) \times (N + 3)$ unknowns. Each set of equations can be reformulated as a block-matrix style shown as below (without causing confusion, since now on we drop coordinate superscript).

$$
\begin{pmatrix}
a_1\Lambda & a_2\Lambda & 0 & 0 & \cdots & 0 & 0 \\
a_0\Lambda & a_1\Lambda & a_2\Lambda & 0 & \cdots & 0 & 0 \\
0 & a_0\Lambda & a_1\Lambda & a_2\Lambda & \cdots & 0 & 0 \\
\vdots & \vdots & \ddots & \ddots & \ddots & \vdots & \vdots \\
0 & 0 & 0 & 0 & \cdots & a_0\Lambda & a_1\Lambda
\end{pmatrix}_{N+3}
\begin{pmatrix} c_{-1} \\ c_0 \\ c_1 \\ \vdots \\ c_{N+1} \end{pmatrix}
=
\begin{pmatrix} d_{-1} \\ d_0 \\ d_1 \\ \vdots \\ d_{N+1} \end{pmatrix}
\tag{5}
$$

where Λ has the tridiagonal structure as Eq. 5, while for the 3D case, the tridiagonal matrix Λ' is nested in the structure of Λ:

$$
\Lambda = \begin{pmatrix}
a_1\Lambda' & a_2\Lambda' & 0 & 0 & \cdots & 0 & 0 \\
a_0\Lambda' & a_1\Lambda' & a_2\Lambda' & 0 & \cdots & 0 & 0 \\
0 & a_0\Lambda' & a_1\Lambda' & a_2\Lambda' & \cdots & 0 & 0 \\
\vdots & \vdots & \ddots & \ddots & \ddots & \vdots & \vdots \\
0 & 0 & 0 & 0 & \cdots & a_0\Lambda' & a_1\Lambda'
\end{pmatrix}_{M+3}
\tag{6}
$$

$$\Lambda' = \begin{pmatrix} a_1 & a_2 & 0 & 0 & \cdots & 0 & 0 \\ a_0 & a_1 & a_2 & 0 & \cdots & 0 & 0 \\ 0 & a_0 & a_1 & a_2 & \cdots & 0 & 0 \\ \vdots & \vdots & \ddots & \ddots & \ddots & \vdots & \vdots \\ 0 & 0 & 0 & 0 & \cdots & a_0 & a_1 \end{pmatrix}_{L+3} \tag{7}$$

3 2D-3D Reconstruction Algorithm

We independently match the femoral and the tibial intensity volumes of the atlas with the input X-ray images. Thus, the 2D-3D reconstruction algorithm as presented below is used for reconstructing both femoral and tibial volumes.

Algorithm (2D-3D Intensity Volume Reconstruction). The following two stages are executed until the convergence of the algorithm.

- Scaled-rigid registration stage: At this stage, at the tth iteration, after applying the 2D-2D image registration-based 3D landmark reconstruction, we will obtain two sets of 3D positions $\{l_f^i\}$ and $\{l_c^{i,t+1}\}$ with known correspondences, which allows us to compute an updated 3D similarity transformation T_g^{t+1} [12].
- Non-rigid registration stage: At this stage, the same 2D-2D image registration-based 3D landmark reconstruction is used in each iteration to obtain two sets of 3D positions with known correspondences. The B-spline interpolation algorithm as described in Sect. 2.2 is used to compute the B-spline coefficients and to further compute a smooth volumetric deformation field T_d^{t+1} to warp the intensity volume at the atlas space to the X-ray image reference space.

4 Experiments and Results

After a local institution review board approval, we designed and conducted experiments on data of 11 cadaveric legs and 10 patients. For each cadaveric leg, we acquired CT data of the full leg with a voxel size of 0.78 mm × 0.78 mm × 1 mm. One of the CT data was randomly chosen to be the atlas for all the 2D-3D reconstruction experiments described in this paper. For the atlas CT data, both femoral and tibial intensity volumes were manually segmented from the associated CT data. We further manually extracted a set of sparse landmarks from the outer surface and the intramedullary canal surface of the associated anatomical structures (we extracted 641 landmarks for femur and 872 landmarks for tibia). For each CT data of the remaining 10cadaveric legs, we generated a pair of simulated X-ray images. The 2D-3D reconstruction of the first experiment was then conducted on the simulated X-ray images. The second experiment was conducted on the patients' data. For each patient, we acquired a pair of X-ray images. The acquired X-ray images were calibrated using the method that we introduced in [13] where a device was designed to immobilize a patient's knee joint and to have a calibration phantom rigidly attached. Additionally, in order to validate the reconstruction accuracy, CT scan around three local joint regions (hip, knee and ankle) are done in one common coordinate system for each patient.

Experiment on Simulated X-ray Images. In this experiment, we take data manually segmented from the associated CT data as the ground truth. We evaluated not only the average surface distance (ASD) but also the intramedullary canal surface distance (Canal ASD) between surface models segmented from the ground truth volumes and the reconstructed volumes. We also estimated the overall Dice overlap coefficients (DICE) between the ground truth volumes and the reconstructed volumes, and the DICE overlap coefficients of the cortical bone regions (Cortical DICE), which were manually segmented from the associated volumes. Measurement differences for functional parameters such as femoral antetorsion (AT) angle, femoral collodiaphyseal (CCD) angle, and leg mechanical axis were also recorded. The quantitative results are shown in Fig. 3, left. Figure 3, right shows a qualitative comparison of the reconstructed volumes with the associated ground truth volumes for both femur and tibia. Overall, the average reconstruction accuracy achieved by our 2D-3D reconstruction technique is 1.5 mm and 1.3 mm for femur and tibia, respectively.

Differences between reconstructed volumes and the ground truth volumes of 10 cadaveric legs

Case	Femur						Tibia				Leg Mechanical Axis (°)
	ASD (mm)	DICE (%)	Canal ASD (mm)	Cortical DICE (%)	AT (°)	CCD (°)	ASD (mm)	DICE (%)	Canal ASD (mm)	Cortical DICE (%)	
#1	1.4	91.4	1.1	82.8	0.2	2.3	1.3	90.7	1.1	79.6	0.2
#2	1.4	91.4	0.9	85.9	0.3	0.4	1.4	90.2	1.0	79.8	0.4
#3	1.4	92.2	0.9	86.1	0.8	4.6	1.4	91.4	1.1	79.9	0.5
#4	1.6	91.7	0.9	86.0	0.9	6.4	1.0	93.6	1.0	82.7	1.5
#5	1.4	91.5	0.9	85.9	3.4	0.3	1.2	93.0	1.0	82	1.1
#6	1.3	92.3	0.9	86.6	1.6	1.0	1.3	91.7	1.1	78	0.1
#7	1.6	91.6	1.3	80.0	1.1	3.5	1.4	91.4	1.4	71.7	0.9
#8	1.9	90.5	1.5	78.6	1.3	2.3	1.7	89.7	1.6	71.6	0.3
#9	1.5	89.1	0.9	83.1	0.6	3.8	1.1	92.2	0.9	78.3	0.4
#10	1.5	89.8	1.1	80.1	5.1	2.7	1.1	91.9	0.9	78.3	0.1
Overall	1.5±0.2	91.2±1.0	1.0±0.2	83.5±3.0	1.5±1.5	2.7±1.9	1.3±0.2	91.6±1.2	1.1±0.2	78.2±3.8	0.6±0.5

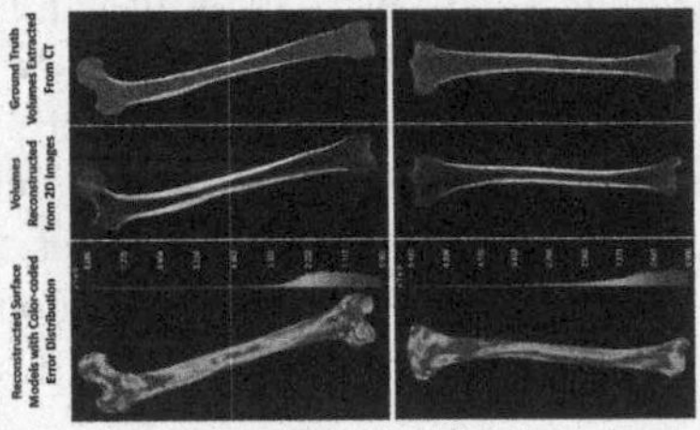

Fig. 3. Results of the experiment conducted on simulated X-ray images. Left: quantitative results; right: a qualitative comparison.

Experiment on 10 Patients' Data. In this experiment, due to the fact that only CT data around three local regions (hip, knee and ankle joints) were available (see Fig. 4, left for an example), the reconstruction accuracies were evaluated by comparing the surface models extracted from the ground truth CT data with those extracted from the reconstructed volumes after rigidly align them together. Similar to what we did in the first experiment, we also computed the measurement differences on functional parameters. The results are shown in Fig. 4, right. Please keep it in mind that here we only evaluated the average surface distances for local regions such as proximal femur (PF ASD), distal femur (DF ASD), proximal tibia (PT ASD) and distal tibia (DT ASD), while in the first experiment, the reconstruction accuracy was evaluated for the complete femur and tibia. An overall reconstruction accuracy of 1.4 mm was found.

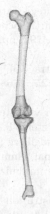

Case	Femur				Tibia		Leg
	PF ASD (mm)	DF ASD (mm)	AT (°)	CCD (°)	PT ASD (mm)	DT ASD (mm)	Mechanical Axis (°)
#1	1.6	1.6	6.3	7.2	1.2	1.3	2.1
#2	1.4	1.7	2.6	3.1	1.1	1.2	7.3
#3	1.0	1.5	2.7	2.7	1.5	1.4	1.1
#4	1.1	1.2	7.7	3.6	1.0	1.4	8.2
#5	1.1	1.7	1.5	7.3	1.4	1.7	6.3
#6	1.1	1.9	3.9	6.2	1.2	1.4	0.9
#7	1.6	2.0	1.6	5.4	2.4	1.6	1.1
#8	1.6	1.6	5.1	5.6	1.4	0.9	7.1
#9	1.4	1.4	4.9	1.5	1.3	1.3	9.4
#10	0.9	1.1	5.2	2.4	1.1	1.4	2.8
Overall	1.3±0.3	1.6±0.3	4.2±2.1	4.5±2.1	1.4±0.4	1.4±0.2	4.6±3.3

Differences between reconstructed volumes and the ground truth CT data of 10 patients

Fig. 4. Results of the experiment conducted on 10 patients' data. Left: an example showing red surface models extracted from ground truth CT data and the green surface models extracted from reconstructed volumes; right: quantitative results. (Color figure online)

5 Conclusions

In this paper, we presented an atlas-based approach for reconstructing 3D volumes of a complete lower extremity (including both femur and tibia) from a pair of calibrated X-ray images. Our method has the advantage of combining the robustness of 2D-3D landmark reconstruction with the global smoothness properties inherent to B-spline parametrization. To the best knowledge of the authors, this is probably the first attempt to derive 3D volumes of a lower extremity from a pair of calibrated X-ray images. Results of experiments conducted on both simulated data and patient data demonstrated the efficacy of the present method.

References

1. Sodickson, A., et al.: Recurrent CT, cumulative radiation exposure, and associated radiation-induced cancer risks from CT of adults. Radiology **251**, 175–184 (2009)
2. Markelj, P., Tomazevic, D., et al.: A review of 3D/2D registration methods for image-guided interventions. Med. Image Anal. **16**, 642–661 (2012)
3. Zheng, G., et al.: A 2D/3D correspondence building method for reconstruction of a patient-specific 3D bone surface model using point distribution models and calibrated X-ray images. Med. Image Anal. **13**, 883–899 (2009)
4. Baka, N., Kaptein, B.L., de Bruijne, M., et al.: 2D-3D reconstruction of the distal femur from stereo X-ray imaging using statistical shape models. Med. Image Anal. **15**, 840–850 (2011)
5. Yao, J., Taylor, R.H.: Assessing accuracy factors in deformable 2D/3D medical image registration using a statistical pelvis model. In: ICCV 2003, pp. 1329–1334 (2003)

6. Sadowsky, O., Chintalapani, G., Taylor, R.H.: Deformable 2D-3D registration of the pelvis with a limited field of view, using shape statistics. In: Ayache, N., Ourselin, S., Maeder, A. (eds.) MICCAI 2007, Part II. LNCS, vol. 4792, pp. 519–526. Springer, Heidelberg (2007)

7. Ahmad, O., et al.: Volumetric DXA (VXA) - a new method to extract 3D information from multiple in vivo DXA images. J. Bone Miner. Res. **25**, 2468–2475 (2010)

8. Zheng, G.: Personalized X-ray reconstruction of the proximal femur via intensity-based non-rigid 2D-3D registration. In: Fichtinger, G., Martel, A., Peters, T. (eds.) MICCAI 2011, Part II. LNCS, vol. 6892, pp. 598–606. Springer, Heidelberg (2011)

9. Yu, W., Zheng, G.: Personalized X-ray reconstruction of the proximal femur via a new control point-based 2D–3D registration and residual complexity minimization. In: VCBM 2014, pp. 155–162 (2014)

10. Mattes, D., Haynor, D.R., Vesselle, H., et al.: PET-CT image registration in the chest using free-form deformations. IEEE Trans. Med. Imaging **22**, 120–128 (2003)

11. Klein, S., Pluim, J.P., Staring, M., Viergever, M.: Adaptive stochastic gradient descent optimization for image registration. Int. J. Comput. Vis. **81**, 227–239 (2009)

12. Challis, J.H.: A procedure for determining rigid body transformation parameters. J. Biomech. **28**, 733–737 (2003)

13. Zheng, G., Schumann, S., Alcoltekin, A., Jaramaz, B.: Patient-specific 3D reconstruction of a complete lower extremity from 2D X-rays. In: Zheng, G., et al. (eds.) MIAR 2016. LNCS, vol. 9805, pp. 404–414. Springer, Heidelberg (2016). doi:10.1007/978-3-319-43775-0_37

3D Fully Convolutional Networks for Intervertebral Disc Localization and Segmentation

Hao Chen[1(✉)], Qi Dou[1], Xi Wang[2], Jing Qin[3], Jack C.Y. Cheng[4], and Pheng-Ann Heng[1]

[1] Department of Computer Science and Engineering,
The Chinese University of Hong Kong, Hong Kong, China
hchen@cse.cuhk.edu.hk
[2] College of Computer Science, Sichuan University, Chengdu, China
[3] School of Nursing, The Hong Kong Polytechnic University, Hong Kong, China
[4] Prince of Wales Hospital, The Chinese University of Hong Kong, Hong Kong, China

Abstract. Accurate localization and segmentation of intervertebral discs (IVDs) from volumetric data is a pre-requisite for clinical diagnosis and treatment planning. With the advance of deep learning, 2D fully convolutional networks (FCN) have achieved state-of-the-art performance on 2D image segmentation related tasks. However, how to segment objects such as IVDs from volumetric data hasn't been well addressed so far. In order to resolve above problem, we extend the 2D FCN into a 3D variant with end-to-end learning and inference, where voxel-wise predictions are generated. In order to compare the performance of 2D and 3D deep learning methods on volumetric segmentation, two different frameworks are studied: one is a 2D FCN with deep feature representations by making use of adjacent slices, the other one is a 3D FCN with flexible 3D convolutional kernels. We evaluated our methods on the 3D MRI data of *MICCAI 2015 Challenge on Automatic Intervertebral Disc Localization and Segmentation*. Extensive experimental results corroborated that 3D FCN can achieve a higher localization and segmentation accuracy than 2D FCN, which demonstrates the significance of volumetric information when confronting 3D localization and segmentation tasks.

1 Introduction

Accurate localization of intervertebral discs (IVDs) is a pre-requisite for quantitative diagnosis and treatment planning of various spinal pathologies [1]. The aim of the localization task is to identify the center of each IVD, while delineating the regions of IVD for the segmentation task. In clinical practice, the IVDs are manually segmented by radiologists thus suffers from the drawbacks of considerable efforts, time-consuming and error-prone [2]. Therefore, automatic approaches are highly demanded to alleviate the workload and improve the efficiency as well

---

H. Chen and Q. Dou—Authors contributed equally.

© Springer International Publishing Switzerland 2016
G. Zheng et al. (Eds.): MIAR 2016, LNCS 9805, pp. 375–382, 2016.
DOI: 10.1007/978-3-319-43775-0_34

as reliability. Nevertheless, the automatic localization and segmentation of IVDs from volumetric images is quite challenging for several reasons. First, IVDs often carry similar morphological appearance due to the repetitive nature of spine, which makes the labeling of individual IVD difficult. Second, the existence of similar anatomical structures or image artifacts would impede the localization and segmentation process. Third, the large shape variations of IVDs among different subjects make the robust localization and segmentation more challenging.

Many researchers have devoted their efforts on this challenging problem. Previous methods commonly utilized hand-crafted features (such as Haar features [14] and HOG [13]) for localizing the IVDs or vertebrae by different classifiers including random forests [6] and Adaboost classifier with geometric constraints [14]. Although considerable progress has been achieved, the employed low-level features are over-specified with a limited representation capability. A joint 2D learning model leveraging feature representations learned from deep convolutional networks was proposed in [3] to localize and identify the centroid of vertebrae from Computed Tomography (CT) data. Recently, 2D fully convolutional networks (FCN) have achieved the state-of-the-art performance on image segmentation tasks [9]. However, 2D FCN may be not optimal for 3D object localization and segmentation tasks from volumetric data, which are common in the field of medical image computing, since limited spatial information is considered.

Inspired by the success of 2D FCN on natural image segmentation tasks and aim to tackle the challenges of 3D object localization and segmentation problems, we propose a novel 3D FCN model for localization and segmentation tasks from high-dimensional volumetric data. We comprehensively studied and compared the 2D and 3D deep learning with end-to-end learning and inference on a challenging medical application. Extensive experiments on the task of IVD localization and segmentation demonstrated that exploring flexible 3D information can achieve more promising performance. In addition, the 3D FCN is overall general and can be readily adapted to other volumetric localization and segmentation tasks.

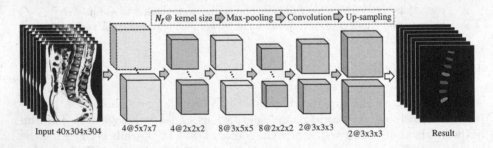

Fig. 1. The illustration of 3D fully convolutional networks.

2   Method

In this section, we present the design and implementation of the proposed end-to-end 3D FCN and explain its advantages over 2D versions. Figure 1 illustrates the overview of the 3D FCN.

2.1   Architecture Design

With the development of imaging technology, volumetric data have been more and more popular in clinical practice, such as the 3D MR images employed in diagnosis and treatment of spinal pathologies. Therefore, researchers attempted to deal with the 3D data by using several adaptations of 2D convolutional neural networks (CNNs) [4,10,11]. However, 2D CNN cannot sufficiently leverage the volumetric information, which is crucial for 3D detection and segmentation tasks. To the best of our knowledge, 3D CNN models have been rarely presented in medical image processing community so far [5,7,12]. Although these models were not trained in an end-to-end way on segmentation tasks, preliminary studies have demonstrated the effectiveness of 3D CNN on volumetric tasks. In this paper, we, for the first time, present an effective and efficient end-to-end trained 3D FCN framework for volumetric data processing. As shown in Fig. 1, our model includes three kinds of layers.

3D Convolutional Layer. In the 3D convolutional layer, a 3D feature volume is produced by convolving the input with 3D kernels, adding a bias term and finally applying a non-linear activation function. Thus, the output is 3D feature volumes (N_f denotes the number of feature volumes) instead of 2D feature maps for 2D CNNs. The 3D feature volumes can be presented as:

$$h_i^l = \sigma \left(b_i^l + \sum_k h_k^{l-1} * W_{ki}^l \right) \tag{1}$$

where h_i^l represents the ith 3D feature volume in the lth layer, W_{ki}^l denotes the 3D convolution kernel connecting the successive feature volumes and b_i^l is the bias term. The $\sigma(\cdot)$ is a non-linear rectifier function [8]. The above operation can be expanded in all three dimensions as:

$$(h_k^{l-1} * W_{ki}^l)[x, y, z] = \sum_m \sum_q \sum_r W_{ki}^l[m, q, r] \, h_k^{l-1}[x - m, y - q, z - r] \tag{2}$$

where $W_{ki}^l[m, q, r]$ and $h_k^{l-1}[x - m, y - q, z - r]$ represent the element-wise values within the 3D convolution kernel and 3D feature volume, respectively. Thus, the 3D kernel is shared within the same feature volume, and the spatial information can be effectively exploited.

3D Max-Pooling Layer. In-between 3D convolutional layers, 3D max-pooling layers are periodically inserted for endowing local invariance. Specifically, max-pooling partitions the input volume into a set of non-overlapping cubes, for each such sub-volume, outputs the maximum value. In this way, the max-pooling operation is performed in a 3D fashion, where activations within a cubic neighborhood are abstracted and promoted to higher layers.

3D Up-Sampling Layer. Due to the utilization of successive down-sampling layers, the output dimensions are typically reduced compared to the original input size. In this regard, we propose a 3D up-sampling layer to bridge the coarse feature volumes into dense predictions. In the up-sampling layer, the dimensions of down-sampled feature volumes are gradually up-sampled to the original input size. Specifically, up-sampling with a factor of d (d was typically set as 2 in our experiments) is achieved by increasing d times convolutions on the coarse feature volumes. While reshaping the neurons into higher resolution feature volumes, a neighboring-like interpolation of cubic neurons was preserved. Note that the up-sampling kernels are not fixed (thus it doesn't have to be bilinear interpolation), but are learned in an end-to-end way. In this way, the network can take a whole volume as input and output the result within a single forward propagation.

2.2 End-to-End Learning and Voxel-Wise Inference

Previous 3D CNN based models were trained on *sub-volume* samples and employed in a sliding window way to generate the segmentation result [12]. Specifically, fixed-sized 3D training sub-volumes were extracted from the volumetric data and utilized to train a classification model. However, these methods suffer from the inefficient testing inference due to the redundant overlapping computations. Compared with previous studies, our method integrated with up-sampling layers can perform end-to-end learning and voxel-wise inference, which significantly improve the efficiency. The network takes the whole volume as input and generates the 3D segmentation mask (the same size of original input) within single forward propagation. Finally, the training of whole network is formulated as a per-voxel classification problem with respect to the ground-truth segmentation mask. By denoting the parameters in the network by $\theta = \{W, b\}$, the optimization objective is to minimize the following negative log likelihood function via standard back-propagation:

$$\mathcal{L}(\mathcal{X}; \theta) = \frac{\lambda}{2}\|W\|_2^2 - \sum_{x \in \mathcal{X}} \sum_{c=1}^{C} y_c^x \log p_c(x; W, b) \tag{3}$$

where the first part is the regularization term and latter one is the fidelity term. The tradeoff of these two terms is controlled by the hyperparameter λ. $p_c(x; W, b)$ denotes the predicted probability of cth class (total C classes) after softmax classification layer for voxel x in volume space $\mathcal{X}$, and $y_c^x \in \{0, 1\}$ is the corresponding label. The parameters $\theta = \{W, b\}$ of our 3D FCN are jointly optimized in an end-to-end way by minimizing the loss function $\mathcal{L}$. In our 3D FCN, each voxel in the 3D image is taken as a training sample to the network. Therefore, the equivalent training database is dramatically enlarged and the risk of over-fitting with the limited medical dataset is effectively alleviated. In addition, with no need to crop overlapped sub-volumes, the learning process is quite efficient.

Finally, we utilized simple post-processing steps to generate local smooth segmentation results. First, we binarized the probability maps by a given threshold after filtering with a small disk. Then the segmentation mask can be obtained by finding the connected component after removing small areas. Furthermore, the center of IVD can be determined as the centroid of the connected component. To this end, the centers and segmentation masks of IVDs (type from $S1$ to $T11$) can be localized and segmented sequentially.

3   Experimental Results

3.1   Dataset and Pre-processing

We evaluated our method on the MICCAI 2015 challenge dataset on *Automatic Intervertebral Disc Localization and Segmentation from MR Images*. The dataset consisted of 25 3D T2-weighted turbo spin echo MR images, which were acquired with the 1.5 Tesla MRI scanner of Siemens Magnetom Sonata. The images were resampled into the resolution of $2 \times 1.25 \times 1.25$ mm^3. A total of 15 3D images with ground-truth annotations were released for training, while testing data was divided into two sections (5 images in test1 for offline evaluation and 5 images in test2 for on-site competition) with ground-truths held out by the challenge organizers for independent evaluation. We pre-processed the data by subtracting the mean value before inputting into the network.

3.2   Implementation Details

The kernels of network were randomly initialized from the Gaussian distribution ($\mu = 0, \sigma = 0.01$). The proposed 3D FCN was implemented with Python based on the Theano library and it took about 0.3 s to process one test image with size $40 \times 304 \times 304$, which was much faster than 2D FCN and methods utilizing the sliding window way [12], which caused a large amount of redundant computations on neighboring voxels.

For comparison, we also implemented a 2D FCN for the processing of volumetric data, where the input is the adjacent slices (3 slices in our implementation and the output is the binary mask of the middle slice.) The 2D FCN was implemented with Matlab and C++ based on the study of [9]. Generally, it took less than 1 min to process one test image with the same size using a standard PC with a 2.50 GHz Intel(R) Xeon(R) E5-1620 CPU and a NVIDIA GeForce GTX X GPU.

3.3   Qualitative Evaluation

Two examples of qualitative localization and segmentation results from different methods can be seen in Fig. 2. We can see that methods including both 2D FCN and 3D FCN can generate visually smooth and accurate segmentation results. As the green crosses shown in the figure, they can successfully localize the centers

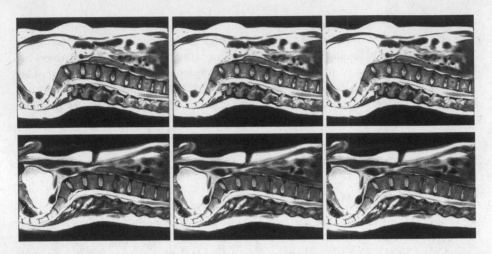

Fig. 2. Examples of localization (the centers of IVDs are marked by green crosses) and segmentation results (the boundaries of segmentation masks are delineated by red lines) of different methods: original images, 2D FCN and 3D FCN (from left to right). (Color figure online)

of IVDs. When comparing the results of 2D FCN and the proposed 3D FCN, it is observed that the 3D FCN can achieve more accurate and smooth results, which is attributed to the advantage of proposed 3D FCN by exploiting large volumetric contextual information.

3.4   Quantitative Evaluation and Comparison

Evaluation Metrics. The evaluation metrics on IVD localization include mean localization distance (MLD) with standard deviation (SD) and successful detection rate P. If the absolute difference between the localized IVD center and the ground truth center is no greater than 2 mm, the localization of this IVD is considered as a correct detection; otherwise, it is considered as a false detection. The evaluation metrics on IVD segmentation include mean dice overlap coefficients (MD) with SD and mean average absolute distance (MAAD) with SD. Larger MD means better segmentation accuracy. MAAD is a metric measuring the average absolute distance between the ground truth disc surface and the segmented surface, hence smaller MAAD means better segmentation accuracy.

Table 1. Results of IVD localization and segmentation on test1 dataset

Method	MLD ± SD (mm)	P (2.0 mm)	MD ± SD	MAAD± SD (mm)
2D FCN	1.07 ± 0.62	91.4 %	83.2 % ± 4.6 %	1.58 ± 0.28
3D FCN	**0.91 ± 0.58**	**94.3 %**	**88.4 % ± 5.3 %**	**1.27 ± 0.26**

Table 2. Results of IVD localization and segmentation on test2 dataset

Method	MLD ± SD (mm)	P (2.0 mm)	MD ± SD	MAAD± SD (mm)
2D FCN	0.89 ± 0.48	**94.3%**	82.2 % ± 6.8 %	1.77 ± 0.29
3D FCN	**0.85 ± 0.52**	**94.3 %**	**89.0 % ± 3.4 %**	**1.22 ± 0.15**

Results of IVD Localization. The quantitative localization results of different methods on test1 and test2 datasets can be seen in Tables 1 and 2, respectively. It is observed that both 3D FCN and 2D FCN can localize the centers of IVD with more than 90 % detection rate, while 3D FCN achieved a higher detection rate (94.3 %) than that of 2D FCN (91.4 %) within range of 2 mm on test1 dataset. In addition, the 3D FCN achieved a smaller MLD with a smaller SD than 2D FCN. The comparison between 2D FCN and 3D FCN demonstrates the efficacy of taking full advantage of 3D volumetric information consistently. The results of our method achieved the best localization results on the onsite competition, outperforming all the other methods.

Results of IVD Segmentation. From the segmentation results of different methods on test1 and test2 datasets, we can see that the 3D FCN achieved much better performance than 2D FCN on different segmentation measurements, highlighting the utility of volumetric information on 3D object segmentation problems. Although without any sophisticated post-processing steps or incorporating explicit shape regression methods (e.g., active shape model), our methods with 3D FCN achieved competitive performance during the challenge on the segmentation task of IVD. To sum up, in comparison of 2D and 3D FCN, we corroborated the significance of volumetric feature representation in 3D object localization and segmentation tasks.

4 Conclusions

In this paper, we propose a novel 3D FCN model with end-to-end learning and inference (i.e., voxel-wise predictions) for intervertebral disc localization and segmentation. We compare the performance of 2D and 3D FCN to validate the efficacy of exploiting volumetric contextual information. Extensive experiments on the 3D T2 MRI data of MICCAI 2015 challenge dataset corroborated that our method achieved the best results on the localization task and competitive performance on the segmentation task. In addition, our approach is general and can be easily extended to other 3D localization and segmentation applications. Future work will include incorporating shape regression methods to further improve the performance and testing our method on a larger dataset with pathological cases included.

Acknowledgements. The work described in this paper was supported by Research Grants Council of the Hong Kong Special Administrative Region (Nos. CUHK 412513 and CUHK 14202514).

References

1. An, H.S., Anderson, P.A., Haughton, V.M., Iatridis, J.C., Kang, J.D., Lotz, J.C., Natarajan, R.N., Oegema Jr., T.R., Roughley, P., Setton, L.A., et al.: Introduction: disc degeneration: summary. Spine 29(23), 2677–2678 (2004)
2. Chen, C., Belavy, D., Yu, W., Chu, C., Armbrecht, G., Bansmann, M., Felsenberg, D., Zheng, G.: Localization and segmentation of 3D intervertebral discs in MR images by data driven estimation. IEEE Trans. Med. Imaging 34(8), 1719–1729 (2015)
3. Chen, H., Shen, C., Qin, J., Ni, D., Shi, L., Cheng, J.C.Y., Heng, P.-A.: Automatic localization and identification of vertebrae in Spine CT via a joint learning model with deep neural networks. In: Navab, N., Hornegger, J., Wells, W.M., Frangi, A.F. (eds.) MICCAI 2015. LNCS, vol. 9349, pp. 515–522. Springer, Heidelberg (2015)
4. Chen, H., Yu, L., Dou, Q., Shi, L., Mok, V.C., Heng, P.A.: Automatic detection of cerebral microbleeds via deep learning based 3D feature representation. In: 2015 IEEE 12th International Symposium on Biomedical Imaging (ISBI), pp. 764–767. IEEE (2015)
5. Dou, Q., Chen, H., Yu, L., Zhao, L., Qin, J., Wang, D., Mok, V.C., Shi, L., Heng, P.A.: Automatic detection of cerebral microbleeds from MR images via 3D convolutional neural networks. IEEE Trans. Med. Imaging 35(5), 1182–1195 (2016)
6. Glocker, B., Zikic, D., Konukoglu, E., Haynor, D.R., Criminisi, A.: Vertebrae localization in pathological Spine CT via dense classification from sparse annotations. In: Mori, K., Sakuma, I., Sato, Y., Barillot, C., Navab, N. (eds.) MICCAI 2013, Part II. LNCS, vol. 8150, pp. 262–270. Springer, Heidelberg (2013)
7. Kamnitsas, K., Chen, L., Ledig, C., Rueckert, D., Glocker, B.: Multi-scale 3D convolutional neural networks for lesion segmentation in brain MRI. In: Ischemic Stroke Lesion Segmentation, p. 13 (2015)
8. Krizhevsky, A., Sutskever, I., Hinton, G.E.: Imagenet classification with deep convolutional neural networks. In: Advances in neural information processing systems, pp. 1097–1105 (2012)
9. Long, J., Shelhamer, E., Darrell, T.: Fully convolutional networks for semantic segmentation. In: Proceedings of the IEEE Conference on Computer Vision and Pattern Recognition, pp. 3431–3440 (2015)
10. Prasoon, A., Petersen, K., Igel, C., Lauze, F., Dam, E., Nielsen, M.: Deep feature learning for knee cartilage segmentation using a triplanar convolutional neural network. In: Mori, K., Sakuma, I., Sato, Y., Barillot, C., Navab, N. (eds.) MICCAI 2013, Part II. LNCS, vol. 8150, pp. 246–253. Springer, Heidelberg (2013)
11. Roth, H.R., Lu, L., Liu, J., Yao, J., Seff, A., Kevin, C., Kim, L., Summers, R.M.: Improving computer-aided detection using convolutional neural networks and random view aggregation. (2015). arXiv preprint arXiv:1505.03046
12. Urban, G., Bendszus, M., Hamprecht, F., Kleesiek, J.: Multi-modal brain tumor segmentation using deep convolutional neural networks. In: Proceedings in MICCAI BraTS (Brain Tumor Segmentation) Challenge, pp. 31–35 (2014)
13. Wang, Z., Zhen, X., Tay, K., Osman, S., Romano, W., Li, S.: Regression segmentation for M3 spinal images. IEEE Trans. Med. Imaging 34(8), 1640–1648 (2015)
14. Zhan, Y., Maneesh, D., Harder, M., Zhou, X.S.: Robust MR spine detection using hierarchical learning and local articulated model. In: Ayache, N., Delingette, H., Golland, P., Mori, K. (eds.) MICCAI 2012, Part I. LNCS, vol. 7510, pp. 141–148. Springer, Heidelberg (2012)

Temporal Prediction of Respiratory Motion Using a Trained Ensemble of Forecasting Methods

Xiaoran Chen, Christine Tanner, Orçun Göksel, Gábor Székely, and Valeria De Luca[✉]

Computer Vision Lab, ETH Zurich, Zurich, Switzerland
vdeluca@vision.ee.ethz.ch

Abstract. Respiratory motion is a limiting factor during cancer therapy. Although image tracking can facilitate compensation for this motion, system latencies will still reduce the accuracy of tracking-based treatments. We propose a novel approach for temporal prediction of the motion of anatomical targets in the liver, observed from ultrasound sequences. The method is based on an ensemble of six prediction models, including neural networks, which are trained on motion traces and images. Using leave-one-subject-out validation on 24 liver ultrasound 2D sequences from the Challenge on Liver Ultrasound Tracking, the best performance was achieved by the linear regression-based ensemble of all methods with an accuracy of 1.49 (2.39) mm for a latency of 300 (600) ms.

Keywords: Image-guided therapy · Temporal prediction · Respiratory motion · Neural networks · Regression

1 Introduction

Intrafraction respiratory motion is a critical limitation in radiation therapy [2,7,11]. Image guidance and tracking allow for the real-time position monitoring of the tumor, which can be used to adjust the treatment beam to the moving target. Yet there is a latency between the target motion and the beam realignment [12]. This latency is mainly due to the image formation and processing (e.g. tracking), and repositioning of the treatment beam, e.g. via dynamic multileaf collimator aperture. The presence of this delay and significant respiratory motion requires temporal prediction of the target position to ensure that the adjusted beam is synchronized to arrive at the actual position of the tumor [7]. Several approaches have been proposed and compared to temporally predict respiratory motion traces [8,9,20]. The most successful and widely used methods include linear prediction [15,19] and neural networks (NNs) [5,15,17]. In addition, the combination [6,13] or decision fusion via median [16] of several

---

V. De Luca—We acknowledge funding from EU's 7th Framework Program under grant no. 611889 (TRANS-FUSIMO).

G. Zheng et al. (Eds.): MIAR 2016, LNCS 9805, pp. 383–391, 2016.
DOI: 10.1007/978-3-319-43775-0_35

prediction strategies has shown promising results. In this work, we propose an ensemble of six predictive methods, namely an adaptive linear filter (LIN), support vector regressor (SVR), kernel density estimator (KDE) and three NNs, trained on different input features to encode different dependencies in the data. The novelties of our approach are (i) the use of several features extracted from motion traces of selected landmarks as network inputs; (ii) additional inclusion of image intensities for predicting the position of the landmarks; and (iii) introduction of a meta-regressor trained to weight the results of the individual predictors.

2   Method

Our method aims to predict the position of a target anatomical location at a time point in the future, given a set of positions (history) of that target. Let $P_{i,s}(t) = [x_1(t), x_2(t)] \in \mathbb{R}^2$ be the tracked position at time t of the i-th anatomical landmark from image $I_s(t)$ in sequence $s \in [1, \ldots, 24]$. The motion traces are up-sampled to 50 Hz via linear interpolation, to increase the number of data points to train the model weights. For each $P_{i,s}(t)$, we aim to predict its position $\hat{P}_{i,s}(t + \Delta t) = [\hat{x}_1(t + \Delta t), \hat{x}_2(t + \Delta t)]$ at time $t + \Delta t$, with Δt being the prediction horizon, equal to the expected latency of the treatment system. The target $\hat{x}_j(t + \Delta t)$ in each of the two image dimensions ($j \in [1, 2]$) is independently predicted from the history window $\bar{\mathbf{x}}_{j,t} = [\bar{x}_j(t - N + 1), \ldots, \bar{x}_j(t)]$ of N time instances, which is smoothed by a low-pass forward-backward filter.

2.1   Existing Models

Following the comparison from [16], we implemented three common existing models, which are here briefly described. These methods take per component K past history windows $\bar{\mathbf{x}}_{j,\tau - \Delta t}$ to learn to predict from these $\hat{x}_j(t + \Delta t)$ for $\tau \in [t - K + 1, \ldots, t]$. The windows are of length $N = \Omega\gamma$, γ is the step size and Ω the number of observations. These parameters were optimized in leave-one-subject-out tests, by taking the median of all sequence-specific parameters (optimized by simulated annealing) not belonging to the left-out subject.

Adaptive Linear Filter (LIN). This filter assumes a linear relationship between $\bar{\mathbf{x}}_{j,\tau - \Delta t}$ and $\hat{x}(t + \Delta t)$, which is determined by minimizing the mean squared errors of the history windows. The optimized median parameters were $\Omega = \{22; 24; 19; 17\}$, $\gamma = \{2; 4; 4; 6\}$ and $K = \{145; 138; 152; 132\}$ for $\Delta t = \{150; 300; 600; 1000\}$ ms.

Support Vector Regressor (SVR). An ϵ-SVR with Gaussian kernels [20] was used to predict a non-linear relationship between past and future observations. Additional parameters are distance ϵ, penalty C and kernel size γ_{SVR}. The median values were $\Omega = \{8; 6; 2; 2\}$, $\gamma = \{20; 10; 10; 8\}$, $K = \{56; 116; 156; 158\}$, $\epsilon = \{0.37; 0.30; 0.23; 0.26\}$, $C = \{3.74; 3.93; 5.14; 5.00\}$ and $\gamma_{SVR} = \{0.98; 0.33; 0.11; 0.11\}$.

Kernel Density Estimation (KDE). The statistics of the relationship between previous and future observations was captured by the KDE method [14]. A probability density function was formed using Gaussian kernels with covariance matrices deduced from the training data. Before the KDE, Principal Components Analysis (PCA) was applied for dimensionality reduction of the input space, covering 90 % cumulative energy. The median parameters were $\Omega = \{16; 2; 5; 15\}$, $\gamma = \{32; 22; 32; 38\}$ and $K = \{244; 478; 420; 215\}$.

2.2 Neural Networks

Features Construction. For each prediction target $\hat{x}_j(t + \Delta t)$, a set of features is extracted from the sliding history window $\bar{\mathbf{x}}_{j,t}$ of length $N = 40$ and step size 1, and results in a feature vector $\mathbf{f}_{j,t} \in \mathbb{R}^{N^{feat}}$. These features are: moving average ($\mu_{j,t}$) and standard deviation ($\sigma_{j,t}$) of window length 3; vector forward differencing ($\delta\hat{x}_j(t) = \hat{x}_j(t) - \hat{x}_j(t-1)$); central first- and second-order differentials ($\bar{\mathbf{x}}'_{j,t}$ and $\bar{\mathbf{x}}''_{j,t}$, respectively); the single-sided power spectral density from the Fast Fourier Transformation ($\mathcal{F}(\bar{\mathbf{x}}_{j,t})$); and the detail coefficients from a single-scale Haar wavelet decomposition ($\mathcal{W}(\bar{\mathbf{x}}_{j,t})$). Let us denote the concatenation of these features by $\mathbf{z}_{j,t} = [\mu_{j,t}, \sigma_{j,t}, \delta\bar{x}_{j,t}, \bar{\mathbf{x}}'_{j,t}, \bar{\mathbf{x}}''_{j,t}, \mathcal{F}(\bar{\mathbf{x}}_{j,t}), \mathcal{W}(\bar{\mathbf{x}}_{j,t})]$.

Organ drift can be observed in several subjects and might affect the prediction accuracy. Hence $\bar{\mathbf{x}}_{j,t}$ is decomposed into de-trended trace $\bar{\mathbf{x}}^{detr}_{j,t}$ and trend $\bar{\Lambda}_{j,t}$ after 20 s ($t \geq 1000$) using locally weighted scatterplot smoothing regression [1]. The trend is extracted from a sliding window of length $N^{tr} \gg N$ to support robustness. $N^{tr} = t$ for $1000 \leq t \leq 2000$ and $N^{tr} = 2000$ otherwise. From $\bar{\mathbf{x}}^{detr}_{j,t}$ we compute the same feature concatenation as before, namely $\mathbf{z}^{detr}_{j,t}$.

To the best of our knowledge, all reported temporal prediction methods are based on motion traces. Yet tracking can have errors, which could affect the prediction accuracy, especially if no confidence values are provided. Hence we propose to incorporate the image appearance in the prediction framework. We assume that the changes of pixel intensities in the US images encode the organ motion. Therefore, we embed the images in a low-dimensional representation via PCA [3]. In details, around a give landmark $P_{i,s}(1)$ we manually select a fixed region of interest $ROI_{i,s} \subset I_s(1)$. For the history window, we first up-sample the US sub-sequence $[ROI(t - N + 1), \dots, ROI(t)]$ to 50 Hz. We then perform PCA on this sub-sequence, resulting in sorted PCA coefficients of the image intensities $\mathbf{V}_{i,t} = [\mathbf{v}_{1,t}, \dots, \mathbf{v}_{L,t}]$, where each l-th coefficient $\mathbf{v}_{l,t} = [v_l(t-N+1), \dots, v_l(t)] \in \mathbb{R}^N$. We selected $L = 4$ to cover at least 90 % cumulative energy.

Network Architecture. The architecture of the proposed NN is illustrated in Fig. 1. A dense input layer takes the input feature vector $\mathbf{f}_{j,t}$ in $n_{in} = N^{feat}$ nodes and passes n_{in} data points to the next layer. The latter is a parametric rectified linear unit (PReLU) [4] activation layer, which outputs the same number of nodes $n_a = n_{in}$. Before the motion traces are de-trended, three fully-connected (dense) layers with linear activation functions follow the activation layer with n_{h1}, n_{h2} and n_{h3} input nodes. Finally, the output layer outputs the target position, $\hat{x}_{j,s}(t + \Delta t) \in \mathbb{R}$. For de-trending, the architecture

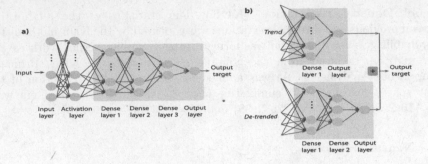

Fig. 1. (a) Initial network for non-de-trended data (NN*notr*). (b) Dense and output NN layers for trend (NN*tr*, top) and de-trended data (NN*detr*, bottom).

of the NN after the activation layer is modified. We employ only two dense layers for the prediction of de-trended motion trace $\hat{x}_j^{detr}(t + \Delta t)$, and one for the prediction of the trend $\hat{\lambda}_j(t + \Delta t)$. The final prediction is then given by $\hat{x}_{j,s}(t + \Delta t) = \hat{x}_j^{detr}(t + \Delta t) + \hat{\lambda}_j(t + \Delta t)$. The parameters and input features of the different networks are summarized in Table 1.

Training the NN consists of learning the set of parameters $\theta = \{\mathbf{w}_{in}; \mathbf{b}_{in}; \mathbf{w}_a;$ $\mathbf{w}_{h_1}; \mathbf{b}_{h_1}; \ldots; \mathbf{w}_{h_k}; \mathbf{b}_{h_k}; \mathbf{w}_{out}; \mathbf{b}_{out}\}$, where $k \in \{1; 2; 3\}$ is the number of dense hidden layers, and $\mathbf{w}$ and $\mathbf{b}$ are the concatenations of the weights and biases of each layer $\in \{in; a; h1; h2; h3; out\}$. The network parameters are learned using the RMSprop optimizer [18], which divides the next gradient by the magnitude of recent gradients so that gradients are normalised. We set a learning rate of 0.0001, damping factor of 10^{-6}, exponential decay rate ρ of 0.9, training mini-batch size of 40 and 150 epochs for NN*tr* and NN*detr* and 500 epochs for NN*notr*.

Table 1. NNs' inputs and parameters. NN: based only on motion traces; NN$_f$: input vector including features extracted from motion traces; NN$_{f+im}$: addition of US image features; *notr*: without de-trend; *detr*: de-trended traces; *tr*: trend.

Model		Input $\mathbf{f}_{i,j,t}$	N^{feat}	Parameters			
				$n_{in} = n_a$	n_{h1}	n_{h2}	n_{h3}
NN	*notr*	$\bar{\mathbf{x}}$	40	40	10	3	2
	detr	$\bar{\mathbf{x}}^{detr}$	40	40	20	3	-
	tr	$\bar{\Lambda}$	40	40	10	-	-
NN$_f$	*notr*	$\{\bar{\mathbf{x}}; \mathbf{z}\}$	360	360	10	3	2
	detr	$\{\bar{\mathbf{x}}^{detr}; \mathbf{z}^{detr}\}$	360	360	20	3	-
	tr	$\bar{\Lambda}$	40	40	10	-	-
NN$_{f+im}$	*notr*	$\{\bar{\mathbf{x}}; \mathbf{z}; \mathbf{V}\}$	520	520	10	3	2
	detr	$\{\bar{\mathbf{x}}^{detr}; \mathbf{z}^{detr}; \mathbf{V}\}$	520	520	20	3	-
	tr	$\bar{\Lambda}$	40	40	10	-	-

2.3   Linear Regression (LR) Ensemble

To learn the most reliable predictors for different Δt and hence achieve higher accuracy and robustness, the outputs of the aforementioned $M = 6$ models (LIN, SVR, KDE, NN, NN$_f$, NN$_{f+im}$) are used to train an LR model, with each training sample containing the prediction of the six models at each time instance as input and the tracked position as target. Based on leave-one-subject-out cross validation, the weights $\mathbf{w} = \{w_m\}$, with $m \in [1, \ldots, M]$, and bias b of the LR ensemble model are optimized to minimize the objective function for dimension $j \in \{1; 2\}$: $L_j(\mathbf{w}) = 1/2 \sum_{n=1}^{T'} (\sum_{m=1}^{M} (w_m \hat{x}_{j,m}(n)) + b - x_j(n))^2$, where T' is the length of the training data, $\hat{x}_{j,m}(n)$ the prediction output of the m-th model on dimension j at time instance n, and $x_j(n)$ the true tracked position. We used ordinary least square with input normalization. The fused prediction at time t for a prediction horizon Δt is then $\hat{x}_j^{LR}(t + \Delta t) = \sum_{m=1}^{M} w_m \hat{x}_{j,m}(t + \Delta t) + b$.

2.4   Evaluation Criteria

A total of 24 2D ultrasound (US) sequences of the liver of 14 subjects under free breathing were obtained from the Challenge on Liver Ultrasound Tracking (CLUST) 2015 test set (http://clust.ethz.ch/) [2]. These have a length of 1–6 min, and temporal and spatial resolution of 11–25 Hz and 0.3–0.7 mm, respectively. A total of 62 manually selected landmarks were provided for time $t = 1$ and accurately tracked using an optical flow-based algorithm [10].

The method was evaluated using leave-one-subject-out cross validation strategy. The RMSE was used to quantitatively evaluate the results on the left-out subject with respect to the tracking results. For each landmark i in sequence s, $\text{RMSE}_{i,s} = \sqrt{1/(T - \Delta t) \sum_{\hat{t}=\Delta t+1}^{T} (\hat{x}_1(\hat{t}) - x_1(\hat{t}))^2 + (\hat{x}_2(\hat{t}) - x_2(\hat{t}))^2}$, where T is the length of the up-sampled sequence. We also computed the overall RMSE by pooling all individual squared differences in one distribution. For baseline comparison, we included the case of no temporal prediction (None), where we assume no motion during Δt: $\hat{x}_j(t + \Delta t) = x_j(t)$. We compared results of: (i) individual models (LIN, SVR, KDE, NN, NN$_f$, NN$_{f+im}$); (ii) ensemble by computing the median of the prediction results of the six models; (iii) state-of-the-art methods, i.e. median ensemble of LIN, second-order polynomial adaptive filter, SVR and KDE (MED) [16], Kalman filter (KF, with dimension of state vector $= 4$) and 1-layer NN (NN$_1$, with $N = 4, n_{h1} = 8$) [15]. In addition, after down-sampling the prediction results to the original temporal resolution, they were submitted to CLUST as if they were tracking results for $t + \Delta t$. The results (mean, standard deviation (std) and 95 % of the Euclidean error with respect to the mean annotation of 3 observers in 10 % of predicted frames [2]) are reported.

3   Results

Table 2 summarizes the prediction results for the proposed approaches. Considering the individual models, for low latencies, the best accuracy is achieved by

Table 2. RMSE (in mm) and run-time (in ms) for the different methods and different latencies Δt (in ms). The best results are in bold face.

Latency	Baseline methods				Individual models						Ensembles	
	None	MED	KF	NN_1	LIN	SVR	KDE	NN	NN_f	NN_{f+im}	Median	LR
150	1.31	1.40	1.54	1.56	0.92	5.34	2.98	1.05	1.10	1.02	0.88	**0.82**
300	2.30	1.54	2.32	2.30	1.63	4.03	1.96	1.70	1.72	1.65	1.54	**1.49**
600	4.02	2.47	3.90	3.83	3.00	3.07	3.37	2.98	2.90	2.75	2.68	**2.39**
1000	5.86	3.45	5.75	5.40	4.91	3.70	4.17	4.07	3.89	3.90	3.38	**3.27**
Run-time	0.00	15.73	1.10	**0.72**	1.51	8.28	4.60	90.12	95.39	114.21	114.30	114.42

the linear method with RMSE = 0.92 (1.63) mm at Δt of 150 (300) ms. On the contrary, neural network models show better performance for $\Delta t \geq 600$ ms with the lowest RMSE = 2.75 mm by NN_{f+im} at 600 ms latency and 3.89 mm by NN_f at 1000 ms. Accuracy is improved for all prediction horizons when fusing the results of the individual models (ensembles). The best results are achieved in all cases by the proposed LR ensemble, for which the RMSE is lowered by 9–16% (3–11%) compared to the best individual models (median ensemble). These improvements are statistically significant (Wilcoxon signed-rank test, $p < 0.01$). NNs and the ensemble methods require a higher run-time (90–114 ms vs. 2 ms for LIN). Combining the fastest 3 individual models with a LR ensemble was statistically significantly worse at high latencies with 2.64 (3.31) mm for 600 (1000) ms, but is an alternative to LIN for 300 ms (1.52 mm). The mean weights assigned to each model in the LR ensemble are summarized in Table 3. For short latencies, high weight is given to the more accurate LIN prediction, while higher weights are given to the feature- and image-based NNs and SVR for long latencies. LR weights show that, out of the 3 NNs, NN is the least important. Figure 2 (left) shows the error statistics over all subjects of LR ensemble vs. the second best individual model for each latency. The std among sequences ranges in [0.39, 1.21] mm for different Δt and increases with latency. Yet this std was the lowest for the LR ensemble. Figure 2 (right) illustrates the predicted motion traces for the sequence with the highest RMSE for the LR ensemble at 300 ms latency. The main source of inaccuracy is a phase shift in the prediction that is present throughout the sequence. In the majority of the sequences, such a shift is not encountered. Amplitude differences between the predicted and original tracking traces were observed due to generally smoother predictions, which stem from smoothing the history windows. The results of None and LR ensemble at a latency of 300 ms were submitted to the official CLUST challenge. The mean (95%) prediction error of LR ensemble resulting from the CLUST evaluation was 1.63 ± 1.99 (4.36) mm. These results were on average 26% better than computing no prediction (None), with prediction error of 2.20 ± 2.04 (5.10) mm. These results cannot be compared to the tracking ones provided by other participants.

All routines are written in Python, using Keras, Theano, Statsmodels, PyWavelets, Butterflow, ffmpeg, Scipy and Scikit-learn. Experiments were

Table 3. Mean weights ± std of individual predictors of the LR ensemble for each Δt (ms). The largest weights are marked in bold face and the lowest underlined.

Latency	Methods (predictors)					
	LIN	SVR	KDE	NN	NN_f	NN_{f+im}
150	**0.67 ± 0.01**	−0.02 ± 0.00	0.05 ± 0.00	0.02 ± 0.00	0.10 ± 0.01	0.23 ± 0.15
300	0.40 ± 0.07	−0.05 ± 0.02	0.10 ± 0.10	0.07 ± 0.10	0.04 ± 0.09	**0.50 ± 0.02**
600	0.13 ± 0.01	0.21 ± 0.02	0.04 ± 0.01	0.08 ± 0.04	0.17 ± 0.02	**0.38 ± 0.01**
1000	0.05 ± 0.01	**0.46 ± 0.04**	0.07 ± 0.02	0.10 ± 0.09	0.27 ± 0.05	0.13 ± 0.01

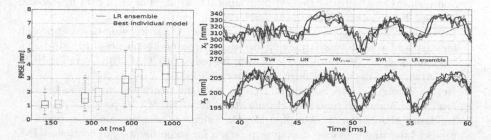

Fig. 2. (Left) Box-plot of $RMSE_{i,s}$ for LR ensemble vs. the best individual model. These are LIN (150 and 300 ms), NN_{f+im} (600 ms), SVR (1000 ms). (Right) Comparison in x_1 and x_2 directions at $\Delta t = 300$ ms for the sequence with the highest RMSE for LR ensemble (3.29 mm). For this case, LIN, SVR, KDE, NN, NN_f and NN_{f+im} have RMSE of 3.49, 6.36, 3.83, 3.75, 3,43 and 3.35 mm, and LR ensemble weight of 0.44, −0.07, 0.03, 0.14, −0.04 and 0.50, respectively.

conducted on two cluster nodes with 12-core Intel Xeon E5-2697v2 processors and 64 GB of memory. The current framework requires around 30 min for feature construction, 5–7 h for training each model and 10 s for training the LR.

4   Conclusion

We described a novel method to compute accurate temporal predictions of liver motion under free breathing from US images and tracked landmarks within these. This method can be used in tracking-based US-guided cancer treatments to compensate for system latencies and enable accurate adjustment of the radiation beam, synchronously with the actual target position. Our approach is based on a trained ensemble of different prediction models, including feature- and image-based neural networks. It achieved a mean accuracy of 1.5 mm for a typical prediction horizon of 300 ms [12]. In addition, the prediction error was always lower than 5 mm, which is clinically acceptable [7]. Yet errors increase with higher latencies. Fusing the results of all models showed to be more accurate and robust than each individual method. The use of feature-assisted NNs significantly improved results. However, their higher computation time suggests the use of the linear adaptive filter for latencies shorter than 150 ms and below, and the use of a LR ensemble of the 3 fastest models for latencies of around 300 ms. The novel use of image information improved the prediction performance and can be applied, and may prove useful, also for other temporal prediction approaches.

References

1. Cleveland, W.S., Devlin, S.J.: Locally weighted regression: an approach to regression analysis by local fitting. J. Am. Stat. Assoc. **83**(403), 596 (1988)
2. De Luca, V., Benz, T., Kondo, S., König, L., Lübke, D., Rothlübbers, S., Somphone, O., Allaire, S., Bell, M.L., Chung, D., et al.: The 2014 liver ultrasound tracking benchmark. PMB **60**(14), 5571 (2015)
3. De Luca, V., Tschannen, M., Székely, G., Tanner, C.: A learning-based approach for fast and robust vessel tracking in long ultrasound sequences. In: Mori, K., Sakuma, I., Sato, Y., Barillot, C., Navab, N. (eds.) MICCAI 2013, Part I. LNCS, vol. 8149, pp. 518–525. Springer, Heidelberg (2013)
4. He, K., Zhang, X., Ren, S., Sun, J.: Delving deep into rectifiers: surpassing human-level performance on ImageNet classification. In: IEEE ICCV, p. 1026 (2015)
5. Isakkson, M., Jaiden, J., Murphy, M.: On using an adaptive neural network to predict lung tumor motion during respiration for radiotherapy applications. Med. Phys. **32**(12), 3801 (2005)
6. Kakar, M., Nyström, H., Aarup, L.R., Nøttrup, T.J., Olsen, D.R.: Respiratory motion prediction by using the adaptive neuro fuzzy inference system (ANFIS). PMB **50**(19), 4721 (2005)
7. Keall, P.J., Mageras, G.S., Balter, J.M., Emery, R.S., Forster, K.M., Jiang, S.B., Kapatoes, J.M., Low, D.A., Murphy, M.J., Murray, B.R., et al.: The management of respiratory motion in radiation oncology report of AAPM Task Group 76. Med. Phys. **33**(10), 3874 (2006)
8. Krauss, A., Nill, S., Oelfke, U.: The comparative performance of four respiratory motion predictors for real-time tumour tracking. PMB **56**(16), 5303 (2011)
9. Lee, S.J., Motai, Y.: Review: prediction of respiratory motion. Prediction and Classification of Respiratory Motion, pp. 7–37. Springer, Heidelberg (2014)
10. Makhinya, M., Goksel, O.: Motion tracking in 2D ultrasound using vessel models and robust optic-flow. In: Proceedings of MICCAI CLUST, p. 20 (2015)
11. O'Shea, T., Bamber, J., Fontanarosa, D., van der Meer, S., Verhaegen, F., Harris, E.: Review of ultrasound image guidance in external beam radiotherapy part II: intra-fraction motion management and novel applications. PMB **61**(8), R90 (2016)
12. Poulsen, P.R., Cho, B., Sawant, A., Ruan, D., Keall, P.J.: Detailed analysis of latencies in image-based dynamic MLC tracking. Med. Phys. **37**(9), 4998 (2010)
13. Putra, D., Haas, O.C., Mills, J.A., Burnham, K.J.: A multiple model approach to respiratory motion prediction for real-time IGRT. PMB **53**, 1651 (2008)
14. Ruan, D.: Kernel density estimation-based real-time prediction for respiratory motion. PMB **55**(5), 1311 (2010)
15. Sharp, G.C., Jiang, S.B., Shimizu, S., Shirato, H.: Prediction of respiratory tumour motion for real-time image-guided radiotherapy. PMB **49**(3), 425 (2004)
16. Tanner, C., Eppenhof, K., Gelderblom, J., Szekely, G.: Decision fusion for temporal prediction of respiratory liver motion. In: IEEE ISBI, p. 698. IEEE (2014)

17. Teo, P., Bruce, N., Pistorius, S.: Application and parametric studies of a sliding window neural network for respiratory motion predictions of lung cancer patients. In: Jaffray, D.A. (ed.) World Congress on Medical Physics and Biomedical Engineering. IFMBE Proceedings, vol. 51, pp. 595–598. Springer, Switzerland (2015)
18. Tieleman, T., Hinton, G.: Lecture 6.5-rmsprop: divide the gradient by a running average of its recent magnitude. COURSERA: Neural Netw. Mach. Learn. **4**, 2 (2012)
19. Vedam, S., Keall, P., Docef, A., Todor, D., Kini, V., Mohan, R.: Predicting respiratory motion for four-dimensional radiotherapy. Med. Phys. **31**(8), 2274 (2004)
20. Verma, P.S., Wu, H., Langer, M.P., Das, I.J., Sandison, G.: Survey: real-time tumor motion prediction for image-guided radiation treatment. Comput. Sci. Eng. **13**(5), 24 (2011)

Automatic Fast-Registration Surgical Navigation System Using Depth Camera and Integral Videography 3D Image Overlay

Cong Ma, Guowen Chen, and Hongen Liao$^{(\boxtimes)}$

Department of Biomedical Engineering, School of Medicine,
Tsinghua University, Beijing, China
liao@tsinghua.edu.cn

Abstract. We propose an automatic fast-registration augmented reality (AR) surgical navigation system for minimally invasive surgery. The system integrates a fast-registration technique with three-dimensional (3D) integral videography (IV) image overlay. The detailed anatomic information generated by IV technique is superimposed to the patient using 3D autostereoscopic images, which reproduce motion parallax with naked eyes. To reduce the patient-3D overlay image registration time and achieve automatic execution, we integrate a 3D image overlay system with a real-time patient tracking system, which utilizes particle filter algorithm and depth camera. Experimental results showed that the system can lower the registration time and the can reach up to 10 frames per second (fps). The 3D overlay image to the patient registration average error is 1.88 mm, with standard deviation of 0.72 mm. Further work for improvement of the depth camera acquisition accuracy and tracking algorithm makes this system more feasible and practical.

Keywords: Minimally invasive surgery · Integral videography · Registration · Particle filter · Depth camera

1 Introduction

Minimally Invasive Surgery (MIS) has been widely utilized, for its minimal invasiveness and smaller wounds, lessening healing time and with a better prognosis for patients [1]. However, one of the major limitations for MIS is the lack of intuitive images for surgical navigation, especially 3D autostereoscopic images [2]. One solution is image-guided surgery (IGS), which offers accurate anatomic information from computed tomography (CT), magnetic resonance imaging (MRI) or other medical data sources. In order to merge virtual scenes with real surgical scenes to assist surgeons in performing operations, augmented reality technology has been applied in IGS, supplying richer surgical navigation content, making surgery much safer, more reliable, and more effective [3].

AR display methods for surgical navigation systems usually include projection displays, head-mounted displays (HMD), operative microscopic displays, and image overlay displays with semi-transparent mirrors. The typical HMD device contains two small display windows, which usually integrates lens, semi-transparent mirrors and

© Springer International Publishing Switzerland 2016
G. Zheng et al. (Eds.): MIAR 2016, LNCS 9805, pp. 392–403, 2016.
DOI: 10.1007/978-3-319-43775-0_36

projectors into a helmet, simulating binocular parallax to generate sense of depth [4]. Surgeons can perform operation with the aid of stereo images containing patients' anatomic structure information [5]. Similarly, to provide 3D perception of the specific anatomic structure information, the microscope-assisted guided interventions (MAGI) project two parallax images into both eyepieces [6].

In order to make image-patient fusion *in situ*, different AR surgical systems employed diverse patient-image registration methods considering various display patterns and practical application scenarios. Sugimoto *et al.* took a markerless registration method in their projection AR surgical system within 5 min [7]. The consistent anatomical landmark was used for registration. Liao *et al.* used a specific stereo pattern to determine the relationship between IV 3D overlay display space and patient space in a 3D image overly AR surgical system [8]. The optical tracking system was utilized into the surgical system to measure the point of reflected stereo pattern one by one. Wang *et al.* chose a stereo camera to capture the calibration model with known geometry [9].

However, one of the challenges with the image-patient process is that it requires a relatively complicated pre-registration procedure, which is time-consuming. The reason for the challenge is that the tracking system used in common AR surgical navigation usually obtains the point information with the markers rather than the surface information. The efficiency of obtaining the spatial information limits the speed of 3D image-patient registration.

To solve the problem, we propose an automatic fast-registration surgical navigation system in this paper. What surgeons need to do is just make the IV 3D overlay image coincide with the patient in the initialization procedure. Furthermore, to collect the complete spatial information effectively, we design a tracking system utilizing the depth camera. It is able to acquire patients' surface information at a high speed. With the acquired surface information, we can track the patient in real-time through a particle filter tracking algorithm. We utilize the parallel processing method to improve the time resolution of the tracking system. Photometric information is also added to enhance the accuracy of registration. We evaluate the feasibility of the proposed system with the phantom experiment.

2 Materials and Methods

2.1 System Configuration

The automatic fast-registration surgical navigation system has some features distinct from the previous AR surgical navigation system: the intuitive 3D image guided for surgery without the hand-eye coordination problem, the simple and fast registration procedure, and the addition of depth information for real-time patient tracking.

The system consists of two main parts: patient tracking and IV 3D image overlay display. The system configuration is shown in Fig. 1. Patient motion tracking is based on a particle filter tracking algorithm with depth and color data. A RGB-D camera is used in the system as the depth and photometric information collection device, which is able to grab depth and photometric data simultaneously. The depth camera is mounted at the patient's side. The distance between the depth camera and patient is about 50 cm. It is used to gather the geometry and photometric information of patients' surface. The IV 3D overlay display device is integrated into a shell with the IV 3D display device and a semi-transparent mirror. The 3D autostereoscopic image is superimposed onto the patient. The IV overlay 3D image can contain not only patients' surface information but also the internal anatomic structure information.

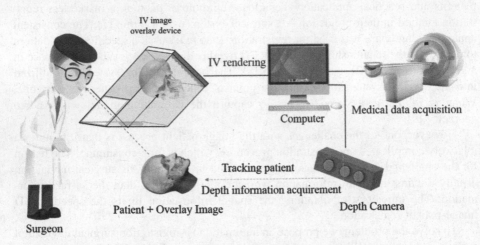

Fig. 1. Configuration of the fast-registration surgical navigation system

Figure 2 shows a flowchart elaborating how the fast-registration surgical navigation system works. First, we need to complete some preoperative preparation procedure, which includes image segmentation, model reconstruction, and surgical planning. Then, two initialization procedures should be finished: (1) Calibrate the position relationship between micro lens array (MLA) and the LCD screen. Through specific image patterns, we can make sure that the IV 3D image won't be deformed because of MLA dislocation. (2) Initialize IV overlay 3D image's position. In order to find the coordinate transformation matrix from depth camera measurement space to IV overlay display space, we need to strictly coincide with the IV overlay 3D image and the real-world object. The software and hardware interfaces have all been designed to ensure coincidence. The surgeon can easily drag the mouse to change the IV overlay 3D image's orientation. At the same time, the IV display device can move within 100 mm range along the linear guide-way to change the display device, and rotate within ±30° around the axis which is 45° to the mirror plane.

After aligning the patient with an IV overlay 3D image, the patient-motion tracking system will be started. The patient position and rotation information will be updated in real-time. The IV overlay 3D image is also updated with the updated transformation matrix to ensure the IV 3D image fuse with patient *in situ*. Therefore, surgeons can perform operation even if the patient has not been strictly stationary during the operation.

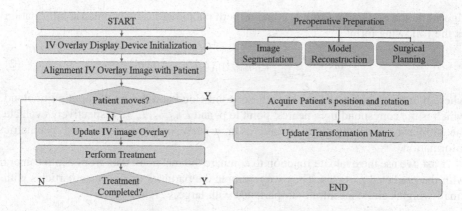

Fig. 2. Flowchart of the system operation

2.2 Patient-Motion Tracking and Fast 3D Image-Patient Registration

The patient-image registration for a common augmented reality surgical navigation system often takes a long time and lots of energy for surgeons to perform. However, in our fast-registration surgical navigation system, the registration procedure has been greatly simplified. What surgeons need to do is ensure that the initial IV overlay 3D image should coincide strictly with the patient. Software and hardware solution for coincidence has been proposed in Sect. 2.1.

The patient-3D overlay image fast registration technique mainly include two procedures: track the patient in real time and obtain the coordinate transformation matrix from patient to depth camera and utilize the obtained transformation matrix to align the IV overlay image to the patient.

The tracking system contains one depth camera, which can acquire depth data and photometric information simultaneously in a high speed. We place the depth camera about half a meter away from the patient, to collect the patients' surface depth data and RGB images. The particle filter tracking algorithm based on Point Cloud Library (PCL) [10] has been employed to calculate the patients' position and rotation.

The particle filter tracking framework has three main steps as Fig. 3 shows: prediction, weighting, and resampling. We denote the particle set state at current time t with X_t, which contains a set of particles. The total number of particles is N. It can be represented as follows:

$$X_t = x_t^{(1)}, x_t^{(2)}, \ldots, x_t^{(N)} \tag{1}$$

The state information of each particle x_t contains two aspects: position and rotation

First, we utilize previously calculated particles' information about position and rotation X_{t-1} to predict particles' information X_t at the current time through random particles. Then, according to the evaluation formula designed, we compute the weights of the particles. In order to improve the feasibility and robustness of the tracking algorithm, the evaluation formula contains both photometric and geometric information as the following form:

$$\omega^{(i)} = \sum_{j=1}^{n} L_{distance}\left(p_j, q_j\right) L_{color}\left(p_j, q_j\right) \tag{2}$$

where p, q means the set of the hypothesis point cloud and the set of input point cloud which is the correspondingly nearest point to p, and $L_{distance}$, L_{color} respectively evaluate the similarity of point cloud p and q in a view of photometric and geometric information.

Last, we use the evaluate function to compare the real point data from depth camera with the predicted particles. Then we resample the particles to eliminate particles with small weights and concentrate on particles with large weights.

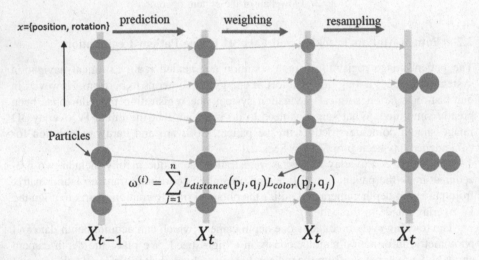

Fig. 3. Particle filter frame work

In our system, we first segment the interested region from the depth data gathered from depth camera as the tracking template. Through the particle tracking algorithm introduced above, we need to calculate the position and rotation of the tracking template to make the likelihood formula reach maximum utility, which means the tracking template aligns with the input cloud data perfectly.

At the same time, to improve the time resolution of the tracking procedure for our system, we have to reduce the computational complexity and raise the computational efficiency. In our system, the computational complexity is related to the number of particles, the data size of the input pointcloud, and segmented tracking template. Therefore, we down sample the input pointcloud and choose a suitable number of particles for tracking. To improve computational efficiency, we utilize the parallel strategy, which includes CPU multi-core acceleration and GPU acceleration. In our system, we use CPU multi-core acceleration strategy called openMP.

The essence of automatic 3D overlay image-patient fast registration is to determine the coordinates transforming relation between the coordinates of the real world where the patient exists and the coordinates of IV display space. We can't find a direct relation between them. Therefore, we use the coordinates of depth camera measurement space as a bridge to connect the coordinates of real world and the coordinates of IV overlay display space. For convenience, we keep the IV overlay device in static. We mark the coordinates of the real world where the patient exists as frame P, the coordinates of depth camera measurement space as frame D, the coordinates of IV overlay display space as frame IV, the coordinates of collected point cloud space as frame C, and coordinates of the reflected IV display space through semi-transparent mirrors as frame R. The coordinates transformation relation is presented in a way of transformation matrix. For example, T_P^{IV} means the transformation matrix from the IV overlay device to the patient. $T_D^{IV}, T_C^D, T_R^{IV}, T_P^C$ are using the same notation. The schematic diagram of coordinates transformation for fast registration shows in Fig. 4.

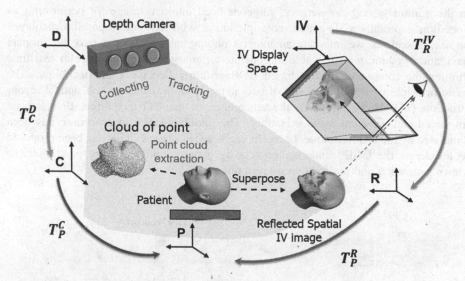

Fig. 4. Coordinates transformation for fast registration

The complete procedure of patient-3D overlay image fast registration is as follows.

(1) We project an IV image of the model of the patient for operation and reflect the 3D image into the real world through semi-transparent mirrors. Rigorous super-position of the IV overlay image and patient must be confirmed. It makes it possible to obtain the precise transformation matrix from the coordinates of IV overlay display space to the coordinates of the reflected spatial IV space marked as T_R^{IV}.

(2) We calibrate the transformation matrix T_D^R. In general cases, we can choose a common camera calibration method for obtaining intrinsic parameters. The depth camera uses low-distortion lenses, so the error can be controlled within a few

pixels. As for extrinsic calibration, we use the OpenNI interface to complete it automatically. Once the procedure of calibration has been completed, the transform matrix from the coordinates of the reflected IV display space to the coordinates of depth camera measurement space will be obtained.

(3) Once the patient is placed at the reflected IV overlay space, we'll get its position and transformation information through a tracking algorithm in real time, producing the transformation T_D^P. Therefore, the transformation from the coordinates of the reflected IV display space, R, to the coordinates of the patient is obtained by the following equation: $T_R^P = T_D^P T_R^D$.

(4) The relation between IV display space and patient space now can be calculated using the previously calculated transformation matrix. With T_P^{IV}, the dynamic updating IV image can be aligned to the patient automatically.

2.3   IV Overlay 3D Image Display System

In the minimally invasive surgery, surgeons need intuitive image for performing an operation, especially a 3D autostereoscopic image with full motion parallax displayed *in situ*. Therefore, we integrate an integral photography technique into the surgical navigation system, which is able to generate an autostereoscopic image in real time through the computer graphics based IP algorithm called the CGIP technique. The basic principle of IP is composed of two steps: IP optical pickup and optical reconstruction [11]. However, given the emergence of the CG technique, IP has been improved and achieved more versatility. The traditional pickup procedure has been simulated by the CG technique. In recent years, a GPU-based CGIP has been proposed to accelerate the CGIP rendering process by a two-round rendering pass: multiple views generation and multiple views resampling [12].

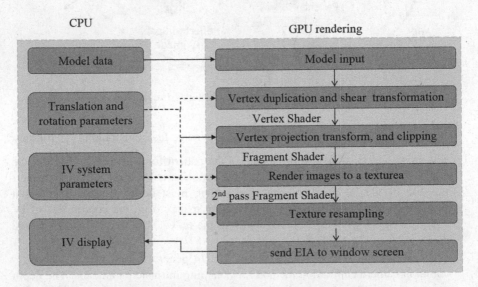

Fig. 5. Flowchart of real-time IV rendering algorithm

Our algorithm for IV generation showed in Fig. 5, which is designed specifically for the fast-registration system. It utilizes GPU-accelerated strategy to improve the speed of autostereoscopic image rendering. The main work for the CPU part is the import of parameters and model data, and the 3D image rendering process is executed in the GPU with a vertex shader and a fragment shader. First, the vertex is duplicated and shored according to multiple viewports. Therefore, when the IV image is translated, it will not cause overlapping artifacts. In vertex shader, vertexes are multiplexed by the projection transform matrix, normalized and clipped. Then, in the fragment shader, we render multiple sheared objects by triangulation and texture mapping in one pass. Lastly, texture resampling and canvas remapping are conducted in the second pass fragment shader to obtain the elemental image array (EIA). The result of EIA will be transmitted to the LCD display by GPU under the display command from the CPU.

The hardware of the IV display system is composed of a high-resolution LCD display device with MLA for 3D autostereoscopic display, a semi-transparent for 3D image overlay, a graphic workstation for IV image generation and an automatic adjustment mechanism for the fine tuning of display depth or degree. The autostereoscopic 3D image is imposed to the patient through a semi-transparent mirror placed in an appropriate degree and display depth.

The 3D medical data source we use to display is often reconstructed from CT, MRI images or any other kinds data source in preoperative examination. The generated IP image is displayed on the LCD behind the microlens array. Behind each lens unit, there is an elemental image. The image and MLA must be placed in a strict congruent configuration, and any misalignment of MLA would cause 3D image deformation. Therefore, it is necessary to execute pixels' adjustment and image correction. Under consistence between hardware setup and rendering setup, IP can reconstruct the light field of expected 3D medical image. The number of viewports is usually set up to the number of pixels of a single elemental image, furthermore, the resolution of autostereoscopic image depends on the density of MLA.

3 Experiments and Results

We fabricated the fast-registration IV overlay surgical system which consisted of a depth camera (Kinect V1, Microsoft Inc., Seattle, America), IV overlay display device and a workstation shown in Fig. 6(a). The depth camera was placed approximately 0.5 meters away from the patient to track its motion. The autostereoscopic image was projected onto the patient *in situ* through the semi-transparent mirror. The motion parallax of the IV image can be perceived by multi observers at the same time. Figure 6 (b) showed the pointcloud collected by the depth camera. The red part is the tracking template and the remaining part is the point cloud of real world. Tracking template always coincided with the phantom in real world. The phantom model was reconstructed from CT image data, which has a resolution 256×256 pixels per slice and a total number of 94 slices. The maximum number of particles for tracking was set up to 500.

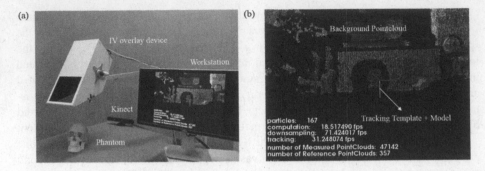

Fig. 6. (a) System configuration; (b) pointcloud capture interface

We also conducted a quantitative evaluation experiment to assess the accuracy of the alignment of IV overlay image and phantom while the patient was moving. The evaluation system showed in Fig. 7(a). The tracking system (POLARIS, Northern Digital Inc., Waterloo, Ontario, Canada) was used to measure the distance between phantom and the IV overlay image through selecting the corresponding point. We moved the phantom to four different positions showed in Fig. 7(b). P1 was located at the center of the IV display window. In the front of P1 was P4 and P3, P4 was located at the left and right of P1.

At each position, we measured 4 different corresponding points of IV overlay image and the phantom. The average distance of the corresponding points, also known as the mean error of the alignment of IV overlay image and patient was assessed. The complete results with average and standard deviation showed in Table 1. Considering all the measured data, the 3D overlay image to the patient registration average error was 1.88 mm, and standard deviation of 0.72 mm. In order to give a more intuitive perception of the effect of IV overlay 3D image-patient registration while patient was moving, we moved phantom to the display boundary. Therefore, there was only some part of 3D image overlaid to the phantom in situ, as showed in Fig. 8.

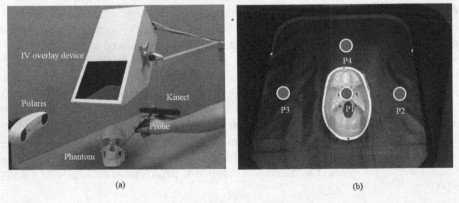

Fig. 7. (a) Evaluation system configuration (b) presenting diagram of measuring positions

The main reason for the errors is the limited accuracy of depth information acquisition equipment. As a pilot study, we used the depth camera in our patient motion tracking system, for which the depth image resolution is just 320 × 240. Another error source is the reduction of computational complexity while utilizing the particle filter tracking algorithm. To track the patient in real time, we have to control the number of particles and choose relatively simple likelihood formula. Furthermore, we need down sample the input cloud and tracking template, which causes the loss of spatial resolution.

Table 1. IV overlay image-patient registration accuracy quantitative evaluation

Tracking position	Mean error/mm	Standard deviation/mm
P1	2.12	0.61
P2	1.47	0.58
P3	2.09	0.61
P4	1.84	0.87
Average result	1.88	0.72

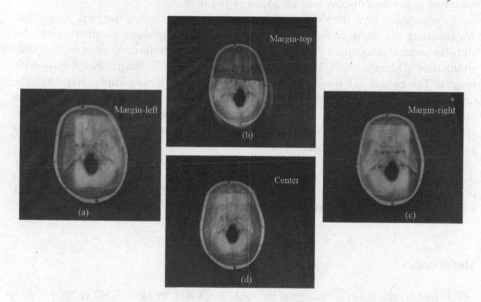

Fig. 8. IV 3D overlaid image at the border and center of display window

4 Discussion and Conclusion

We propose a fast-registration surgical navigation system using depth camera and integral videography overlay. The autostereoscopic image generated by integral videography technique is superimposed onto the patient through a semitransparent mirror. The depth camera and particle filter tracking algorithm are used to track patient motion and align the

IV overlay image with the patient. Phantom experiments demonstrate that our system is feasible with the IV overlay technique and fast registration technique. The mean error of the patient-image fast registration is 1.88 mm, and the standard deviation is 0.72 mm. The precisions of the tracking system can be improved by choosing a more accurate depth acquisition equipment. At the same time, improvements for the tracking algorithm is also considered, which includes increasing the number of particles, adopting a more efficient likelihood formula, and enhancing the efficiency of the algorithm.

Since there is a limit to the working distance of the depth camera, we have to place it at least 0.5 m away from the patient. The overlay device has to be static, therefore, causing a limited viewing area. The solution to the problem is to just switch to a lower working distance depth camera and equip it on the overlay display device. The depth camera moves or rotates with the overlay device, which can change the interested area. Another solution is multiple-object tracking. The tracking system has to track the patient and overlay device simultaneously. Both solutions can determine the transformation matrix from the IV overlay device to the tracking system, whether the overlay device moves or not.

Also, the depth data of patient's surface collected by the depth camera can be used for more than just tracking. The preoperative reconstructed model fused with intraoperative depth data display will be added in future work.

In conclusion, we developed an automatic fast-registration surgical navigation system using the depth camera and IV image overlay technique to superimpose the autostereoscopic image onto the patient to assist surgeons performing an operation with an intuitive 3D image guide. Even if the patient moves, the 3D image always fuses with patient. The patient-3D image registration procedure is quite simple. Experimental results show that the system can help the surgeons during an operation. We believe the improvement of depth camera collection accuracy and tracking algorithm will make the system more reliable. Therefore, the system can be applied in minimally invasive surgery and other medical applications.

Acknowledgments. This study was supported in part by National Natural Science Foundation of China (Grant Nos. 81427803, 61361160417, 81271735), Grant-in-Aid of Project 985, and Beijing Municipal Science & Technology Commission (Z151100003915079).

References

1. Jaffray, B.: Minimally invasive surgery. Arch. Dis. Child. **90**(5), 537–542 (2005)
2. Hamad, G.G., Curet, M.: Minimally invasive surgery. Am. J. Surg. **199**(2), 263–265 (2010)
3. Grimson, W.E.L., Kikinis, R., Jolesz, F.A., et al.: Image-guided surgery. Sci. Am. **280**(6), 54–61 (1999)
4. Sutherland, I.E.: A head-mounted three dimensional display. In: Fall Joint Computer Conference, pp. 757–764. ACM (1968)
5. Keller, K., State, A., Fuchs, H.: Head mounted displays for medical use. J. Disp. Technol. **4**(4), 468–472 (2008)

6. Edwards, P.J., King, A.P., Maurer, J.C.R., et al.: Design and evaluation of a system for microscope-assisted guided interventions (MAGI). IEEE Trans. Med. Imaging **19**(11), 1082–1093 (2000)
7. Sugimoto, M., Yasuda, H., Koda, K., et al.: Image overlay navigation by markerless surface registration in gastrointestinal, hepatobiliary and pancreatic surgery. J. Hepato-Biliary-Pancreatic. Sci. **17**(5), 629–636 (2010)
8. Liao, H., Inomata, T., Sakuma, I., et al.: 3-D augmented reality for MRI-guided surgery using integral videography autostereoscopic image overlay. IEEE Trans. Biomed. Eng. **57**(6), 1476–1486 (2010)
9. Wang, J., Suenaga, H., Hoshi, K., et al.: Augmented reality navigation with automatic marker-free image registration using 3-D image overlay for dental surgery. IEEE Trans. Biomed. Eng. **61**(4), 1295–1304 (2014)
10. Aldoma, A., Marton, Z.C., Tombari, F., et al.: Point cloud library. IEEE Robot. Autom. Mag. 1070(9932/12) (2012)
11. Lippmann, G.: La photographie integrale. C.R. Acad. Sci. **146**, 446–451 (1908)
12. Wang, J., Suenaga, H., Liao, H., et al.: Real-time computer-generated integral imaging and 3D image calibration for augmented reality surgical navigation. Comput. Med. Imaging Graph. **40**, 147–159 (2015)

Patient-Specific 3D Reconstruction of a Complete Lower Extremity from 2D X-rays

Guoyan Zheng[1]([✉]), Steffen Schumann[1], Alper Alcoltekin[1],
Branislav Jaramaz[2], and Lutz-P. Nolte[1]

[1] Institute for Surgical Technology and Biomechanics,
University of Bern, Bern, Switzerland
guoyan.zheng@istb.unibe.ch
[2] Blue Belt Technolgies, Inc., 2828 Liberty Avenue, Pittsburgh, PA 15222, USA

Abstract. This paper introduces a solution that can robustly derive 3D models of musculoskeletal structures from 2D X-ray Images. The present method, as an integrated solution, consists of three components: (1) a musculoskeletal structure immobilization apparatus; (2) an X-ray image calibration phantom; and (3) a statistical shape model-based 2D-3D reconstruction algorithm. These three components are integrated in a systematic way in the present method to derive 3D models of any musculoskeletal structure from 2D X-ray Images in a functional position (e.g., weight-bearing position for lower limb). More specifically, the musculoskeletal structure immobilization apparatus will be used to rigidly fix the X-ray calibration phantom with respect to the underlying anatomy during the image acquisition. The calibration phantom then serves two purposes. For one side, the phantom will allow one to calibrate the projection parameters of any acquired X-ray image. For the other side, the phantom also allows one to track positions of multiple X-ray images of the underlying anatomy without using any additional positional tracker, which is a prerequisite condition for the third component to compute patient-specific 3D models from 2D X-ray images and the associated statistical shape models. Validation studies conducted on both simulated X-ray images and on patients' X-ray data demonstrate the efficacy of the present solution.

1   Introduction

The common approach to derive three-dimensional (3D) model is to use imaging techniques such as computed tomography (CT) or magnetic resonance imaging (MRI). These have the disadvantages that they are expensive and/or induce high-radiation doses to the patient. An alternative is to reconstruct surface models from two-dimensional (2D) X-ray or C-arm images. Although single X-ray or C-arm image based solutions have been presented before for certain specific applications [1,2], it is generally agreed that in order to achieve an accurate surface model reconstruction, two or more images are needed. For this purpose, one

© Springer International Publishing Switzerland 2016
G. Zheng et al. (Eds.): MIAR 2016, LNCS 9805, pp. 404–414, 2016.
DOI: 10.1007/978-3-319-43775-0_37

has to solve three related problems, i.e., patient tracking/immobilization, image calibration, and 2D-3D reconstruction. Depending on the applications, different solutions have been presented before, which will be reviewed below.

Patient tracking/immobilization means to establish a coordinate system on the underlying anatomy and to co-register the acquired multiple images with respect to this common coordinate system. In the literature, both external positional tracker based solutions and calibration phantom based solutions have been introduced [3–8]. The methods in the former categories usually require a rigid fixation of the so-called dynamic reference base (DRB) onto the underlying anatomy, whose position can be tracked in real-time by using an external positional tracker [3–5]. In contrast, the methods in the latter categories eliminate the requirement of using an external positional tracker [6–8]. In such a method, the calibration phantom itself acts as a positional tracker, which requires the maintenance of a rigid relationship between the calibration phantom and the underlying anatomy during image acquisition. Although not mentioned in the context of 2D-3D reconstruction, immobilization solutions [9,10] have been developed before to maintain such a rigid fixation.

The second related problem is image calibration, which means to determine the intrinsic and extrinsic parameters of an acquired image. The image is usually calibrated with respect to the common coordinate system established on the underlying anatomy. When an external positional tracker is used, this means the coordinate system established on the DRB [3–5]. When a calibration phantom acts as a positional tracker, this usually means a coordinate system established on the phantom itself [6,8]. Another issue is how to model the X-ray projection, which determines the way how the imaging parameters are calculated. No matter what kind of model is used, a pre-requisite condition before the imaging parameters can be calculated is to establish correspondences between the 3D fiducials on the calibration phantom and their associated 2D projections.

The third problem is related with the methods used to compute 3D models from 2D calibrated X-ray images. The available techniques can be divided into two categories: those based on one generic model [11,12] and those based on statistical shape and/or appearance models (SSM) [13–16]. The methods in the former categories derive a patient-specific 3D model by deforming a generic model while the SSM-based methods use a SSM to produce only the statistically likely types of models and to reduce the number of parameters to optimize. Hybrid methods, which combine the SSM-based methods with the generic model-based methods, have also been introduced. For example, Zheng et al. [17] presented a method that combines SSM-based instantiation with thin-plate spline based deformation.

The contribution of this paper is a method that can robustly derive 3D models of musculoskeletal structures from 2D X-ray Images. We are aiming to develop a solution that will address all three problems as we mentioned above. Our method, as an integrated system, consists of three components: (1) a musculoskeletal structure immobilization apparatus; (2) an X-ray image calibration phantom; and (3) a statistical shape model-based 2D-3D reconstruction algorithm.

These three components are integrated in a systematic way in the present method to derive 3D models of any musculoskeletal structure from 2D X-ray Images in a functional position (e.g., weight-bearing position for lower limb). More specifically, the musculoskeletal structure immobilization apparatus will be used to rigidly fix the X-ray calibration phantom with respect to the underlying anatomy during the image acquisition. The calibration phantom then serves for two purposes. For one side, the phantom will allow one to calibrate the projection parameters of any acquired X-ray image. For the other side, the phantom also allows one to track positions of multiple X-ray images of the underlying anatomy without using any additional positional tracker, which is a prerequisite condition for the third component to compute patient-specific 3D models from 2D X-ray images and the associated statistical shape models. In principle, our method can be applied to any musculoskeletal structure. In this paper, the reconstruction of patient-specific 3D models of the complete lower extremity (both femur and tibia) is used to demonstrate the efficacy of the present method.

The paper is organized as follows. Section 2 presents the materials and methods. Section 3 describes the experimental results, followed by discussions and ·conclusions in Sect. 4.

2   Materials and Methods

A schematic view of the complete pipeline of the present method is shown in Fig. 1. It starts with the immobilization of the image calibration phantom with respect to the underlying anatomy (both femur and tibia), followed by patient tracking and calibration of each acquired image, and ended by computing patient-specific 3D models from the calibration X-ray images. Below a detailed description about each component will be given.

2.1   Immobilization

It is important to maintain the rigid relationship between the calibration phantom and the underlying anatomy. Without such a fixed relationship, the relative movement between the calibration phantom and the underlying anatomy will lead to inconsistent correspondences between the projections of the same anatomical features in different images such that a reconstruction of the 3D models of the underlying anatomy will not be able to achieve. When multiple anatomical structures around a joint are involved, such as the situation when one would like to derive 3D models of the complete extremity, all the involved anatomical structures around a joint have to be maintained rigidly with respect to the image calibration phantom throughout the complete image acquisition procedure. Thus, due to the mobility of a joint, the conventional way of using a belt or a jacket to fix the calibration phantom to a patient cannot guarantee no relative movement between the calibration jacket and the underlying anatomy during the image acquisition.

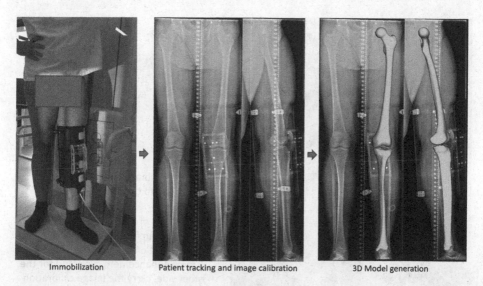

Fig. 1. A schematic view of the present invention. From left to right: immobilization, patient tracking and image calibration, and 3D model generation.

In this paper we developed a new way of immobilizing all the involved anatomical structures as well as the calibration phantom. Our immobilization device is a two-layer construction. See Fig. 2 for a prototype. The inner layer comprises a bag filled with a granular material with an encapsulated shell to which the bag is mounted. Furthermore, between the encapsulated shell and the bag a hollow space is formed for receiving pressured air in order to produce a force on the bag to immobilizing a knee joint. The inner layer is then further enhanced with the introduction of an outer layer of hard shell which can add further force to the inner layer fixation with 4 force enhancement clips, a mechanism that has been widely used in designing ski boots. A second purpose of the outer layer of hard shell is to rigidly carry the image calibration phantom such that all the involved underlying anatomical structures can be maintained rigidly with respect to the calibration phantom.

2.2 Patient Tracking and Image Calibration

The aim of the X-ray image calibration is to compute both the intrinsic and the extrinsic parameters of an acquired image. This is achieved by developing a mobile phantom as shown in Fig. 3. There is a total of 16 sphere-shaped fiducials embedded in this phantom: 7 big fiducials with diameter of 8.0 mm and 9 small fiducials with diameter of 5.0 mm. The 16 fiducials are arranged in three different planes: all 7 big fiducials are placed in one plane and the rest 9 small fiducials distributed in other two planes. Furthermore, the 7 big fiducials are arranged to form three line patterns as shown in Fig. 3, left. Every line pattern consists of three fiducials $\{M_i^1, M_i^2, M_i^3\}, i = 1, 2, 3$ with different ratios

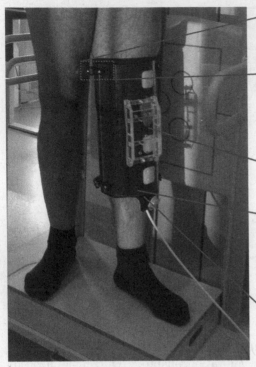

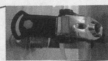

Force enhancement clip

Image calibration object rigidly attached to the outer layer

Outer layer of hard shell, which, for one side, can further enhance the immobilization of the inner layer with 4 force enhancement clips, and for the other side, carry the image calibration phantom

Inner layer, which immobilizes the underlying anatomical structures with pressured air and granular materials

Fig. 2. The immobilization device when applied to the knee joint. It is a two-layer construction with force enhancement mechanism.

$\{r_i = |M_i^1 M_i^2|/|M_i^2 M_i^3|\}$. The exact ratio for each line is used below to identify which line pattern has been successfully detected.

After an X-ray image is acquired, we first extract the sub-region containing the phantom projection. We then apply a sequence of image processing operations to the image. As those fiducials are made from steel, a simple threshold-based method is first used to segment the image. Connected-component labeling is then applied to the binary image to extract a set of separated regions. Morphology analysis is further applied to each label connected-component to extract two types of regions: candidate regions from big fiducial projections and candidate regions from small fiducial projections. The centers of these candidate regions are regarded as projections of the center of a potential fiducial. Due to background clutter, it is possible that some of the candidate projections are outliers and that we may miss some of the true fiducial projections. Furthermore, to calculate both the intrinsic and the extrinsic parameters, we have to detect the phantom in the image. Here phantom detection means to establish the correspondences between the detected 2D fiducial projection centers and their associated 3D coordinates in the local coordinate system of the phantom. For this purpose, a robust simulation-based method as follows is proposed. The pre-condition to use this method to build the correspondences is that one of the

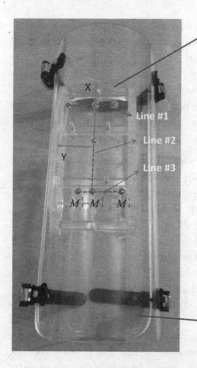

Calibration phantom with 16 fiducials (7 big and 9 small). The 7 big fiducials are arranged to form three lines with uniquely identified ratios between the fiducial distances. Such a design enables the automatic detection and 2D-3D correspondence establishment between the 2D projections of all 16 fiducials and the associated 3D fiducials. As soon as such correspondences are established, we can calculate both the intrinsic and extrinsic calibration parameters of each acquired image. The extrinsic calibration parameters allow us to track the relative motion between the imaging device and the underlying anatomical structures across multiple acquired images.

Outer layer, which is a hard shell construction

Fig. 3. The calibration phantom attached on the outer layer of our immobilization device. The calibration phantom is designed for both patient tracking and image calibration.

three line patterns has been successfully detected. Due to the fact that these line patterns are defined by big fiducials, chance to missing all three line patterns is rare.

We model the X-ray projection using a pin-hole camera.

$$\alpha[I_x, I_y, 1]^T = \mathbf{K}(\mathbf{R}[x, y, z]^T + \mathbf{T}) = \mathbf{P}[x, y, z, 1]^T \tag{1}$$

where α is the scaling factor, $\mathbf{K}$ is the intrinsic calibration matrix, $\mathbf{R}$ and $\mathbf{T}$ are the extrinsic rotation matrix and translational vector, respectively. Both the intrinsic and the extrinsic projection parameters can be combined into a 3-by-4 projection matrix $\mathbf{P}$ in the local coordinate system established on the mobile phantom.

The idea behind the simulation-based method is to do a pre-calibration to compute both the intrinsic matrix $\mathbf{K}$ as well as the extrinsic parameters $\mathbf{R}_0$ and $\mathbf{T}_0$ of the X-ray image acquired in a reference position. Then, assuming that the intrinsic matrix $\mathbf{K}$ is not changed from one image to another (we only use this assumption for building the correspondences), the projection of an X-ray image acquired at any other position with respect to the phantom can be expressed as

$$\alpha[I_x, I_y, 1]^T = \mathbf{K}(\mathbf{R}_0(\mathbf{R}^x \mathbf{R}^y \mathbf{R}^z[x, y, z]^T + \mathbf{T}) + \mathbf{T}_0) \tag{2}$$

where $\mathbf{R}^x$, $\mathbf{R}^y$, $\mathbf{R}^z$ and $\mathbf{T}$ are the rotation matrices around three axes (assuming the z-axis is in parallel with the view direction of the calibration phantom at the reference position, see the middle column of Fig. 3 for details) and the translation vector from an arbitrary acquisition position to the reference position, respectively, expressed in the local coordinate of the mobile phantom. To detect the phantom projection when an image is acquired in a new position, the simulation-based method consists of two steps.

Image Normalization. The purpose of this step is to remove the influence of the parameters $\mathbf{R}^z$, α, and $\mathbf{T}$ on the phantom detection by normalizing the image acquired at the new position as follows. Assuming that we know the correspondences of fiducials on one line pattern, which is defined by 3 landmarks M_1, M_2, M_3 with their correspondent projections at IM_1, IM_2, IM_3, we can define a 2D coordinate system based on IM_1, IM_2, IM_3, whose origin O is located at $(IM_1 + IM_2)/2$ and the x-axis is defined along the direction $O \rightarrow IM_3$. Accordingly a 2D affine transformation $T_{normalize}$ can be computed to transform this line pattern based coordinate system to a standard 2D coordinate system with its origin at $(0, 0)$ and x-axis along direction $(1, 0)$ and at the same time to normalize the length of the vector $IM_1 \rightarrow IM_3$ to 1. By applying $T_{normalize}$ to all the fiducial projections, it can be observed that for a pair of fixed $\mathbf{R}^x$ and $\mathbf{R}^y$, we can get the same normalized image no matter how the other parameters $\mathbf{R}^z$, α, and $\mathbf{T}$ are changed because the influence of these parameters is just to translate, rotate, and scale the fiducial projections, which can be compensated by the normalization operation. Therefore, the fiducial projections after the normalization will only depend on the rotational matrices $\mathbf{R}^x$ and $\mathbf{R}^y$.

Normalized Image Based Correspondence Establishment. Since the distribution of the fiducial projections in the normalized image only depends on the rotation matrices $\mathbf{R}^x$ and $\mathbf{R}^y$, it is natural to build a look-up table which up to a certain precision (e.g., 1°) contains all the normalized fiducial projections with different combination of $\mathbf{R}^x$ and $\mathbf{R}^y$. This is done off-line by simulating the projection operation using Eq. (1) based on the pre-calibrated projection model of the X-ray machine at the reference position. For an image acquired at position other than the reference, we apply the normalization operation as described above to all the detected candidate fiducial projections. The normalized candidate fiducial projections are then compared to those in the look-up table to find the best match. Since the items in the look-up table are generated by a simulation procedure, we know exactly the correspondence between the 2D fiducial projections and their corresponding 3D coordinates. Therefore, we can establish the correspondences between the candidate fiducial projections and the fiducials embedded in the phantom.

Once the correspondences are established, we can further fine-tune the fiducial projection location by applying a cross-correlation based template matching. After that, the direct linear transformation algorithm [18] is used to compute the projection matrix $\mathbf{P}$.

2.3   2D-3D Reconstruction

After image calibration, we independently match the femoral and the tibial SSMs with the input X-ray images. The 2D-3D reconstruction algorithm as introduced in [17] is used for reconstructing both femoral and tibial models.

3   Experimental Setup

We conducted two studies to validate the efficacy of the present method, with one based on simulated X-ray images and the other based on clinical X-ray images.

CT data of 12 cadavers (24 legs) were used in the first study. For each leg, two digitally reconstructed radiographs (DRRs), one from the antero-posterior (AP) direction and the other from the later-medial (LM) direction, were generated and used as the input to the iLeg software. In generating the DRRs, we set the distance from the focal point to film as 2000 mm and the pixel resolution in the range of 0.20 to 0.25 mm. The purpose of the first study was designed to validate the accuracy of the 2D-3D reconstruction algorithm when applied to reconstruction of 3D models of the complete lower extremity. Thus, for each leg, the two DRRs were used as the input to the 2D-3D reconstruction algorithm to derive patient-specific 3D models of the leg. In order to evaluate the 2D-3D reconstruction accuracy, we conducted a semi-automatic segmentation of all CT data using the commercial software Amira (Amira 5.2, FEI Corporate, Oregon, USA). The reconstructed surface models of each leg were then compared with the surface models segmented from the associated CT data. Since the DRRs were generated from the associated CT data, the surface models were reconstructed in the local coordinate system of the CT data. Thus, we can directly compare the reconstructed surface models with the surface models segmented from the associated CT data, which we took as the ground truth. Again, we used the software Amira to compute distances from each vertex on the reconstructed surface models to the associated ground truth models.

The full leg 2D-3D reconstruction validation results of 24 legs are shown in Table 1. When the reconstructed models were compared with the surface models segmented from the associated CT data, a mean reconstruction accuracy of 1.07 ± 0.19 mm, 1.05 ± 0.23 mm, 1.07 ± 0.21 mm and 1.07 ± 0.19 mm was found

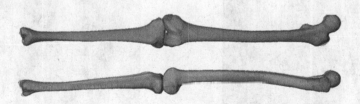

Fig. 4. Comparison of reconstructed surface models (grey solid) with the surface models segmented from the associated CT data (red transparent). Top: AP view; bottom: LM view. (Color figure online)

for left femur, right femur, left tibia and right tibia, respectively. When looking into the reconstruction of each subject, we found an average reconstruction accuracy in the range of 0.8 mm to 1.3 mm. Overall, the reconstruction accuracy was found to be 1.06 ± 0.20 mm. Figure 4 shows an example of comparison

Table 1. Full leg 2D-3D reconstruction accuracy (mm).

Subject	Femur		Tibia		Average
	Left	Right	Left	Right	
#1	1.5	1.2	1.1	1.1	1.2
#2	1.0	1.0	1.0	0.9	1.0
#3	0.9	0.8	1.1	0.8	0.9
#4	1.2	1.3	1.1	1.2	1.2
#5	1.2	1.4	0.7	0.9	1.1
#6	1.0	1.1	1.4	1.2	1.2
#7	1.0	1.3	0.9	0.9	1.0
#8	1.0	0.9	0.8	1.0	0.9
#9	1.2	1.2	1.3	1.4	1.3
#10	1.1	0.9	1.3	1.3	1.2
#11	0.8	0.7	0.9	0.9	0.8
#12	0.9	0.8	1.2	1.2	1.0
Overall	1.1	1.1	1.1	1.1	1.06 ± 0.20

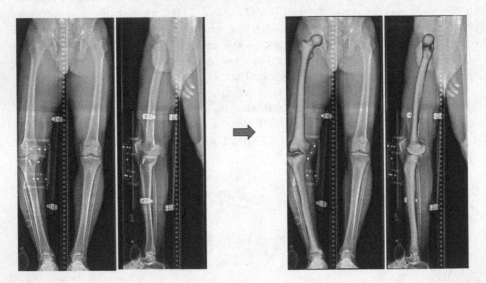

Fig. 5. An example of reconstructing patient-specific 3D models of the lower extremity from 2D X-ray images.

of reconstructed surface models (grey solid) with the surface models segmented from the associated CT data (red transparent).

The second study was a clinical feasibility study designed to evaluate the clinical usability of the present solution. In this study, we evaluated our complete solution on 5 patients (6 trials). At each trial, we recorded the immobilization device mounting time and acquired two images of a patient, one from the AP direction and the other from a roughly LM direction. As there is no ground truth CT scan of the patient, we cannot validate the reconstruction accuracy and we just check whether the immobilization is loosed. If loosing happens, then the two acquired images after calibration will not be in a common space, leading to unsuccessful reconstruction.

It was found that the immobilization device mounting time ranged from 1 to 5 min and there was no device loosing. All 2D-3D reconstructions were successful. Figure 5 shows a reconstruction example.

4 Discussions and Conclusions

In this paper, we presented an integrated solution addressing three challenges in deriving 3D patient specific models from 2D X-ray images, i.e., patient tracking/immobilization, image calibration, and 2D-3D reconstruction. Although there exist large number of work addressing either one of the three problems, there is only few work targeting for solving all three problems. Chriet et al. [7] proposed to use a calibration jacket based solution for the 3D reconstruction of the human spine and rib cage from biplanar X-ray images. However, only using a calibration jacket is hard to prevent the relative movement between the calibration jacket and the underlying anatomy during image acquisition. An alternative solution is to develop a specialized X-ray imaging device, as exemplified by the development of the EOS imaging system [19], where two images are simultaneously acquired, thus eliminating the requirement of patient tracking. However, due to the relative high acquisition and maintenance costs, the EOS imaging system at this moment is only available in a few big clinical centers and is not widely available.

References

1. Novosad, J., et al.: Three-dimensional 3-D reconstruction of the spine from a single X-ray image and prior vertebra models. IEEE Trans. Biomed. Eng. **51**(9), 1628–1639 (2004)
2. Zheng, G.: Statistically deformable 2D/3D registration for estimating postoperative cup orientation from a single standard AP X-ray radiograph. Ann. Biomed. Eng. **38**(9), 2910–2927 (2000)
3. Yaniv, Z., Joskowicz, L., Simkin, A., Garza-Jinich, M., Milgrom, C.: Fluoroscopic image processing for computer-aided orthopaedic surgery. In: Wells, W.M., Colchester, A.C.F., Delp, S.L. (eds.) MICCAI 1998. LNCS, vol. 1496, pp. 325–334. Springer, Heidelberg (1998)

4. Hofstetter, R., et al.: Fluoroscopy as an imaging means for computer-assisted surgical navigation. Comput. Aided Surg. **4**(2), 65–76 (1999)

5. Livyatan, H., Yaniv, Z., Joskowicz, L.: Robust automatic C-arm calibration for fluoroscopy-based navigation: a practical approach. In: Dohi, T., Kikinis, R. (eds.) MICCAI 2002, Part II. LNCS, vol. 2489, pp. 60–68. Springer, Heidelberg (2002)

6. Jain, A., Fichtinger, G.: C-arm tracking and reconstruction without an external tracker. In: Larsen, R., Nielsen, M., Sporring, J. (eds.) MICCAI 2006. LNCS, vol. 4190, pp. 494–502. Springer, Heidelberg (2006)

7. Cheriet, F., et al.: A novel system for the 3-D reconstruction of the human spine and rib cage from biplanar X-ray images. IEEE Trans. Biomed. Eng. **54**(7), 1356–1358 (2007)

8. Schumann, S., et al.: Calibration of C-arm for orthopedic interventions via statistical model-based distortion correction and robust phantom detection. In: Proceedings of the ISBI 2012, pp. 1204–1207 (2012)

9. Carter, C.R., Hicken, G.J.: Device for immobilizing a patient and compressing a patient's skeleton, joints and spine during diagnostic procedures using an MRI unit, CT scan unit or X-ray unit. US Patent 6,860,272 (2005)

10. Schmit, B.P., Keeton, M., Babusis, B.: Restraining apparatus and method for use in imaging procedures. US Patent 6,882,878 (2005)

11. Mitton, D., et al.: 3D reconstruction method from biplanar radiography using non-stereocorresponding points and elastic deformable meshes. Med. Biolo. Eng. Comput. **38**(2), 133–139 (2000)

12. Yu, W., Zheng, G.: Personalized X-ray reconstruction of the proximal femur via a new control point-based 2D–3D registration and residual complexity minimization. VCBM **2014**, 155–162 (2014)

13. Sadowsky, O., Chintalapani, G., Taylor, R.H.: Deformable 2D-3D registration of the pelvis with a limited field of view, using shape statistics. In: Ayache, N., Ourselin, S., Maeder, A. (eds.) MICCAI 2007, Part II. LNCS, vol. 4792, pp. 519–526. Springer, Heidelberg (2007)

14. Ahmad, O., et al.: Volumetric DXA (VXA) - a new method to extract 3D information from multiple in vivo DXA images. J. Bone Miner. Res. **25**, 2468–2475 (2010)

15. Baka, N., Kaptein, B.L., de Bruijne, M., et al.: 2D–3D reconstruction of the distal femur from stereo X-ray imaging using statistical shape models. Med. Image Anal. **15**, 840–850 (2011)

16. Zheng, G.: Personalized X-ray reconstruction of the proximal femur via intensity-based non-rigid 2D-3D registration. In: Fichtinger, G., Martel, A., Peters, T. (eds.) MICCAI 2011, Part II. LNCS, vol. 6892, pp. 598–606. Springer, Heidelberg (2011)

17. Zheng, G., et al.: A 2D/3D correspondence building method for reconstruction of a patient-specific 3D bone surface model using point distribution models and calibrated X-ray images. Med. Image Anal. **13**, 883–899 (2009)

18. Hartley, R., Zisserman, A.: Multiple View Geometry in Computer Vision, 2nd edn. Cambridge Univeristy Press, Cambridge (2004)

19. Wybier, M., Bossard, P.: Musculoskeletal imaging in progress: the EOS imaging system. Joint Bone Spine. **80**(3), 238–243 (2013)

Cross-Manifold Guidance in Deformable Registration of Brain MR Images

Jinpeng Zhang[1], Qian Wang[1], Guorong Wu[2], and Dinggang Shen[2]([✉])

[1] Med-X Research Institute, School of Biomedical Engineering,
Shanghai Jiao Tong University, Shanghai 200030, China
[2] Department of Radiology and BRIC,
University of North Carolina at Chapel Hill, Chapel Hill, NC 27599, USA
dgshen@med.unc.edu

Abstract. Manifold is often used to characterize the high-dimensional distribution of individual brain MR images. The deformation field, used to register the subject with the template, is perceived as the geodesic pathway between images on the manifold. Generally, it is non-trivial to estimate the deformation pathway directly due to the intrinsic complexity of the manifold. In this work, we break the restriction of the single and complex manifold, by short-circuiting the subject-template pathway with routes from multiple *simpler* manifolds. Specifically, we reduce the anatomical complexity of the subject/template images, and project them to the virtual and simplified manifolds. The projected simple images then guide the subject image to complete its journey toward the template image space step by step. In the final, the subject-template pathway is computed by traversing multiple manifolds of lower complexity, rather than depending on the original single complex manifold only. We validate the cross-manifold guidance and apply it to brain MR image registration. We conclude that our method leads to superior alignment accuracy compared to state-of-the-art deformable registration techniques.

1 Introduction

The task of deformable image registration computes a deformation pathway to align the subject to the template images. As registration enables individual images to be quantitatively compared within the common space, the technique is fundamentally important to many brain studies based on magnetic resonance (MR) imaging. Conventionally image registration is regarded as an optimization problem, in which the deformation field is estimated to maximize the similarity between the warped subject and the template. The optimization, often cursed by the high dimensionality of both the images and the deformation fields, is difficult to solve especially when there are large shape/appearance differences between the two images. Many efforts have thus been devoted to improve image registration by incorporating (1) more accurate image similarity or voxel correspondence estimator [1, 2], (2) robust deformation modeling [3–5], and (3) high-performance optimizer [6, 7].

Recent studies show that, within an image collection, the subject may utilize other *intermediate* images as the bridges to fill in the gaps along its deformation pathway

© Springer International Publishing Switzerland 2016
G. Zheng et al. (Eds.): MIAR 2016, LNCS 9805, pp. 415–424, 2016.
DOI: 10.1007/978-3-319-43775-0_38

toward the template [8, 9]. That is, the intermediate images can provide guidance by partitioning the subject-template deformation pathway into several short and easy-to-estimate deformation segments. Even though the entire subject-template deformation pathway is difficult to estimate directly, it can be concatenated from several relatively easy-to-estimate deformations that correspond to individual segments of the pathway.

The guidance in image registration can be interpreted by the image *manifold*, which is often used to describe the distribution of the high-dimensional image data [10]. In general, similar images distribute closely on the manifold, and their in-between pathways encode their respective deformations. Given a certain subject whose appearance is significantly different from the template, an intermediate image can be selected if (1) it is spatially close to the subject on the manifold and (2) its deformation pathway toward the template is easier to estimate. In this way, a set of intermediate images can be determined recursively, such that the subject-template pathway is decomposed into several segments for robust and accurate estimation of the deformation fields.

However, it might be insufficient for the aforementioned single manifold to guide brain MR image registration [11]. In order to identify the optimal intermediate images, the manifold has to be learned from a lot of individual images to account for the high dimensionality of the images and their distribution. Meanwhile, for each segment of the subject-template pathway, the deformation is often estimated through state-of-the-art registration methods. That is, the resulted deformation pathway is located on the manifold of high dimensionality and thus cursed by the complexity of neural anatomies. In general, the concatenated subject-template deformation pathway is far from being perfect inevitably.

In this work, we introduce the cross-manifold guidance for brain MR image registration. Given the subject and the template images, we *first* reduce their anatomical complexity by smoothing their inner/outer cortical surfaces. The smoothing process yields *simpler* subject/template images, which are projected from the original image manifold to a new manifold of less anatomical complexity. The simplified images *then* provide intermediate guidance. That is, the subject and the template detour their in-between pathway by estimating the deformation fields toward the smoothed images and travelling to the simplified manifold, respectively. Meanwhile, the deformation pathway between the smoothed subject and template images, which can be further decomposed recursively, becomes much easier to estimate than the original subject-template deformation. *Finally*, the subject is registered with the template by concatenating all individual segments that traverse multiple manifolds, each of which encodes relatively low anatomical complexity.

The cross-manifold guidance makes our method unique among state-of-the-art methods, in which the deformation field is often regarded as the (geodesic) pathway on the manifold. Specifically, we take the shortcuts of the simplified (virtual) manifolds to reduce the subject-template variation, thus getting rid of the single complex manifold that is usually insufficient to encode all anatomical complexity of human brains. At the same time, the concatenation of the subject-template pathway provides two registration modes, varying according to the destination of the subject:

1. In the *intrinsic* mode, the subject image is warped back to the *intrinsic* space of the template image, by tracing the cross-manifold pathway travelled by the template inversely;
2. In the *virtual* mode, the subject image ends with being aligned to the simplified template image that is projected on the *simple* and *virtual* manifold.

We will provide details of our method in Sect. 2. Then, we will validate our method quantitatively and compare the two registration modes in Sect. 3. This work will be concluded in Sect. 4.

2   Method

We presume that the subject-template deformation pathway becomes easier to estimate, when the two images are projected from their intrinsic and complex manifold to the simplified manifold. Given the subject S and the template T in Fig. 1, we first segment their white matter (WM) and grey matter (GM) tissues by FSL [12] (c.f. S_1 and T_1 in the figure). The cortex is highly convoluted, implying that the two images are distributed upon a high-dimensional and complex manifold. Therefore, it is challenging to directly estimate the deformation pathway (denoted by ϕ_1) on the first (intrinsic) manifold. Alternatively, we reduce the complexity of S_1 and T_1 in our method, by projecting them to S_2 and T_2 on the second simplified manifold. Then, ϕ_1 is decomposed into three segments (c.f. ψ_{S_2}, ϕ_2, $\psi_{T_2}^{-1}$), each of which is relatively easier to compute. Essentially, our method can recursively decompose the challenging registration task into a series of (1) inter-manifold registration between the same subject/template images of different

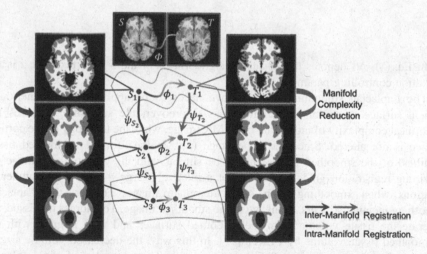

Fig. 1. By manifold complexity reduction, the subject/template images (i.e., S and T) are projected to the simplified manifolds that encode less complex convolution patterns of cortex. The subject-template pathway (e.g. ϕ_i) is recursively decomposed into the inter-manifold deformations ($\psi_{S_{i+1}}$ and $\psi_{T_{i+1}}^{-1}$) and the intra-manifold deformation (ϕ_{i+1}).

complexity ($\psi_{S_{i+1}}$ and $\psi_{T_{i+1}}^{-1}$) and (2) intra-manifold registration between simplified subject and template after complexity reduction (ϕ_{i+1}). Implementation details for our method will be provided in the next. For convenience, the notations used in this paper are summarized in Table 1.

Table 1. Summary of important notations in this paper.

Variable	Note
S, T	The subject and the template images
Φ, Φ^{-1}	The deformation field from S to T, and the inverse field from T to S
S_i, T_i	The projected subject/template images on the i-th manifold
ψ_{S_i}, ψ_{T_i}	The deformation fields from S_{i-1} to S_i, and from T_{i-1} to T_i
ϕ_i	The deformation field from S_i to T_i

2.1   Manifold Complexity Reduction

The key point of our method relies on the reduction of manifold complexity, since we expect that the guidance from the simplified manifold can help register the complex subject/template images. We associate the anatomical complexity with the highly convoluted patterns of the cortical surfaces, as all images are segmented into WM/GM tissues already. Triangular meshes are then reconstructed from the segmented tissue volumes to represent the inner and the outer cortical surfaces, respectively.

We apply the Laplacian smoothing upon the cortical surface mesh to reduce the anatomical complexity. With $\mathbf{x}_i$ to represent the location of the i-th vertex of the mesh of inner/outer cortical surface, its new coordinate after smoothing is defined as

$$\mathbf{x}_i := \alpha\mathbf{x}_i + (1 - \alpha)\frac{\sum_{j\in\mathcal{N}_i}\mathbf{x}_j}{|\mathcal{N}_i|}. \tag{1}$$

In Eq. (1), $\mathcal{N}_i$ denotes the adjacent neighborhood of the i-th vertex, and α is the relaxation controlling parameter.

The Laplacian smoothing in the above needs to be applied to the inner/outer cortical surface mesh for several iterations. Moreover, the smoothing reduces the anatomical complexity of individual brain MR image, while the topology of the cortical surface is not altered. Since the appearance (i.e., in the form of segmented tissue volumes) of the smoothed image should be similar with the unsmoothed image for providing registration guidance, we adopt a relatively large α and small number of iterations when smoothing each subject/template image. Further, the Laplacian smoothing inevitably incurs shrinkage to the smoothed image. To address this issue, we generate the tissue volume from the smoothed surfaces and then align it with the unsmoothed tissue volume by FLIRT [12]. In this way, the decreased volume size of the smoothed image can be effectively corrected. The examples of the Laplacian smoothing can be found in Fig. 1.

2.2 Inter- and Intra-Manifold Registration

The Laplacian smoothing reduces the image complexity and projects the subject/template image from its intrinsic space to the new space on the simplified manifold. To provide guidance for registration, the subject/template should be well registered with the smoothed image on the simplified manifold, which is referred by inter-manifold registration. Also, the concatenation of the subject-template pathway requires a connection between the smoothed subject and template images on the simplified manifold, which is named as intra-manifold registration. Specifically, given the subject S_i and the template T_i tentatively on the i-th manifold, the registration task is decomposed into three segments, corresponding to two inter-manifold pathways between the subject/template and their respective smoothed counterparts, and one intra-manifold pathway between the two smoothed images, respectively:

$$\phi_i = \psi_{S_{i+1}} \circ \phi_{i+1} \circ \psi_{T_{i+1}}^{-1}. \tag{2}$$

The inter-manifold registration is relatively easy to complete as we require the appearance of the smoothed image to be similar with the unsmoothed image in Sect. 2.1. Meanwhile, the intra-manifold registration can be further recursively decomposed following Eq. (2), such that the direct intra-manifold registration happens between very simple and similar images only.

Considering time efficiency, we choose diffeomorphic Demons to complete the direct registration of similar images [13], which also guarantees the invertibility of the inter-manifold registration. Besides, diffeomorphic Demons also avoids changing the topology of the anatomy during inter-manifold registration. Taking S_{i-1} and S_i for example, we solve for the deformation field ψ_{S_i} by

$$\psi_{S_i} = \left\| \arg\min_{\psi_{S_i}} G_o(S_i) - G_\sigma\left(S_{i-1}\left(\psi_{S_i}\right)\right) \right\|^2 + \mathrm{Reg}\left(\psi_{S_i}\right). \tag{3}$$

Here, $G_\sigma(\cdot)$ is a Gaussian smoothing operator as both S_{i-1} and S_i are represented by binary tissue segmentation. The term $\mathrm{Reg}(\cdot)$ enforces diffeomorphic constraint upon the resulted deformation field. ψ_{T_i} and ϕ_i can be estimated in the same way.

2.3 Intrinsic and Virtual Registration Modes

After projecting the subject/template to multiple manifolds of reduced complexities and connecting them through inter-/intra-manifold registration, we compute the entire subject-template pathway in the final to attain the intrinsic registration. The algorithm to recursively solve for the subject-template deformation (i.e., $\Phi = \phi_1$) is summarized in the next. After each manifold complexity reduction, we first estimate the inter-manifold deformations $\psi_{S_{i+1}}$ and $\psi_{T_{i+1}}$. Then, the subject and the template are warped accordingly (c.f. Line 5). The newly updated S_{i+1} and T_{i+1} (instead of those after complexity reduction in Line 2) are used as the intermediate images for S_i and T_i. Once finishing the recursive decomposition and the concatenation of the subject-template deformation (Lines 6–7), we further refine the tentative estimation of ϕ_i (Line 8). That is, we apply the intra-manifold registration to align S_i and T_i directly, by initiating with the tentative ϕ_i and running only a few iterations of optimization.

Algorithm: ϕ_i = Cross-Manifold_Registration(S_i, T_i, i)
1   **if** $i <$ MAX
2   S_{i+1} = Complexity_Reduction(S_i), T_{i+1} = Complexity_Reduction(T_i);
3        $\psi_{S_{i+1}}$ = Inter-Manifold_Registration(S_i, S_{i+1});
4        $\psi_{T_{i+1}}$ = Inter-Manifold_Registration(T_i, T_{i+1});
5        $S_{i+1} \leftarrow S_i \circ \psi_{S_{i+1}}$, $T_{i+1} \leftarrow T_i \circ \psi_{T_{i+1}}$;
6   ϕ_{i+1} = Cross-Manifold_Registration($S_{i+1}, T_{i+1}, i+1$);
7        $\phi_i = \psi_{S_{i+1}} \circ \phi_{i+1} \circ \psi_{T_{i+1}}^{-1}$;
8   ϕ_i = Deformation_Refinement(S_i, T_i, ϕ_i);
9   **else**
10   ϕ_i = Intra-Manifold_Registration(S_i, T_i);
11   **end if**
12   **return** ϕ_i.

The above algorithm belongs to the *intrinsic* mode, since the subject is warped to the intrinsic image space of the template following the resulted deformation field in the final. Similarly, the subject may also end within the image space that corresponds to the projected template on the more simplified manifold. Since the smoothed template is artificially created, we designate it as the *virtual* image space in this paper. The *intrinsic* algorithm in the above can be easily converted to the *virtual* mode, by replacing Line 7 with $\phi_i = \psi_{S_{i+1}} \circ \phi_{i+1}$ and then changing the refinement target in Line 8 accordingly. Note that the virtual space only depends on the template image and the degree of manifold complexity reduction. With a specific template, all subject images can be aligned to the same virtual template space and quantitatively compared.

3   Experimental Results

In this section, we apply our method to two brain MR image datasets (i.e., NIREP NA0 and ADNI) and validate its performance. All images are pre-processed necessarily, including bias correction, skull-stripping, and affine registration to a common space. For corresponding anatomical regions-of-interest (ROIs) in the registered subject and the template, we compute the Dice ratio to measure their overlapping. Note that the Dice ratio is a typical indicator of image registration accuracy [14].

Since diffeomorphic Demons is used as a tool to complete inter- and intra-manifold registration in our method, we compare our method with it in the experiments. In particular, we adopt the three-level multi-scale multi-resolution framework, as well as the recommended parameters, for direct registration of diffeomorphic Demons. The same settings are also applied when calling diffeomorphic Demons in our cross-manifold guidance framework, except that fewer iterations of optimization are used (c.f. Lines 3–4, 6, 8 in the listed algorithm in Sect. 2.3). The inversion and composition of deformations are implemented by ITK (itk.org). Considering efficiency, we adopt two levels of manifold complexity reduction to demonstrate the capability of our method.

3.1 NIREP NA0 Dataset

There are 16 images in the NIREP NA0 dataset, each of which carries 32 ROI labels mainly covering the cortical area. We choose one template image in turn, and then register all other images with the template. The overall Dice ratios, averaged over all registration tasks and ROIs, are summarized in Table 2. As mentioned previously, there are two registration modes for our method. In the intrinsic mode, the Dice ratios are evaluated in the intrinsic image space of the template; while in the virtual mode, the Dice ratios are computed from the space of the projected template in the (most) simplified manifolds. We also compare our method with two direct registration schemes by diffeomorphic Demons. In particular, Demons-I indicates that the intensity images of the subjects are registered with the template, while Demons-S indicates registration of the segmented subject and template images. Note that both of the two direct registration tasks are conducted in the multi-scale and multi-resolution scheme.

Table 2. The Dice ratios of the NIREP NA0 dataset yielded by different registration schemes.

Demons-I	Demons-S	Intrinsic mode	Virtual mode
69.0 ± 1.30 %	70.3 ± 0.97 %	72.3 ± 0.98 %	73.2 ± 0.91 %

In the intrinsic mode, the overall Dice ratio for our method is 72.3 %, which is higher than the two direct registration schemes (+3.3 % compared to Demons-I and +2.0 % for Demons-S). Paired t-tests show that the improvement of our method is statistically significant over all registration tasks ($p < 0.001$ compared to both Demons-I and Demons-S). The results confirm that our method estimates the subject-template pathways more accurately. Moreover, the virtual mode achieves even higher Dice ratio than the intrinsic mode, implying that the subject images are better aligned with the smoothed templates. Therefore, we argue that the smoothed template on the simplified manifold might be a better choice for morphologic analysis to brain MR images.

Among all 32 ROIs, our method achieves higher improvement on L/R occipital lobe, L/R superior frontal gyrus, L/R middle frontal gyrus, L/R superior partial lobule and L/R inferior parietal lobule (+4.2 % for intrinsic mode versus Demons-I and +2.9 % versus Demons-S), which are close to cortical surfaces. In contrast, the improvement is relatively limited on L/R cingulate gyrus, L/R insula gyrus, and L/R parahippocampal gyrus (+1.6 % for intrinsic mode versus Demons-I and +0.8 % versus Demons-S), which are far away from the cortical surfaces. For visualization of the difference, we show one exemplar registration task in Fig. 2. It is clear that the regions near the cortical surfaces are better aligned by our methods (e.g., zoomed in by red boxes). This observation is related to the fact that we associate the manifold complexity with the cortical convolution patterns. In manifold complexity reduction, the regions near the cortical surfaces are simplified most, where the accuracy of subsequent image registration is thus significantly increased.

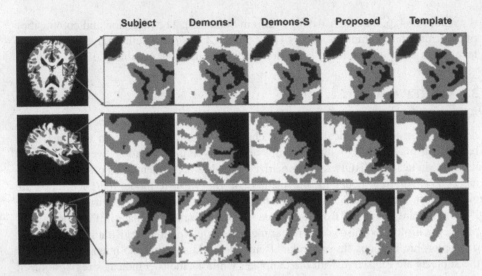

Fig. 2. Visualization of the exemplar registration result. The zoom-in views (from left to right) are available for the subject, the result of Demons-I, the result of Demons-S, the result of the proposed method, and the template. Better alignment can be observed by comparing the proposed method with Demons-I and Demons-S. (Color figure online)

3.2   ADNI Dataset

We use the Alzheimer's Disease Neuroimaging Initiative (ADNI) data to further verify the capability of handling pathologic images for our method. To this end, we randomly select 20 normal control (NC) and 20 Alzheimer's disease (AD) subjects from ADNI. All 40 subjects are registered with another NC template image. After registration, we compute the Dice ratios of brain tissues (i.e., WM and GM), which are used as the indicators of registration quality. The results are shown in Table 3.

Table 3. The Dice ratios of the ADNI dataset yielded by different registration schemes.

		Demons-I	Demons-S	Intrinsic mode	Virtual mode
AD	GM	61.7 ± 12.1 %	75.1 ± 3.7 %	84.8 ± 1.8 %	85.1 ± 1.9 %
	WM	75.8 ± 6.0 %	85.1 ± 2.6 %	91.2 ± 1.2 %	95.6 ± 0.6 %
NC	GM	65.2 ± 9.3 %	78.6 ± 1.6 %	86.7 ± 0.9 %	87.0 ± 0.9 %
	WM	80.0 ± 4.0 %	87.3 ± 1.2 %	92.3 ± 0.6 %	96.2 ± 0.3 %

In the intrinsic mode, it is clear that our method can increase the Dice ratios of WM/GM significantly, compared to the direct registration of the subjects to the template. Note that, in the direct registration, the Dice ratios for the AD subjects are lower than the NC subjects, partly due to the fact that the AD images are less similar with the NC template in appearances. However, with our method, the Dice ratios increase more for the AD subjects than the NC subjects, indicating that our method can better handle the challenging cases of registration. At the same time, similar to the results on NIREP

NA0 dataset, the Dice ratios in the virtual mode of our method are higher than the intrinsic mode. The results confirm again that the smoothed template space on the simplified manifold might be a better choice for analyzing the selected AD/NC subject images.

4 Conclusion and Discussion

We have proposed the cross-manifold guidance to brain MR image registration in this work. The method projects the subject/template image to the simplified manifolds. Even though the subject and the template vary a lot regarding their appearances, they may become similar enough once being projected to a certain simplified manifold. In this way, the subject-template pathway can be decomposed into several segments, each of which corresponds to an easy-to-estimate deformation field. In general, our method can register the subject with the template more accurately, as confirmed by the experiments.

We also propose that the smoothed template space on the simplified manifold might be a better choice for analyzing the large-scale collection of brain MR images. The ultimate goal for image registration is to align corresponding anatomical structures in the common space to facilitate subsequent quantitative comparisons. As the anatomical complexity of the template is much reduced, the alignment of individual images with the simplified template becomes easier and more accurate. It thus implies that the simplified template may introduce fewer errors to the image-based statistical analyses in the process of image registration.

Though sharing similar idea with the popular multi-resolution multi-scale registration framework (i.e., in terms of reducing registration complexity), our method is unique as we seek for the cross-manifold guidance by smoothing the cortical surfaces and reducing the anatomical complexity of the subject/template images. Specifically, in the conventional multi-resolution registration framework, images are down-sampled for the estimation of the low-resolution deformation field. The field is later up-sampled and further optimized at the high resolution. In our method, however, the inter-manifold registration directly estimates the deformation field of the same resolution with the subject/template images. Meanwhile, the intra-manifold registration is only performed between the simplified images, as their anatomical complexity is reduced to the minimum. Note that the intra- and inter-manifold registration in our method is implemented in the multi-resolution multi-scale fashion. To this end, the guidance from the simplified manifolds is robust and accurate for the estimation of the deformation pathway upon the highly complex image manifold. Our experiments confirm that the proposed method yields superior registration quality regarding the alignment of corresponding anatomical areas between the subject and the template images. In general, the experiments prove that our method can outperform conventional multi-scale multi-resolution direct registration schemes.

There are several issues to address in our future work. First, it is hard to determine the optimal manifold for registering the projected subject and template. Second, the smoothing upon the cortical surface for manifold complexity reduction not only is time-consuming, but also restricts our method to be applied to segmented brain MR images only. Currently we adopt two levels of complexity reduction. We will investigate the effect of better ways and configurations to project the image manifold in future. We will also seek for more generalized solution of manifold complexity reduction such that our method can be applied to intensity images directly.

References

1. Shen, D., Davatzikos, C.: HAMMER: hierarchical attribute matching mechanism for elastic registration. IEEE Trans. Med. Imaging 21, 1421–1439 (2002)
2. Viola, P., Wells III, W.M.: Alignment by maximization of mutual information. Int. J. Comput. Vis. 24, 137–154 (1997)
3. Rueckert, D., Sonoda, L.I., Hayes, C., Hill, D.L.G., Leach, M.O., Hawkes, D.J.: Nonrigid registration using free-form deformations: application to breast MR images. IEEE Trans. Med. Imaging 18, 712–721 (1999)
4. Beg, M.F., Miller, M.I., Trouvé, A., Younes, L.: Computing large deformation metric mappings via geodesic flows of diffeomorphisms. Int. J. Comput. Vis. 61, 139–157 (2005)
5. Paquin, D., Levy, D., Schreibmann, E., Xing, L.: Multiscale image registration. Math. Biosci. Eng. 3, 389–418 (2006)
6. Avants, B.B., Epstein, C.L., Grossman, M., Gee, J.C.: Symmetric diffeomorphic image registration with cross-correlation: evaluating automated labeling of elderly and neurodegenerative brain. Med. Image Anal. 12, 26–41 (2008)
7. Maes, F., Vandermeulen, D., Suetens, P.: Comparative evaluation of multiresolution optimization strategies for multimodality image registration by maximization of mutual information. Med. Image Anal. 3, 373–386 (1999)
8. Jia, H., Yap, P.-T., Shen, D.: Iterative multi-atlas-based multi-image segmentation with treebased registration. Neuroimage 59, 422–430 (2012)
9. Wang, Q., Kim, M., Shi, Y., Wu, G., Shen, D.: Predict brain MR image registration via sparse learning of appearance and transformation. Med. Image Anal. 20, 61–75 (2015)
10. Aljabar, P., Wolz, R., Rueckert, D.: Manifold learning for medical image registration, segmentation, and classification. In: Machine Learning in Computer-Aided Diagnosis: Medical Imaging Intelligence and Analysis. IGI Global (2012)
11. Ye, D.H., Hamm, J., Kwon, D., Davatzikos, C., Pohl, K.M.: Regional manifold learning for deformable registration of brain MR images. In: Ayache, N., Delingette, H., Golland, P., Mori, K. (eds.) MICCAI 2012, Part III. LNCS, vol. 7512, pp. 131–138. Springer, Heidelberg (2012)
12. Jenkinson, M., Beckmann, C.F., Behrens, T.E.J., Woolrich, M.W., Smith, S.M.: FSL. Neuroimage 62, 782–790 (2012)
13. Vercauteren, T., Pennec, X., Perchant, A., Ayache, N.: Diffeomorphic demons: efficient non-parametric image registration. NeuroImage 45, S61–S72 (2009)
14. Klein, A., Andersson, J., Ardekani, B.A., Ashburner, J., Avants, B., Chiang, M.-C., Christensen, G.E., Collins, D.L., Gee, J., Hellier, P., Song, J.H., Jenkinson, M., Lepage, C., Rueckert, D., Thompson, P., Vercauteren, T., Woods, R.P., Mann, J.J., Parsey, R.V.: Evaluation of 14 nonlinear deformation algorithms applied to human brain MRI registration. Neuroimage 46, 786–802 (2009)

Eidolon: Visualization and Computational Framework for Multi-modal Biomedical Data Analysis

Eric Kerfoot[1(✉)], Lauren Fovargue[1], Simone Rivolo[1], Wenzhe Shi[2], Daniel Rueckert[2], David Nordsletten[1], Jack Lee[1], Radomir Chabiniok[1,3], and Reza Razavi[1]

[1] Division of Imaging Sciences and Biomedical Engineering,
King's College London, London, UK
eric.kerfoot@kcl.ac.uk
[2] Department of Computing, Imperial College London, London, UK
[3] Inria and Paris-Saclay University, Palaiseau, France

Abstract. Biomedical research, combining multi-modal image and geometry data, presents unique challenges for data visualization, processing, and quantitative analysis. Medical imaging provides rich information, from anatomical to deformation, but extracting this to a coherent picture across image modalities with preserved quality is not trivial. Addressing these challenges and integrating visualization with image and quantitative analysis results in **Eidolon**, a platform which can adapt to rapidly changing research workflows. In this paper we outline **Eidolon**, a software environment aimed at addressing these challenges, and discuss the novel integration of visualization and analysis components. These capabilities are demonstrated through the example of cardiac strain analysis, showing the **Eidolon** supports and enhances the workflow.

1 Introduction

A growing area of current biomedical research involves the computational analysis of multi-modal imaging data (MRI, CT, etc.) to extract a greater understanding of biological behaviour and the nature of pathologies. For example, in cardiovascular research, different imaging sequences of a patient provide pieces of an overall picture, such as geometry, 3D motion, or scar and fibrosis. Although there have been considerable advances in correcting motion artefacts in acquisition, the current state of the art still requires substantial post-processing for the detailed quantification needed in biomedical engineering. Done correctly, this can result in the characterization of patient-specific properties or the derivation of innovative biomarkers, giving a deeper understanding of disease than can be achieved by visual assessment of the images.

Visualization is a key component in this process, used to verify the correctness of image reconstruction, image fusion, quantification, and to display the results of simulations or other derived calculations. This requires a visualization environment which can seamlessly render multiple time-dependent image or geometry

G. Zheng et al. (Eds.): MIAR 2016, LNCS 9805, pp. 425–437, 2016.
DOI: 10.1007/978-3-319-43775-0_39

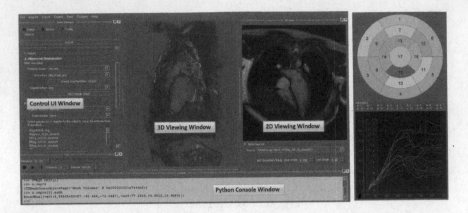

Fig. 1. Screenshot of the **Eidolon**'s user interface. Left image illustrates the control interface, 3D view, 2D view, and Python console. Here three different representations of the left ventricle (LV) are shown, two image sequences and one geometric mesh. Right image illustrates the analysis pane, an alternative to the 2D viewing window, showing calculated strains in AHA regions of the LV.

objects simultaneously in a single scene. Data processing and computation is a second component in the process which is necessary to manipulate datasets, automate common tasks in a workflow, and otherwise prototype the research activities. Thus, exposing data processing functionality through an interactive programming interface is a necessary tool for these activities. As a result there exists a compelling need for an integrated environment where visualization, data processing, and prototyping are presented through a common graphical and programming interface.

In this paper we present our software, **Eidolon**, which addresses these requirements with a unique integrated visualization and computing application, shown in Fig. 1. The important advantage for our software is the integration of an image processing and quantitative analysis environment with visualization components specifically tailored to bioengineering applications of medical image data. This allows users to rapidly process and experiment with data in a way more general tools cannot support. Moreover, it bridges the gap between biomedical engineers and clinicians by providing a common platform, used by the former for developing workflows and by the latter for multi-modal imaging patient evaluations.

This visualization component is implemented in C++ and based on the Ogre3D engine (http://www.ogre3d.org). The majority of **Eidolon** however is implemented in the Python language (http://www.python.org) using the SciPy library stack (http://www.scipy.org) to include a significant amount of the processing and computational facilities. **Eidolon** is thus built upon large open-source projects and is itself open source.

Initially the paper will describe how **Eidolon** is tailored to biomedical research and the features designed to facilitate research activities. Next, the utilization of

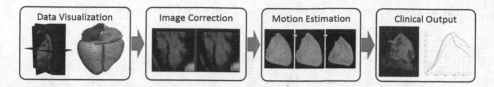

Fig. 2. Illustration of overall workflow for biomedical engineers assessing image motion derived outputs.

Eidolon will be illustrated through a specific research workflow (strain evaluation for a patient with dyssynchronous heart failure), followed by a concluding discussion and future work.

2   Method

For biomedical engineers focused on using multi-modal imaging for the derivation of clinically relevant indicators, the overall workflow can be broken into four main stages, illustrated in Fig. 2. Image data is firstly acquired and visualized, correction operations are then applied to the data to account for acquisition motion error. Subsequently, parameters such as regional strain and torsion are estimated from time-dependent images, and clinical assessment is made.

In this section we outline how **Eidolon** is specifically tailored to this workflow by providing integrated imaging processing functionality, i.e. image registration and alignment with motion tracking, and comprehensive visualization features. **Eidolon** implements much of its image reconstruction features with the Image Registration Toolkit (IRTK) [8,12], creating an accessible GUI designed for a non-technical clinician audience.

Other visualization and biomedical platforms exist to address similar requirements (compared in Table 1), however for the purposes of medical imaging and biomedical engineering **Eidolon** provides the most comprehensive functionality in a single environment. Combining these features with an user-friendly interface results in a tool which maximizes the efficiency of the biomedical workflow illustrated above.

Unlike the other tools compared in Table 1, **Eidolon** is primarily implemented in the Python language with C++ reserved for the critical rendering facilities only. This allows **Eidolon** to take advantage of the dynamic and malleable software environment Python provides through the nature of the language itself, and integrate with the very large standard library the Python runtime includes and numerous other third party packages. This capability will ensure **Eidolon** users are using the most state-of-the art algorithms in image correction.

2.1   Image Correction

A significant component of data processing involves the spatio-temporal correction of image data through alignment and registration. IRTK is an open-source

Table 1. Comparison of major biomedical software libraries and applications

	Mesh Render	2D Image Render	3D Image Render	Mesh/Image Overlay	Image Alignment	Image Registration	Motion Tracking	Plugin Interface	Image Segmentation	User Programming
ParaView	✗	✗	✗	✗	·	·	·	✗	·	✗
Osirix	·	✗	✗	·	·	·	·	✗	·	·
medINRIA	✗	✗	✗	✗	·	✗	·	✗	✗	·
3D Slicer	·	✗	✗	·	·	·	·	✗	✗	·
MITK	✗	✗	✗	✗	·	·	·	✗	✗	·
MeVisLab	✗	✗	✗	✗	·	✗	·	✗	✗	✗
cmgui	✗	✗	·	·	·	·	·	·	·	✗
ITK-Snap	✗	✗	·	·	·	·	·	·	✗	·
GIMIAS	✗	✗	✗	✗	·	·	·	✗	·	·
Seg3D	·	✗	✗	·	·	·	·	✗	✗	·
Eidolon	✗	✗	✗	✗	✗	✗	✗	✗	✗	✗

library of algorithms which achieves the main post-processing tasks: rigidly registering one image series to another, and correcting alignment of the individual slices of a multi-slice sequence (e.g. short axis Cine stack). This ability to align data is especially critical for quantitative analyses, where continuous and smooth spatial descriptions are needed. **Eidolon** provides a graphical user interface for these algorithms, allows researchers and clinicians to easily utilize this functionality, where alternative GUI options are limited.

Figure 3 illustrates an example of rigid registration between two different image sequences. Figure 3a shows a long axis 2D image on the left and 3D volume on the right, both representing the left ventricle of the same subject. Although the two images are acquired as different series, they are part of one study and so should correlate in space. However they are clearly misaligned, a common issue due to breathold variation or patient movement. To compensate, IRTK's rigid registration is applied to correctly re-align the images, giving more continuous data as shown in Fig. 3b.

Figure 3c shows the alignment of different slices on a single image series, the cardiac Cine MRI short axis. This is a sequence of 5–10 mm thick images which spatially and temporally cover the heart's ventricles. The acquisition of the series requires multiple breatholds by the patient and thus variability in chest position causes misalignment, as seen here in the jagged appearance of the blood pool. Post-processing through **Eidolon** can easily correct this misalignment with the wrapped IRTK functionality as shown in Fig. 3d.

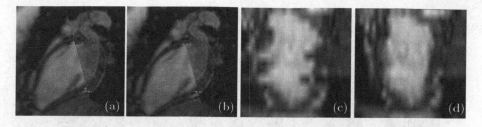

Fig. 3. Example of image registration and alignment: (a) misalignment of two different left ventricle images, (b) rigid registration of images showing alignment, (c) short axis stack of the left ventricle (bright blood pool) where slices are misaligned due to respiratory motion, (d) re-aligned short axis stack.

Visualizing the results of these reconstruction operations is a necessary component of ensuring data correctness as automatic registration algorithms do not always produce optimal results. **Eidolon** allows for easy observation of the results in three dimensions and time, providing a level of user feedback two dimensional and single image viewing tools do not.

2.2 Motion Estimation

Motion estimation from time-dependent images is performed using IRTK's built-in routines [1,11] based on non-rigid registration. This results in deformation fields which are applied to a user-specified geometric mesh giving quantitative motion data.

The motion tracking process is procedurally more complicated than rigid registration and is time-intensive. To manage this process, and automate the deformation of geometry using these files, **Eidolon** includes the module and UI support for invoking IRTK correctly. Within a single environment, the user can import and prepare motion image data, extract motion, and apply the resulting deformation to geometry without having to translate IRTK specific outputs.

Figure 4 shows the result of this process done with the motion extracted from a 3D Tagged MRI [9] sequence of a healthy left ventricle applied on its mesh. This particular type of image is rich in 3D motion information and used by engineers, discussed further in the results. The 2D and 3D viewing windows of **Eidolon** provides different but necessary views for researchers to interpret the derived motion.

2.3 Clinical Output

Deriving clinically-relevant results from the motion geometry is the final stage of the biomedical workflow. Strain, average displacement, wall thickness, volume changes, and other indicators can be calculated from the left ventricle geometry mesh, which are relevant to assessing cardiac function. Additionally, these are the

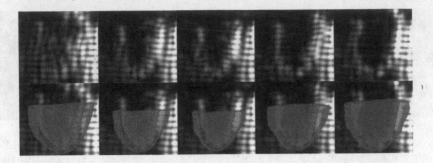

Fig. 4. Deformation of a healthy left ventricle with motion estimation from a 3D Tagged MRI sequence. The top pictures hows the image itself, while the bottom overlays the geometric mesh.

type of image derived metrics that can help stratify patients in disease groups, a common technique for understanding aetiology and potential treatment efficacy.

Eidolon simplifies and streamlines how the tasks leading to these results are carried out by enabling complex operations through simple interfaces, and providing rapid assessment of results through its visualization features. Some of the derived clinical quantities are more sensitive to noise, however the ability to pre-process the data in **Eidolon** alleviates some of that burden.

2.4   3D Visualization

Multi-sequence imaging data represents information captured in specified areas of 3D space (at a particular time) from a common spatial origin. A single 2-dimensional image includes spatial transformation data placing each captured pixel in a 3D position. Typically such transformations are in a coordinate system relative to the acquiring scanner (for scanner modalities), therefore multiple acquisition sequences can be expected to exist in the same space. This allows visualization of multiple image series concurrently, however certain considerations must be taken to ensure any image renderings compose together correctly, compose coherently with geometry data, and align in time. Figure 5 illustrates the types of image data which must be rendered together to allow different image acquisition series to be compared.

Rendering images as individual planes in space is a simple matter of representing each image as a quadrilateral with a texture. Intersecting geometry renders correctly together if totally opaque, however applied transparency may introduce artefacts if the order of rendering is incorrect. Rendering a 2D image with 3D volume (Fig. 5(c)) must also take the order into account, however the important issue is how the textured quad is composited with the volume.

Our solution is to employ a volume-slicing technique [2,4] for representing volume objects. Image series are converted into 3D textures and associated with a rendering object which generates geometry planes bisecting the image volume. These planes are parallel with the view direction and slice through the volume

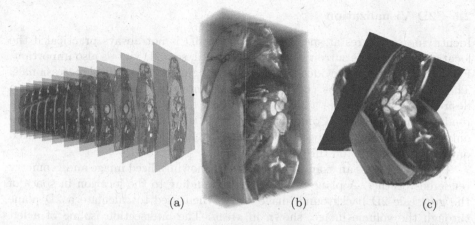

Fig. 5. Example time-dependent MR images: (a) 3D image stack represented as 2D planes uniformly spaced apart and aligned with the LV axis (short axis), (b) the same stack data represented as a 3D volume, (c) 2D plane intersecting 3D volume.

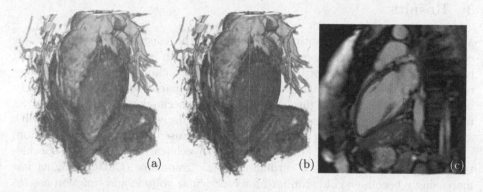

Fig. 6. Image volume of left ventricle, (a) MR image only, (b) LV segmentation mesh, (c) 2D image (greyscale) with sliced volume (green) and sliced mesh (red). (Color figure online)

at regular intervals. Texture coordinates are assigned to these planes so that they represent the equivalent slice through the texture space. By rendering this geometry back-to-front a volume is built up which will composite with other geometry in the standard way defined by the rendering pipeline.

A volume image can be combined with 2D images (Fig. 5(c)) and with geometry meshes (Fig. 6). The latter figure illustrates a left ventricle mesh derived from an automated segmentation [3] of the image it overlays. The ability to render both multiple images and geometries together is important for assessing the alignment of images which represent the same structures, verifying the segmentation meshes were generated in the correct space, or otherwise visually assessing the correctness of data.

2.5 2D Visualization

Identifying structures at specific locations in 3D is not always practical if the location of interest is surrounded by other detail, so a 2D view is also important. Further, the 2D view provides a familiar data alignment for medical professionals. The slicing approach has the additional advantage in that a single slice on a desired view plane within a 3D volume can be taken from the volume and then rendered in a 2D view. Computationally this is a cheap calculation, requiring only a small geometric object to be created, and when rendering shaders need only calculate values on this geometry.

Figure 6(c) gives an example of a 2D view showing sliced image and geometry rendered together. A plane is chosen corresponding to the location in space of the greyscale 2D background image and is then used to calculate a 2D plane through the volume image, shown in green. The intersection isoline of a left ventricle segmentation geometry with the plane is shown in red, validating that the geometry is a correct segmentation at this location.

3 Results

Myocardial strain is a quantity that indicates the effectiveness of ventricular contractions and thus cardiac health. In patients with heart failure, quantifying how synchronously the ventricle contracts is a key clinical metric for therapy response. Further, investigating this quantity compared to the motion seen in healthy subjects can shed light on overall disease mechanisms. Thus, researchers utilizing **Eidolon** are interested in strain metrics derived from MR images with an ultimate goal of assessing if these metrics can be used for patient stratification.

Historically, strain has been assessed with echocardiography (by speckle-tracking techniques), however cardiac magnetic resonance (CMR) imaging has increasingly become a gold standard for ventricular volume and function assessment [5]. With CMR, 3D Tagged MRI is the preferred sequence for strain measurements, as it provides rich three dimensional deformation data [9]. Cine MRI is a commonly used sequence in the clinical scenario due to its relatively high spatio-temporal resolution [13]. Unfortunately the two dimensional nature of the image modality, and fundamental difficulty in tracking actual material points, limits its capability to capture complex myocardial motion. **Eidolon** is used to comparatively render different meshes to assess the difference in calculating strain from Cine MRI versus 3D Tagged MRI.

The synergy of multi-modal images and computational geometry provided by **Eidolon** is shown in Fig. 7. By viewing these datasets together with different renderings in space and time, researchers can quickly assess the resulting mesh's quality and ensure the derived strain values accurately characterize the subject.

Figure 8 demonstrates a typical global strain pattern for healthy individuals in the cardiac cycle starting in diastole from 3D Tagged MRI and Cine MRI

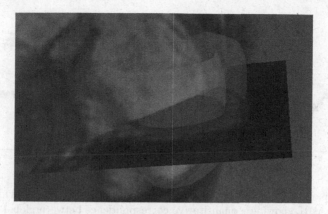

Fig. 7. Visualization of 3D Tagged MRI (green), Cine MRI (black and white) and geometric meshes (red) used for strain analysis in **Eidolon**. This highlights the image registration and correction capabilities of **Eidolon** as multi-modal images and computational meshes are made spatially consistent. (Color figure online)

data preprocessed by **Eidolon**. The global radial strain has a positive peak since the myocardium is thickening during the cardiac cycle. Conversely, both the circumferential and longitudinal strains exhibit negative peaks, capturing the cavity volume reduction and axial shortening respectively. The difference in strain calculated from the two modalities clearly shows how Cine MRI lacks longitudinal shortening information as it inaccurately gives a non-physiological strain.

Comparing the strain pattern between a healthy volunteer and dyssynchronous heart failure patient (Fig. 9) highlights the significant difference in the peak global strain measures (over 50 %), revealing the inefficient contraction pattern of the patient. The reason behind this decrease is better portrayed in Fig. 10 where the global circumferential strain is broken into its mid-ventricle regional components for both the healthy subject and patient. In the healthy subject, the circumferential strain is consistently negative during systole and the peak strain of each region occurs at approximately the same time, which demonstrates synchronicity of contraction. Conversely, the patient's ventricle does not have the same synchronous contraction pattern as evidenced by the spread in circumferential strain across positive and negative values. Thus, the global sum of regional strain is negative when adding strictly negative regional values, whereas the mismatched positive and negative regional patient strains sum closer to zero. The ability to look reliably in more depth at the data, from global to regional quantities, is made possible by the resulting data quality from the **Eidolon**'s preprocessing capabilities.

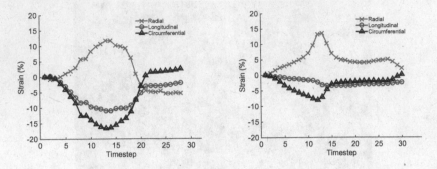

Fig. 8. Comparison of global strain measurements derived from (a) 3D tagged MRI and (b) Cine MRI, showing a quantitative correspondence between global radial strain and a qualitative correspondence in circumferential strain, both in terms of the peak strain and peak timing. However, it is clear that the two dimensional nature of Cine MRI fails to capture the shortening and thus the resulting longitudinal strain.

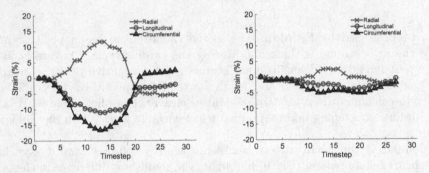

Fig. 9. Comparison of the global strain patterns between a healthy subject (left) and patient with dyssynchronous heart failure (right), showing a significant difference in magnitude for each strain component. This data was calculated from 3D tagged MR images.

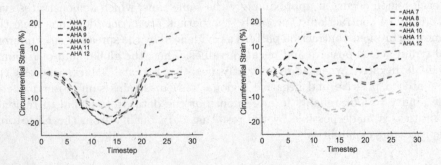

Fig. 10. Dissection of strain values into regional components for a healthy volunteer (left) and patient with dyssynchronous heart failure (right), for AHA regions 7–12.

4   Discussion

We have described our visualization software **Eidolon** and demonstrated its use within the context of a research workflow. The visualization component has been specifically targeted at biomedical applications with a volume rendering approach which emphasizes suitability for 3D as well as 2D rendering of time-resolved image sequences, and a simple accessible underlying implementation.

This approach contrasts with GPU-based raycasting techniques [6,10] which have been the subject of much current research. Although raycasting has certain advantages both aesthetically and in some cases in terms of performance, compositing with arbitrary geometry is not a simple adaptation to the technique. Our slicing implementation uses Cg [7] shader programs to implement a color transfer function and other features including slicing. Combining these shaders, which are applied to geometry as well as image objects, with a raycasting volume object would also involve a complex implementation.

By using Python, **Eidolon** can access the wide range of modules which come with the language's runtime, from general purpose application support to user interface creation. **Eidolon** integrates a command console which allows user access to the internal code and data structures of the visualization module, as well as data processing algorithms. The SciPy libraries, which include image processing and data analysis, are accessible through this console, allowing users to interact with image and geometry data loaded in **Eidolon**, define new algorithms, generate data, and immediately visualize results within a single interface.

This concept of an all-inclusive environment, made interactive through a programming language, is similar in notion to the IPython (http://www.ipython.org) or the MATLAB environment. Although separate tools exist to perform these functions, our experience has been that the cyclic workflow of data processing, visualization, adjusting parameters, and then repeating, is best enabled by an integrated tool specifically targeted at biomedical research.

In terms of limitations, **Eidolon** must rely on a multi-language implementation since critical algorithms must be implemented in C++ for speed. Due to the renderer not being compatible with other visualization libraries, functionality for implementing visualizations or interfaces cannot be directly used but must be to some degree re-implemented in Python.

5   Conclusion and Future Work

We have presented **Eidolon** and discussed the critical role an integrated visualization and computational environment plays in biomedical engineering research. Visualizing multiple images with geometry data is shown here to be an important aspect in this research, as a tool for analysis and validation, and the specific properties of our approach best suits research workflows.

Currently, **Eidolon** is being used in a large research project, VP2HF (http://vp2hf.eu), which aims to better understand why only 66 % of heart failure patients respond to CRT treatment. Additionally, a current prospective clinical trial aims to perform predictive patient-specific modeling within a decision timeframe of two weeks. Without the integration and computation facilities of **Eidolon**, adhering to this timeline would be difficult. In other ways we intend to extend the framework **Eidolon** represents to encompass a greater scope of visualization and computational tasks inherent in these efforts, including visualization of velocity fields and image reconstruction from acquired raw data.

Acknowledgements. This research was partly supported by the National Institute for Health Research (NIHR) Biomedical Research Centre (BRC), and by the NIHR Healthcare Technology Co-operative for Cardiovascular Disease, both at Guy's and St Thomas' NHS Foundation Trust. The research leading to these results has received funding from the EU FP7 for research, technological development and demonstration under grant agreement VP2HF (no 611823), and from BHF New Horizons grant NH/11/5/29058. Views expressed are those of the authors and not necessarily of the NHS, the BHF, the NIHR, or the Department of Health.

References

1. Chandrashekara, R., Mohiaddin, R.H., Rueckert, D.: Analysis of 3D myocardial motion in tagged MR images using nonrigid image registration. IEEE Trans. Med. Imaging **23**(10), 1245–1250 (2004)
2. Cullip, T.J., Neumann, U.: Accelerating volume reconstruction with 3D texture hardware. Technical report, Chapel Hill, NC, USA (1994)
3. Groth, A., Weese, J., Lehmann, H.: Robust left ventricular myocardium segmentation for multi-protocol MR. In: Medical Imaging 2012: Image Processing, vol. 8314, p. 83142S, February 2012
4. Hibbard, W., Santek, D.: Interactivity is the key. In: Proceedings of the 1989 Chapel Hill Workshop on Volume Visualization, VVS 1989, pp. 39–43. ACM, New York (1989)
5. Keenan, N.G., Pennell, D.J.: CMR of ventricular function. Echocardiography **24**(2), 185–193 (2007)
6. Kruger, J., Westermann, R.: Acceleration techniques for GPU-based volume rendering. In: Proceedings of the 14th IEEE Visualization 2003 (VIS 2003), p. 38. IEEE Computer Society, Washington, DC (2003)
7. Mark, W.R., Glanville, R.S., Akeley, K., Kilgard, M.J.: Cg: a system for programming graphics hardware in a C-like language. ACM Trans. Graph. **22**(3), 896–907 (2003)
8. Rueckert, D., Sonoda, L.I., Hayes, C., Hill, D.L., Leach, M.O., Hawkes, D.J.: Nonrigid registration using free-form deformations: application to breast MR images. IEEE Trans. Med. Imaging **18**(8), 712–721 (1999)
9. Rutz, A., Ryf, S., Plein, S., Boesiger, P., Kozerke, S.: Accelerated whole-heart 3D CSPAMM for myocardial motion quantification. Magn. Reson. Med. **59**, 755–763 (2008)
10. Scharsach, H.: Advanced GPU raycasting. In: Proceedings of CESCG 2005, pp. 69–76 (2005)
11. Shi, W., Zhuang, X., Wang, H., Duckett, S., Luong, D., Tobon-Gomez, C., Tung, K., Edwards, P., Rhode, K., Razavi, R., Ourselin, S., Rueckert, D.: A comprehensive cardiac motion estimation framework using both untagged and 3D tagged MR images based on non-rigid registration. IEEE Trans. Med. Imaging **31**(6), 1263–1275 (2012)

12. Studholme, C., Hill, D., Hawkes, D.: An overlap invariant entropy measure of 3D medical image alignment. Pattern Recogn. **32**(1), 71–86 (1999)
13. Walsh, T.F., Hundley, W.G.: Assessment of ventricular function with cardiovascular magnetic resonance. Magn. Reson. Imaging Clin. N. Am. **15**(4), 487–504 (2007)

Erratum to: Medical Imaging and Augmented Reality

Guoyan Zheng[1(✉)], Hongen Liao[2], Pierre Jannin[3], Philippe Cattin[4], and Su-Lin Lee[5]

[1] Institute for Surgical Technology, University of Bern, Bern, Switzerland
guoyan.zheng@istb.unibe.ch
[2] Department of Biomedical Engineering, School of Medicine, Tsinghua University, Beijing, China
[3] Faculte de Medicine, Universite de Rennes 1, Rennes Cedex, France
[4] University of Basel, Allschwil, Switzerland
[5] Hamlyn Centre, Imperial College London, London, UK

Erratum to:
G. Zheng et al. (Eds.)
Medical Imaging and Augmented Reality
DOI: 10.1007/978-3-319-43775-0

The affiliation of Hongen Liao was incorrect.
The correct affiliation should read as below:
Hongen Liao
Tsinghua University
Department of Biomedical Engineering
School of Medicine
Beijing, China

The updated original online version for this Book can be found at 10.1007/978-3-319-43775-0

© Springer International Publishing Switzerland 2016
G. Zheng et al. (Eds.): MIAR 2016, LNCS 9805, p. E1, 2016.
DOI: 10.1007/978-3-319-43775-0_40

Author Index

Printed in the United States
By Bookmasters